Pharmaceutical Science: Drug Discovery and Formulation

Pharmaceutical Science: Drug Discovery and Formulation

Editor: John Jensen

FOSTER ACADEMICS

www.fosteracademics.com

www.fosteracademics.com

FOSTER ACADEMICS

Cataloging-in-Publication Data

Pharmaceutical science : drug discovery and formulation / edited by John Jensen.
p. cm.
Includes bibliographical references and index.
ISBN 978-1-63242-946-9
1. Drugs. 2. Pharmacology. 3. Pharmacy. 4. Drugs--Design.
5. Pharmaceutical chemistry. I. Jensen, John.
RM301 .P43 2020
615.1--dc23

Foster Academics,
118-35 Queens Blvd., Suite 400,
Forest Hills, NY 11375, USA

ISBN 978-1-63242-946-9 (Hardback)

Printed and bound in China.

Contents

Preface

Pharmaceutical science is an amalgamation of several interdisciplinary fields that are concerned with the design, discovery, action and disposition of drugs. It is a broad field with several branches, such as pharmacology, pharmaceutics, pharmacognosy and pharmaceutical chemistry. Drug discovery and drug formulation are two important areas of pharmaceutical science that are constantly evolving. Natural products or extracts, and small synthetic molecules are subject to screening in cells or whole organisms for identifying substances with therapeutic effect. Due to the advent of high throughput screening and sequencing of the human genome, large compounds libraries are now screened against biological targets. Hits that are shown to be disease-modifying are then tested in cells and in animals to determine their efficacy. In pharmaceutical formulation, different chemical substances and the active drug are combined to create the final medicinal product, which is both stable and acceptable. To achieve this, factors such as polymorphism, article size, solubility and pH are considered. The drug form developed also depends on the route of administration, such as capsules, pills and tablets. This book traces the progress of pharmaceutical science and highlights some of its key principles and practices. It discusses the fundamentals as well as modern approaches of drug discovery and drug formulation. The extensive content of this book provides the readers with a thorough understanding of the subject.

The researches compiled throughout the book are authentic and of high quality, combining several disciplines and from very diverse regions from around the world. Drawing on the contributions of many researchers from diverse countries, the book's objective is to provide the readers with the latest achievements in the area of research. This book will surely be a source of knowledge to all interested and researching the field.

In the end, I would like to express my deep sense of gratitude to all the authors for meeting the set deadlines in completing and submitting their research chapters. I would also like to thank the publisher for the support offered to us throughout the course of the book. Finally, I extend my sincere thanks to my family for being a constant source of inspiration and encouragement.

Editor

1

Prescription drug coverage in Canada: a review of the economic, policy and political considerations for universal pharmacare

Jaden Brandt[1*], Brenna Shearer[1,2] and Steven G. Morgan[3]

Abstract

Background: Canadians have long been proud of their universal health insurance system, which publicly funds the cost of physician visits and hospitalizations at the point of care. Prescription drugs however, have been subject to a patchwork of public and private coverage which is frequently inefficient and creates access barriers to necessary medicine for many Canadians.

Methods: A narrative review was undertaken to understand the important economic, policy and political considerations regarding implementation of universal prescription drug access in Canada (pan-Canadian pharmacare). PubMed, SCOPUS and google scholar were searched for relevant citations. Citation trails were followed for additional information sources. Published books, public reports, press releases, policy papers, government webpages and other forms of gray literature were collected from iterative internet searches to provide a complete view of the current state on this topic.

Main findings: Regarding health economics, all five of the reviewed pharmacare simulation models have shown reductions in annual prescription drug expenditure. However, differing policy and cost assumptions have resulted in a wide range of cost-saving estimates between models. In terms of policy, a single-payer, 'first-dollar' coverage model, using a minimum national formulary, is the model most frequently advocated by the academic community, healthcare professions and many public and patient groups. In contrast, a multi-payer, catastrophic 'last-dollar' coverage model, more similar to the current "patchwork" state of public and private coverage, is preferred by industry drug manufacturers and private health insurance companies. Primary concerns from the detractors of universal, single-payer, 'first-dollar' coverage are the financing required for its implementation and the access barriers that may be created for certain patient populations that are not majorly present in the current public-private payer mix.

Conclusion: Canada patiently awaits to see how the issue of prescription drug coverage will be resolved through the work of the Advisory Council on the Implementation of National Pharmacare. The overarching and ongoing discourse on policy and program implementation may be construed as a political debate informed by divergent public and private interests.

Keywords: Pharmacare, Canada, Prescription drugs, Health insurance, Health policy, Healthcare economics, Politics

* Correspondence: umbrand2@myumanitoba.ca
[1]College of Pharmacy, Rady Faculty of Health Sciences, University of Manitoba, Winnipeg, MB, Canada
Full list of author information is available at the end of the article

Background

Canadians have long been proud of their universal health insurance system, "Canadian Medicare" as it is affectionately known [1]. This system of public health insurance, coordinated between the provinces and the federal government through the *Canada Health Act*, keeps Canadians comforted in the knowledge that medically necessary physician visits, diagnostic tests and hospitalizations will be "taken care of" as a matter of course regardless of their age, income, or province of residence [2]. However, the benefits of Canada's universal public health insurance system stop at the community pharmacy, where uninsured costs of medications result in financial hardship for many Canadians [3, 4]. This makes Canada unique insofar as it is the only high-income country with a universal health insurance system that does not provide universal coverage of prescription drugs.

Canada's system of universal health insurance was not supposed to exclude prescription drugs. Canadian Medicare was a national health insurance system built in stages through conditional grants from the federal government to the provinces that are ultimately responsible for health care administration [5]. Since the outset of Canadian Medicare, national commissions have repeatedly recommended that universal public drug coverage – universal "Pharmacare" as that vision is often called in Canada – be part of Canada's universal public health insurance system [6–9]. The topic of universal pharmacare has waxed and waned in past policy debates, often in accordance with the publication of reports by national commissions on Canada's health care system [10]. Despite these brief windows of attention in the past, universal pharmacare has not been implemented in prior eras owing to various political and economic constraints [11]. Factors which have historically impeded progress on this front range from the large implementation cost that would be incurred by government, misalignment of views between policy actors at different levels and the historical lack of electoral incentives to make pharmacare an issue worthy of attention at the highest levels of political campaigning [11]. Nonetheless, recently pharmacare has become a central topic of national health policy debate and the gap between policy discourse and policy action appears to be narrowing as evidenced by the federal government's creation of an Advisory Council on the Implementation of National Pharmacare in 2018 [12].

In this paper, we provide a narrative review and commentary on three major issues relevant to the current topic of universal pharmacare in Canada; the economics, policy options and political considerations of such a system. It is meant to provide an accessible summary of the complexities of Canada's ongoing efforts to achieve a system of universal drug coverage. Beyond this, we believe it offers a compelling case-study (especially for those new to pharmaceutical policy) which details the multiple variables and factors that must be considered for policy decision making and program implementation at the highest levels of public health. For the reader wholly unfamiliar with the different entities operating in Canada's pharmaceutical market environment, supplemental Additiional file 1 provides a brief overview that may be useful before proceeding into the following sections of the article.

Methods

This narrative review was informed by a structured search strategy applied to PubMed, SCOPUS and google scholar using combinations of the terms: 'pharmacare', 'Canada', 'Canadian', 'prescription drug', 'drug coverage', 'policy', 'formulary', 'provincial', 'national'. Citation trails were also followed from bibliographies to accumulate more information sources. Lastly, published books, public reports, press releases, policy papers, government webpages and other forms of gray literature were collected from iterative google searches to provide a complete view of the current state on this topic. There were no date restrictions, though preference was given where possible to newer information sources.

While the lack of a reproducible, systematic search strategy may be seen as a significant limitation of this review, we maintain that combining the various aspects of the pharmacare topic (economics, policy and politics) into a coherent work was more amenable to a realist, narrative strategy rather than a rigorous systematic approach. Lastly, all authors, having varying levels of professional experience relating to pharmaceutical policy in Canada were engaged in formulating the structure of the review to ensure its appropriate breadth and depth of content.

Current prescription drug coverage in Canada

In contrast with its universal Medicare system, Canada's system of prescription drug coverage involves a complex and largely uncoordinated mix of public and private insurance plans that differ in terms of eligibility, patient charges, and drugs covered (i.e., formularies) [13]. Though there are no national standards for public drug programs in Canada, each province offers some form of public subsidy for prescription drugs. These programs evolved beginning in the 1960s and 1970s, and traditionally provided relatively comprehensive public drug insurance for select population groups: specifically, persons on social assistance and persons over the age of 65 [14]. Today, the public drug plans offered by provinces vary more dramatically in terms of who is covered because some provinces – notably Manitoba and British Columbia – no longer provide comprehensive coverage for older residents. The greatest differences in public drug coverage in Canada are differences in drug benefits available for residents who are not on social assistance and age 65 or older. As summarized in Table 1, no province provides universal, comprehensive

Table 1 – Provincial Drug Coverage Programs for General Population (non-senior and non-social assistance)

	Patient Eligibility	Coverage Details
British Columbia	No restrictions	Catastrophic coverage with deductibles up to 3% of annual income, then patient pays 30% co-insurance.
Alberta	No restrictions	Voluntary coverage with premiums, then patient pays 30% co-insurance.
Saskatchewan	No restrictions	Catastrophic coverage with deductibles at 3.4% annual income, then patient pays 35% co-insurance.
Manitoba	No restrictions	Catastrophic coverage with deductibles up to 6.97% annual income, then full coverage of eligible drugs.
Ontario	No restrictions	Catastrophic coverage with deductibles at approximately 4% of annual income, then patient pays $2 fixed co-payment.
Quebec	Restricted to those not eligible for private insurance	Mandatory coverage with premiums and a $19.90 monthly deductible, then patient pays 34.9% co-insurance.
Newfoundland	No restrictions	Catastrophic coverage with out-of-pocket payments ranging from 5 to 10% of income
Nova Scotia	No restrictions	Catastrophic coverage with deductibles up to 20% of annual income, then patient pays 20% co-insurance.
New Brunswick	No restrictions	Voluntary coverage with premiums, then co-payments of $5 to $30 per eligible prescription, depending on income.
Prince Edward Island	No restrictions	Catastrophic coverage with deductibles up to 12% of annual income, then full coverage of eligible drugs.

Source [93]: Authors summary of information in CIHI (1028) National Prescription Drug Utilization Information System Plan Information Document, July 2018 supplemented by information from public drug plan websites, where necessary

public coverage for this general population group.[1] Instead, most provinces offer the general population coverage against "catastrophic costs" that exceed deductibles set as a percentage of household income. The percentages of household income used to define deductibles vary considerably across provinces that offer these catastrophic coverage programs. After a deductible limit is met, the government pays for all or a significant portion of the cost for eligible drug products.

Two provinces, Alberta and New Brunswick, offer the general population the option to purchase premium-based public drug coverage, which is subject to co-insurance on prescriptions filled. One province, Quebec, requires that all residents not eligible for private insurance, by way of their occupation, to purchase premium-based public drug coverage, which is subject to monthly deductibles and co-insurance on prescriptions filled.

Many Canadians have private insurance for prescription drugs. In Quebec, private insurance has been mandatory since 1997 for employees who qualify for extended health benefits as part of their compensation packages [15]. In all other provinces, private insurance is available on a voluntary basis and generally obtained only through extended health benefits as part of compensation packages negotiated between employers and unions. It is estimated that approximately two-thirds of Canadian workers have private insurance coverage [16]. Employees who work full-time, earn over $30,000, and over the age of 25 are more likely to have access to such private insurance coverage than part-time workers, those earning lower wages, and those under age 25 [16]. In 2016, 59% of Canadians reported having some form of private drug coverage [17]. Deductibles in private insurance plans are rare, applying to plans for just 11% of privately insured Canadians; however, most citizens who have private drug insurance pay co-insurance (67% of all beneficiaries) or fixed co-payments (17% of beneficiaries) [18].

Overall the "patchwork" system of private and public drug coverage in Canada leaves approximately one in five Canadians reporting that they have no coverage for their prescriptions [17]. Several surveys conducted over the past 15 years have found that approximately one in ten Canadian patients do not fill prescriptions written for them as a consequence of out-of-pocket costs [17, 19–22]. International comparisons have shown that, although access to medicines is higher in Canada than the United States, Canadians experience higher rates of cost-related non-adherence to medications (10.2%) than do residents in comparable high-income countries with universal drug coverage (average of 3.7%) [23]. This is estimated to result in hundreds of premature deaths annually in Canada, relative to the health outcomes that would be achieved if Canada had the same rates of cost-related non-adherence to medications as is found in comparable countries with universal drug coverage [24].

Pharmacare economic considerations

Being informed on the economics of universal pharmacare requires, first and foremost, an overview of current prescription drug expenditure trends in Canada. Following this, an analysis of previous pharmacare simulations and their associated fiscal projections will provide an important summary when looking to the future on this topic.

Current prescription drug expenditures in Canada

Canadians spent approximately C$33.9 billion on prescription pharmaceuticals in 2017, or C$926 per capita [25]. Prescription drugs accounted for 14.0% total healthcare spending in Canada in 2017, the third largest category of expenditure after hospital costs at 28.3% and physician services at 15.4% [25]. Over the past 30 years, total prescription drug expenditure in Canada has grown at an average annual rate of 8.1% while physician and hospital expenditures have trailed behind at average annual increases of 5.6% and 4.4% respectively [25]. And while growth of pharmaceutical expenditure slowed from 2011 to 2014, prescription drug costs still outpace the cost of physicians' services and hospital care: prescription drug costs grew by 5.5% in 2017 while physician and hospital costs grew 4.4% and 2.9% respectively [25].

Part of the reason pharmaceutical costs have outgrown other major health expenditures in Canada stems from global changes in the availability and price of prescription drugs since the 1980s [26]. Another contributing factor is the difference in its system of financing medicines versus how it financed medical and hospital care. Canada's system of universal, comprehensive, public insurance for medical and hospital care publicly finances 98% of all expenditures on physician services and 90% of all expenditures on hospital care [25]. In contrast, only 42% of total prescription drug expenditures are financed by public programs in Canada [25]. The balance of prescription expenditures in Canada are financed by private insurance plans (35%) and by out-of-pocket payment by patients (23%).

Provincial drug plans apply a variety of tools to control the expenditures under their programs. All provinces apply generic substitution policies or generic reference-based reimbursement policy, and a few provinces apply therapeutic reference-based reimbursement policies [27]. For example, in regards to therapeutic reference based compensation, the public plan may pay the cost of the lowest-cost Angiotensin Converting Enzyme inhibitor and allow patients to pay additional costs if they would prefer another molecule. Over the past decade, provinces have also increasingly used confidential rebate negotiations to obtain better prices for patented drugs than the manufacturer would allow them to obtain in a transparent fashion [28].

In 2010, Canada's provinces and territories began to jointly negotiate brand-name prices and jointly set terms for generic drug pricing through the pan-Canadian Pharmaceutical Alliance [29, 30]. These negotiations set out the pricing terms in a mutually agreed upon letter of intent between governments and a drug's manufacturer. Because final decisions regarding drug coverage reside in the individual provinces, manufacturers are not necessarily guaranteed coverage under all public drug plans in Canada even if pricing terms are agreed upon by the pan-Canadian Pharmaceutical Alliance [31]. This, combined with the fact that provincial drug plans finance less than half of all expenditures on prescriptions in Canada limits the power and impact of these negotiation processes.

As such, it is partially the uncoordinated mix of prescription drug financing that has resulted in less favorable conditions for controlling drug spending than are found in other high-income countries with universal drug coverage [32]. In 2015, for example, total per capita expenditure on pharmaceuticals in Canada was 43% higher than the average for the Organization for Economic Cooperation and Development (OECD) countries, surpassed only by the multi-payer systems of the United States and Switzerland [33]. Despite that Canada has a slightly younger population than some comparable countries (such as France, the Netherlands, Sweden, and the United Kingdom) [34], it spends more on medications per capita than these nations [35]. Research indicates that more coordinated systems of drug financing, particularly those that consolidate purchasing power in price negotiations with drug manufacturers, achieve lower prescription drug expenditures through lower prices and more cost-conscious prescribing patterns than Canada achieves [36, 37].

Simulated pharmacare models

A number of recent studies have attempted to quantify the potential savings that a single-payer pharmacare program would provide Canada [38–43]. Published studies have indicated that a single-payer system could generate between $4 billion and $11 billion in annual savings for Canada [42–44]. These simulated results prompted Canada's parliamentary Standing Committee on Health to commission the Parliamentary Budget Officer of Canada to produce government estimates of such a program [18]. In 2017, the Parliamentary Budget Officer estimated net annual cost reductions of $4.2 billion annually, or approximately 17% [18]. Importantly, these estimated savings also take into account the prospect of increased utilisation among those who currently lack coverage. The Parliamentary Budget Officer, for example, estimated that there would be more than 50 million additional prescriptions filled in Canada under a universal pharmacare program [18].

A number of proposals arguing for the enactment of particular policy frameworks for universal pharmacare, put forward by various sources in recent years, have enabled some political traction on the issue [38–43]. Five of the most recent pharmacare simulation models, with their associated cost reduction estimates, are briefly summarised in Table 2.

Gagnon et al. made the economic case for universal pharmacare in 2010 which was later updated in 2014 [42, 43]. He asserts that a universal 'first-dollar' model would save between $2.7 and $11.5 billion annually, dependent upon whether favorable pricing reforms were implemented in

Table 2 – Pan-Canadian Pharmacare Models and Associated Fiscal Projections

	Data Sources	Type of Coverage	Model Assumptions	Financing Source	Net Difference in Total System Expenditures
Morgan et al. (2015) [40]	-Canada Rx Atlas 2012/2013 for drug utilisation data [94] -International drug pricing data from PMPRB	-Public Universal 'First Dollar'	-Competitive pricing estimates as per singe-payer bulk-purchasing arrangement	-Federal/Provincial/Territorial (F/P/T) Government funding (tax based) -Small patient co-payments based on tiered national formulary	-Annual expense reduction of $4.2 to $9.4 billion
Gagnon and Canadian Federation of Nurses Unions (2014) [43][a]	-Canada Rx Atlas for drug utilisation data -International drug pricing data from PMPRB	-Public Universal 'First-Dollar'	-Competitive generic pricing estimates as per singe-payer bulk-purchasing arrangement –10% increase in base-expenditures due to higher utilisation -Improved evidence-based formulary management –2% reduction in dispensing fees -PMPRB pricing reform	-F/P/T Government (tax-based) -Small patient co-payments based on tiered national formulary	-Annual expense reduction of $2.7 to $11.5 billion
PDCI Market Access inc. (2016) [41][a]	-Canadian Drug Claims Database -International pricing data from PMPRB	-Varies ranging from fully public to fully private	-Numerous assumptions dependent upon model	-F/P/T Government funding (tax-based) -Private plan premiums -Patient co-payments	-$1.92 billion in annual expense reductions or up to $350 million in increased annual expenses
Canadian Centre for Policy Alternatives & Canadian Doctors for Medicare (2017) [38][a]	Canadian Institute for Health Information (CIHI) and previous studies	-Public Universal 'First-Dollar'	-Unclear -Data derived from various sources for approximate calculation	-F/P/T Government funding (tax-based)	-approximately $30 billion in total savings (unspecified time period)
Parliamentary Budget Officer (2017) [18]	-CIHI datasets -Quintile IMS datasets	-Public Universal 'First-Dollar'	-Competitive generic pricing estimates as per singe-payer bulk-purchasing arrangement -Quebec drug formulary	-F/P/T Government funding (tax-based) -$5 co-payments (on patented products)	-annual expense reduction: $4.2 billion

[a]Commissioned report from external stakeholder

tandem by the Patented Medicine Prices Review Board (PMPRB) [43]. Morgan et al., in a 2015 simulated cost study found that, even in their "worst-case" scenario model, $4.2 billion would be saved overall on prescription drug spending with implementation of universal 'first-dollar' pharmacare [44]. A 2017 study comparing 10 developed nations lend further support to these findings, showing that countries utilising single-payer models with evidence-based drug coverage criteria had lower average drug expenditures over countries with multiple payers [36]. The most recent iteration of a universal pharmacare proposal from Morgan and Gagnon et al. is their pharmacare 2020 proposal, which, though remaining otherwise consistent with previous publications, recommends federal assistance to each province in the form of an additional funding transfer to cover 25% of the added public expenses for universal pharmacare [45].

Contending the findings of Morgan et al., PDCI Market access inc. released a report, commissioned by the Canadian Pharmacists Association, which claimed that "existing proposals for national, exclusively publicly funded, pharmacare programs are impractical, disruptive, and overstated in regards to cost-savings"[42(pg 4)] Instead, their analysis consisted of a number of models based on differing co-pay structures and population coverage (funding only the uninsured or all Canadians) [41]. Models that varied the patient co-payment, based on a publicly funded first-dollar universal model, all produced the same modest estimate of ~$1 billion in cost-savings. This represented a reduction in savings of over $3 billion from Morgan et al.'s 'worst-case' model. PCDI instead favor an approach where coverage is expanded for the under-insured population who currently lack equitable drug access, while maintaining the public-private insurer mix. This drug coverage strategy supposedly offers net cost-differences from current baseline spending ranging from a ~$2 billion surplus to a $350 million spending deficit, depending on the model [41]. However, given the commissioned nature of this report and its seemingly unverifiable methodology, it is best understood in the broader political context as informed by external stakeholder interests.

Perhaps the most definitive report so far on the costs and economic outlook of pan-Canadian pharmacare comes from the parliamentary budget officer of Canada [18]. The parliamentary budget office estimated net annual cost reductions of 17%, amounting to projected savings of ~$4.2 billion annually [18]. This was an important finding from government because it is largely in accordance with previous estimates from the academic community involved in health economic policy research (i.e Morgan, Gagnon et al.). Furthermore, the transparent methodology and reporting was accompanied by an exploration of various assumptions through sensitivity analysis. Although, the sensitivity analysis demonstrated the volatility of estimates under varying model assumptions.

Combined with the gaps in access to medicines within and across Canada, the evidence of poor cost-control under Canada's patchwork system of private and public drug coverage has been a key motivation behind the recommendations by various government commissions that Canada adopt a universal system of pharmacare – including the 2018 recommendation of the Standing Committee on Health that the government act on implementing a pharmacare model consistent with the one costed by the Parliamentary Budget Officer [9].

Pharmacare policy considerations

As Canada considers implementing some form of universal prescription drug coverage, there are several logical issues to consider. Among the most important policy questions are which drugs would be covered, who will be covered, what level of coverage will be offered, and who will administer the program?

What drugs will be covered?

A system of universal drug coverage for Canada requires, first and foremost, the determination of the medicines that every Canadian will have coverage for. This will require a national formulary, a common list of eligible drugs for coverage, with or without additional drug-specific coverage criteria, that defines the minimum benefits that all Canadians would be entitled to. There have been several studies of existing public drug plan formularies in Canada, the most recent of which has demonstrated that there already exists an "implicit" national formulary by way of the extensive overlap of drugs listed in major therapeutic categories [46, 47]. The areas where there is already agreement among the provincial public drug plans in Canada may become the starting point for a national formulary under a universal pharmacare program.

A national formulary might, alternatively, approximate an "essential medicines" list for Canada. Essential medicines lists, such as the model list of the World Health Organization, comprise drugs selected as "...those that satisfy the priority healthcare needs of a population." [48] Canadian clinicians and researchers have created a Canadian essential medicine list that comprises 125 medications that suit the majority of prescribing needs in Canada's primary health care system [49]. Economic analysis suggest that universal coverage of that list would be a small but pragmatic step toward more comprehensive universal pharmacare, one that could generate $4.27 billion in annual savings for patients and private drug plan sponsors, at an incremental government cost of $1.23 billion per year [50].

An important distinction in the discussion of a national drug formulary is whether the concept implies a "minimum" standard for coverage within each of Canada's provinces and territories. This idea of a minimum standard has been mentioned in some policy documents, including the 2018 report of the Standing Committee on Health [9]. In this context, "minimum" implies that provinces and territories can retain partial autonomy by having the freedom to go beyond the required drug listing, according to their own assessment of factors within their respective jurisdictions. In other words, while provincial/territorial drug program administrators would not be able to de-list drugs from the national formulary within their jurisdiction, they would be permitted to add drugs at their own discretion. If the national formulary was only to comprise an essential medicines list, it would be likely that most provinces would add to it. However, it is possible that a comprehensive national formulary would include more drugs than some provinces currently provide coverage for, making coverage beyond that list unlikely.

Whether the national formulary is to be comprehensive or narrow, it would likely be created by way of modifications of existing health technology assessment processes at the Canadian Agency for Drugs and Technologies in Health and the price negotiation processes of the pan-Canadian Pharmaceutical Alliance. The former agency provides formulary listing recommendations to provincial members of the latter, in the form of clinical and cost-effectiveness assessments, via their Common Drug Review and pan-Canadian Oncology Drug Review services [51, 52]. However, currently the individual provincial policy-makers are under no obligation to accept the recommendations coming from reviews of the Canadian Agency for Drugs and Technologies in Health. A recent high-level government advisory committee has recommended that the roles and responsibilities of such pan-Canadian agencies be aligned with the vision of creating and maintaining an evidence-based national formulary for a universal pharmacare program for Canada [53]. This would not necessarily increase public administration costs nor necessarily preclude agencies from doing some technology assessment and price negotiations for consideration on a case-by-case and province-by-province basis.

Who will be covered?

The concept of "universal" pharmacare self-evidently suggests that all Canadian citizens and permanent residents be granted the same treatment under any future coverage framework. Thus, the precedent that has long been established by the *Canada Health Act* is probably the best indicator for predicting who would be covered. However, the question remains as to how the policy framework would be resolved to address the status of other persons residing in Canada such as refugees, permanent residency applicants, extended travellers and undocumented persons.

As alluded to in the case of permanent residents, the Government of Canada has previously entitled this group of persons to the same level of universal "medically necessary" coverage as Canadian citizens [54]. As such, it would be unexpected for any future pharmacare plan to exclude permanent residents as this would be an unequal extension of the already existent universal coverage. Likewise, for those not meeting permanent resident status, the benefits that fall temporarily under the Interim Federal Health Program (which are very similar to coverage for citizens) may be extended and re-organized to reflect any new, universal pharmacare program [55]. Regardless of whether prescription drug coverage changes for this group, the separation of the Interim Federal Health Program from the conventional "medicare" system covering citizens will likely remain, if only for epidemiological government data collection purposes.

What level of coverage will be offered?

Canadian Medicare is a 'first-dollar' health insurance program. Essentially, the healthcare provider or institution bills the province/territory for the cost of goods and services rendered, at no direct cost to the patient. This is in accordance with the principles of the *Canada Health Act*, which provinces are obliged to adhere to if they wish to receive federal government funding in the form of the federal health transfer [56]. Several commissions and government reports have recommended that a national formulary of medicines be added to the *Canada Health Act*, which would appear to imply that similar prohibitions on prescription user-charges would apply [6–9]. This would make Canada not unlike that of the United Kingdom nations; Wales, Scotland and Northern Ireland (but not England) where prescription charges were incrementally abolished by the National Health Service throughout the 2000's [57]. But such a program would be a radical transformation of existing public drug plans in Canada, virtually all of which employ deductibles, co-insurance, and/or fixed co-payments for eligible beneficiaries.

At the other extreme in terms of benefit designs under universal pharmacare would be to set the national standard at the level of catastrophic coverage against high costs. Given that such 'last-dollar' coverage is commonplace in the provinces, designing universal pharmacare in Canada around this option would be a national move to establish uniform catastrophic thresholds. This may result in an increase or decrease in what patients already must pay depending on their province of residence and the agreed upon national threshold. Furthermore, nationalizing catastrophic coverage as the standard of public drug benefits in Canada may not address the goals of improving access to medicines since the province wherein such a 'last-dollar' coverage model is applied universally (British Columbia) experiences the highest rates of cost-related non-adherence to medications in Canada [17].

Last-dollar coverage is, however, appealing to industry interests, which could reduce the political costs of program implementation. Drug manufacturers prefer this model of coverage because it makes the government plan a payer of last resort only, rather than the single-payer for covered drugs. Under those circumstances, a majority of drug purchases by a majority of patients will be below deductible, meaning the patients will have to pay for them whether they are on the national formulary or not. This diminishes the negotiating power of the public plan because it reduces the impact on demand of a positive formulary listing [58]. Private insurers also prefer a 'last-dollar' model for universal public pharmacare because it leaves considerable room for them to sell private insurance for costs not covered by the public plan. This is because private insurance generally will offer some level of immediate and perceived financial benefit to the enrollee which is otherwise not realised for many patients under 'last-dollar' public coverage alone. Additionally, a 'last-dollar' model of pharmacare leaves private insurers with a market for covering routine operating expenses while eliminating their exposure to the highest cost medicines (i.e., the catastrophic expenses that would be incurred by government).

Who will administer the plan?

A final consideration is who will administer universal pharmacare? There are two dimensions to this question in the Canadian federation. First, will the program be run as a public program or will private insurers be providers of the pharmacare plan? Second, will the public portion of the program be provincially or federally administered?

If universal pharmacare in Canada is to be a catastrophic, 'last-dollar' model of public drug coverage, then there will remain a major role for private insurers to provide plans for those interested and able to cover expenses below their annual deductibles and for medicines not on the national formulary. This is a form of complementary private insurance wherein the core, universal benefit of protection against catastrophic drug costs would remain a public responsibility. Because most provinces already offer catastrophic drug coverage for most or all of their populations, this would imply little or no change in the role of the private insurance sector in Canada's system. Administration costs would therefore likely remain as they are in both the private and public sector; higher in the private than public sphere [59]. Also, purchasing power would likely remain fragmented and therefore limited by comparison to a single-payer system.

If universal pharmacare in Canada is to be a more comprehensive benefit for medicines on the national formulary, it is possible that such a program could be a single-payer public plan for such medications or a mandatory private plan for such medications. Universal drug coverage can be achieved in a manner like Quebec has had since 1997. In their system, private insurers are the primary providers of drug benefits in the sense that all employees who qualify for private insurance for prescription drugs as part of their compensation packages must have such private insurance. This program limited the public sector cost of implementing universal drug coverage; however, it also limited both incentives and capacity for cost control, which has resulted in far higher prescription drug costs in Quebec than in the rest of Canada [15].

If pharmacare is to be implemented as a single-payer system for drugs on a national formulary, such a system will have significant purchasing power and superior administrative efficiency [38, 39, 59]. It also has the benefit of achieving greater equity and efficiency in revenue collection, which can come from changes to existing sources of government general revenues (such as incremental increases in personal and corporate income taxes). These are among the reasons that a single-payer model has been recommended by major commissions and government committees. Under such circumstances, private insurance would likely remain for individuals who wished to have choices beyond the drugs listed on the national formulary, and possibly for those who wished to have pre-payment plans for the co-payments or co-insurance that the universal public benefit might still have.

Even if there is to be a single-payer, public model of pharmacare for the drugs on a national formulary, a final question would remain: would the program be run by provinces or by the federal government. Because the *Canadian Constitution Act*, in conjunction with the *Canada Health Act*, assigns provinces primary responsibility for matters related to health care administration, it is likely that universal pharmacare would be run by individual provinces but held to national standards established by federal legislation. This legislation would define the terms by which it would grant funding to support the pharmacare program(s). As an aside, how the pharmacare framework is legislatively enacted, be it through changes to the existing *Canada Health Act* or by the drafting of a new statute is an important topic, but one that goes beyond the scope of our review. For the interested reader, this legislative issue has recently been taken up in detail elsewhere [60].

Regardless of the legislative operationalization of the policy framework, universal pharmacare, under the aforementioned assumptions, would be tantamount to how Canadian medicare is run and could be a viable option if the federal government was willing to put sufficient funding into the system. As the provinces currently spend over $12 billion per year on their existing public drug plans, it is likely that the federal government would have to come up with most, if not all, of the incremental public expenditure needed to make those programs compliant with a national standard for universal pharmacare. Based on the estimates of the Parliamentary Budget Officer, that would require $7 billion or more in federal funding – though it is worth noting that the Parliamentary Budget Officer estimates that the net benefit to taxpayers would be a $4 billion savings [18].

Pharmacare political considerations

The federal government's recent creation of an Advisory Council on the Implementation of National Pharmacare in 2018 suggests that some form of pharmacare may be forthcoming, likely after the 2019 election campaign in which promises of universal pharmacare may be a differentiating factor between conservative and progressive political parties [12]. Political considerations are therefore paramount at this point in the policy development cycle. To what extent is the promise of a universal pharmacare program something that will help the current federal government get re-elected or an opposition party elected? As this is a major health care issue, an important political consideration is the support or opposition from health professional groups, health charities, industry and patient organizations.

Health professionals

Among professionals, physicians and nurses have become increasingly vocal advocates for a universal, comprehensive pharmacare program. The most vocal physicians have been the members of Canadian Doctors for Medicare, an organization that has actively campaigned for universal pharmacare on the grounds that such a program would increase access to medicines, improve patient outcomes, reduce administrative burden on physicians, and save money through bulk purchasing [38, 61]. The Canadian Medical Association has taken a more tentative stance, however, arguing that universal coverage is necessary but that it need not be comprehensive nor fully funded through public financing [62].

Nurses have also been active in advocating for national pharmacare [43]. Since 1991, the Canadian Federation of Nurses Unions have campaigned for universal pharmacare through a variety of organizational activities [39, 43, 63, 64]. Their campaigning is based on similar logic as that of the Canadian Doctors for Medicare; however, the nurses unions enjoy the support of other nursing organizations, such as the Registered Nurses Association of Ontario, who have added their voice to the call for universal, comprehensive, public pharmacare [65].

On behalf of the pharmacy profession, the Canadian Pharmacists Association has been the leading voice in the pharmacare dialogue. They have regularly updated their views and recommendations on this issue over the years as the policy discourse has developed [66–70]. In the past, they have commissioned an external report on pharmacare costing to assist in informing their economic position [41]. Overall, they have been more conservative than other health profession groups; cautioning government about the potential for health system efficiency issues that may arise from universal 'first-dollar' coverage implementation such as drug shortages, interrupted access to medicines no longer covered, and potentially inappropriate drug prescribing choices [67]. However, the Canadian Pharmacists Association has consistently advocated for reinvestment of cost-savings from potential lost dispensing fee revenue back into pharmacy business in the form of funding for clinical pharmacy services; an argument based on the cost-effectiveness of improved health outcomes resulting from pharmacist intervention [67, 69].

The conservative position of the Canadian Pharmacists Association may be reflective of the significant and precarious state imposed on pharmacy business from pharmaceutical market reform (increasing drug genericization and provincial policy responses) that have resulted in reduced revenue from dispensing fees and product mark-ups. How much influence large, corporate, chain-drug stores have had on forming the Canadian Pharmacists Association's position (directly or indirectly) is debatable but worthy of consideration. This speculation is based on past observation of opposition by corporate chain-pharmacy to Quebec's proposed public prescription drug funding which occurred in the 1990's [15, 71]. Importantly, as payment mechanisms have always been dependent on provision of pharmaceuticals as the core service, there has been a somewhat silent struggle by pharmacists, largely unbeknownst to the public and other health professions, to rectify the smaller patchwork of clinical pharmacy service remuneration simultaneously with the drug coverage patchwork [72]. Nonetheless, this revenue-based concern is largely exempt for hospital pharmacists, who are not reliant on dispensing fees for their income. Perhaps this explains why their representative organization, the Canadian Society for Hospital Pharmacists, has advocated instead for a universal pharmacare framework that appears closer to that of other healthcare groups in the nursing and medical professions [73].

Public opinion and representation

A groundswell of major national public interest groups, consisting of diverse representation ranging from charities, advocacy organizations and academia to labour unions and retiree associations, have added their voices to the pharmacare debate in recent years. Among these groups, the Health Charities Coalition of Canada, the Canada Health Coalition, Canada Labour Congress, the Canadian Association for Retired Persons and 'Pharmacare 2020' (health affiliated research professors) have come out in support of universal pharmacare [45, 74–79]. Nevertheless, the extent of their involvement and the content of their policy prescriptions have varied considerably. Beyond organized advocacy, polling data and focus groups such as the Citizens' Reference Panel on Pharmacare have backed the need for implementation of universal pharmacare [80, 81].

Other patient advocacy groups, such as the Canadian Organization for Rare Disorders, while in support of universal pharmacare in principle, have raised concerns about access limitations to expensive, rarely used agents that may ensue after program implementation [82]. These concerns stem justifiably from fear that a restricted minimum national formulary, nested in a single-payer model, may radically disrupt pre-existing financial support arrangements in the form of private payer insurance.

In spite of the widespread support for universal pharmacare, there remains staunch opposition from some conservative political think tanks such as the Fraser Institute and the Taxpayers Federation [83, 84]. Essentially at odds with the socialist principles underlying a universal 'first-dollar' pharmacare model, their foremost considerations are limiting the financial burden to the taxpayer while preserving the market for private competition.

Industry

The interests of the Canadian pharmaceutical industry have been prominently represented by Innovative Medicines Canada, who represent more than 45 drug manufacturer members [85]. In attempts to remain 'politically correct' in their positions, they have been openly supportive of a national pharmacare strategy, albeit with the important caveat that any decided solution not limit the current insurable coverage situation of any Canadian [86, 87]. The motivating interest underlying this position is to maintain the ongoing operation of private insurance company formularies, which often cover patented drug products that are not eligible benefits under public plans. And so, a switch to a universal 'first-dollar' public plan, based on rigorous cost-effectiveness assessment, would potentially exclude expensive industry products where sales figures were previously disproportionately reliant on private plan coverage.

The Canadian Life and Health Insurance Association, as the voice of private insurers, has been diligent in issuing press releases and responses to various reports and news developments related to universal pharmacare [88–92]. Echoing that of the pharmaceutical manufacturers, the private insurance industry position has strongly maintained that a universal pharmacare plan should co-exist with private third parties and not threaten the holdings of beneficiaries of private insurance [92]. To this end, they have invoked the existence of their ~ 26 million beneficiaries, who they claim generally receive broader and more extensive coverage than public plans, to imply the potential entailment of negative consequences on the Canadian public from a radical change to existing coverage arrangements. Essentially, they contend that, should the federal government implement single-payer, 'first-dollar', universal coverage, an estimated \$14–20 billion would need to be immediately earmarked for public drug expenditure that was previously reimbursed privately [88, 91].

Conclusion

After more than 60 years of recommendations from national commissions and government committees, Canada appears poised to implement some form of universal pharmacare, likely in the government mandate that would start after the federal election in late 2019. Many stakeholder groups, academic experts, and government committees have more or less agreed on many of the major framework characteristics. Namely, universal pharmacare in Canada would, ideally, involve a reasonably comprehensive, evidence-based national formulary that is covered by a single-payer public program involving limited direct charges to patients. Private insurance would be a voluntary and complementary option for covering additional drug choices and prepaying any user charges that the universal public system may entail.

But the policy process isn't over until it is over. The concept of a universal, single-payer pharmacare program in Canada looms as a significant threat to the interests of industry; private insurers and drug manufacturers who stand to lose the most from the program. There is also opposition from citizens concerned about tax increases, even if such increases produce net savings to taxpayers, and those who simply do not wish to have the role of government expanded within Canada's health care system.

Whether Canada moves forward on reforms will therefore depend on voter mobilization. This will be influenced, in part, by the work of the Advisory Council on the Implementation of National Pharmacare. If the panel develops a proposal that resonates with government and, importantly, the public, it may become a roadmap and touchstone in public debate and form the basis of the current government's 2019 election platform. However, policy development will also depend on the balance of political power of groups involved in the sector. The stakeholders who stand to lose revenues and profits under a universal pharmacare program have more concentrated interests than those who stand to gain; as such, it is possible that those opposed to major policy reforms may be able to launch marketing campaigns that change the narrative in ways that may make it difficult for reforms to take place. Time will tell.

Endnotes

[1]We have excluded Canada's territories from table 1 because of the greater reliance on federal drug program funding in the territories and their relatively small share of the Canadian populations (the three territories combined account for less than 1% of Canada's total population).

Acknowledgements
JB extends his gratitude to Prof. Les Carrothers for whom this manuscript would not exist were it not for his encouragement, insight and classroom instruction.

Authors contributions
JB conceived the paper, wrote the first draft and added revisions to the later drafts. BS provided edits, comments and updates to the contents of all drafts. SM provided additional citation material and major edits to the final draft. All authors approved the final version of the manuscript.

Competing interests
JB has served as Vice-President of Pharmacists Manitoba (professional advocacy body).

Author details
[1]College of Pharmacy, Rady Faculty of Health Sciences, University of Manitoba, Winnipeg, MB, Canada. [2]Pharmacists Manitoba, Winnipeg, MB, Canada. [3]School of Population and Public Health, Faculty of Medicine, University of British Columbia, Vancouver, BC, Canada.

References
1. Soroka SN. Health Council of Canada. Toronto: Canadian Perceptions of the Health Care System: A Report to the Health Council of Canadians; 2007. http://www.queensu.ca/cora/_files/PublicPerceptions.pdf
2. Martin D, Miller AP, Quesnel-Vallée A, Caron NR, Vissandjée B, Marchildon GP. Canada's universal health-care system: achieving its potential. Lancet. 2018;391(10131):1718–35. https://doi.org/10.1016/S0140-6736(18)30181-8.
3. Caldbick S, Wu X, Lynch T, Al-Khatib N, Andkhoie M, Farag M. The financial burden of out of pocket prescription drug expenses in Canada. Int J Heal Econ Manag. 2015;15(3):329–38. https://doi.org/10.1007/s10754-015-9171-3.
4. McLeod L, Bereza BG, Shim M, Grootendorst P. Financial burden of household out-of-pocket expenditures for prescription drugs: cross-sectional analysis based on national survey data. Open Med. 2011;5(1):e1–9 http://www.ncbi.nlm.nih.gov/pubmed/22046212%5Cnhttp://www.pubmedcentral.nih.gov/articlerender.fcgi?artid=PMC3205811.
5. Marchildon G. Canada: health system review. Health Syst Transit. 2013;15(1):1–179.
6. Government of Canada. Royal Commission on Health Services; 1964.
7. Government of Canada. Canada Health Action. Ottawa: Building on the Legacy; 1997.
8. Government of Canada. Building on Values. Saskatoon: The Future of Health Care in Canada - Final Report; 2002.
9. Government of Canada. Pharmacare Now: Prescription Medicine Coverage for All Canadians. Ottawa; 2018. http://publications.gc.ca/collections/collection_2018/parl/xc62-1/XC62-1-1-421-14-eng.pdf.
10. Daw JR, Morgan SG, Thomson PA, Law MR. Here today, gone tomorrow: the issue attention cycle and national print media coverage of prescription drug financing in Canada. Health Policy (New York). 2013;110(1):67–75. https://doi.org/10.1016/j.healthpol.2013.01.006.
11. Morgan SG, Boothe K. Universal prescription drug coverage in Canada: long-promised yet undelivered. Healthc Manag Forum. 2016;29(6):247–54. https://doi.org/10.1177/0840470416658907.
12. Government of Canada. Towards Implementation of National Pharmacare - Discussion Paper. Ottawa; 2018. https://www.canada.ca/content/dam/hc-sc/documents/corporate/publications/council_on_pharmacare_EN.PDF.
13. Daw JR, Morgan SG. Stitching the gaps in the Canadian public drug coverage patchwork? A review of provincial pharmacare policy changes from 2000 to 2010. Health Policy (New York). 2012;104(1):19–26. https://doi.org/10.1016/j.healthpol.2011.08.015.
14. Grootendorst P. Beneficiary cost sharing under Canadian provincial prescription drug benefit programs: history and assessment. Can J Clin Pharmacol. 2002;9(2):79–99.
15. Morgan SG, Gagnon MA, Charbonneau M, Vadeboncoeur A. Evaluating the effects of Quebec's private-public drug insurance system. CMAJ. 2017; 189(40):E1259–63. https://doi.org/10.1503/cmaj.170726.
16. Barnes S, Anderson L. Low earnings, Unfilled Prescriptions: Employer-Provided Health Benefit Coverage in Canada.; 2015. http://www.wellesleyinstitute.com/wp-content/uploads/2015/07/Low-Earnings-Unfilled-Prescriptions-2015.pdf.
17. Law MR, Cheng L, Kolhatkar A, et al. The consequences of patient charges for prescription drugs in Canada: a cross-sectional survey. CMAJ open. 2018; 6(1):E63–70. https://doi.org/10.9778/cmajo.20180008.
18. Office of the Parliamentary Budget Officer. Federal Cost of a National Pharmacare Program. Ottawa; 2017. https://www.pbo-dpb.gc.ca/web/default/files/Documents/Reports/2017/Pharmacare/Pharmacare_EN_2017_11_07.pdf.
19. Kennedy J, Morgan S. A cross-national study of prescription nonadherence due to cost: data from the joint Canada-United States survey of health. Clin Ther. 2006;28(8):1217–24. https://doi.org/10.1016/j.clinthera.2006.07.009.
20. Kennedy J, Morgan S. Cost-related prescription nonadherence in the United States and Canada: a system-level comparison using the 2007 international health policy survey in seven countries. Clin Ther. 2009;31(1):213–9. https://doi.org/10.1016/j.clinthera.2009.01.006.
21. Law MR, Cheng L, Dhalla IA, Heard D, Morgan SG. The effect of cost on adherence to prescription medications in Canada. CMAJ. 2012;184(3):297–302. https://doi.org/10.1503/cmaj.111270.
22. Lee A, Morgan S. Cost-related nonadherence to prescribed medicines among older Canadians in 2014: a cross-sectional analysis of a telephone survey. C open. 2017;5(1):E40–4. https://doi.org/10.9778/cmajo.20160126.
23. Canadian Institute for Heallth Information. How Canada Compares: Results from the Commonwealth Fund's 2016. Ottawa: International Health Policy Survey of Adults in 11 Countries; 2017.
24. Lopert R, Docteur E, Morgan SG. Body Count: The Human Cost of Financial Barriers to Prescription Medications. Ottawa; 2018.
25. Canadian Institute for Health Information. National Health Expenditure Trends, 1975 to 2017. Ottawa, ON: CIHI; 2017. https://doi.org/10.1007/s10916-010-9605-x.
26. Belloni A, Morgan D, Paris V. Pharmaceutical expenditure and policies: past trends and future challenges. Paris. 2016. https://doi.org/10.1787/5jm0q1f4cdq7-en.
27. Canadian Health Services Research Foundation. Reference-based drug insurance policies can cut costs without harming patients *CHSRF - Evid Boost*. 2005;(June). https://www.cfhi-fcass.ca/migrated/pdf/mythbusters/boost2_e.pdf.
28. Morgan SG, Friesen MK, Thomson PA, Daw JR. Use of product listing agreements by Canadian provincial drug benefit plans. Healthc Policy. 2013; 8(4):45–55.
29. Husereau D, Dempster W, Blanchard A, Chambers J. Evolution of drug reimbursement in Canada: the Pan-Canadian pharmaceutical alliance for new drugs. Value Heal. 2014;17(8):888–94. https://doi.org/10.1016/j.jval.2014.08.2673.
30. IBM Canada Ltd. Pan Canadian Drugs Negotiations Report; 2014. https://canadaspremiers.ca/wp-content/uploads/2013/12/pan_canadian_drugs_negotiations_report_march22_2014.pdf.
31. Morgan SG, Thomson PA, Daw JR, Friesen MK. Inter-jurisdictional cooperation on pharmaceutical product listing agreements: views from Canadian provinces. BMC Health Serv Res. 2013;13(1):1–6. https://doi.org/10.1186/1472-6963-13-34.
32. Morgan SG, Daw JR, Thomson PA. Pharmaceuticals. In: Marchildon GP, Di Matteo L, editors. Bending the Cost Curve in Health Care: Canada's Provinces in International Perspective. 1st ed: University of Toronto Press; 2015. p. 113–37.
33. Candian Institute for Health Information. Drug Spending at a Glance – Information Sheet; 2017. p. 1–2. https://www.cihi.ca/sites/default/files/document/nhex2017-drug-infosheet-1-en.pdf
34. Department of Economic and Social Affairs. United Nations. Changing Population Age Structures and Sustainable Development. Vol E/CN.9/201; 2017. https://doi.org/10.1017/S0020818300006640.

35. Organization for Economic Cooperation and Development. OECD publishing. In: Health at a Glance 2017 OECD Indicators; 2017. Doi:10.1787/health_glance-2017-en.
36. Morgan SG, Leopold C, Wagner AK. Drivers of expenditure on primary care prescription drugs in 10 high-income countries with universal health coverage. CMAJ. 2017;189(23):E794–9. https://doi.org/10.1503/cmaj.161481.
37. Law MR, Morgan SG. Purchasing prescription drugs in Canada: hang together or hang separately. Healthc Policy. 2011;6(4):22–6. https://doi.org/10.1300/J104v17n03_07.
38. Canadian Doctors for Medicare, Canadian Centre for Policy Alternatives. Cost Savings Resulting from a National Pharmacare Program. 2017;(September):1–9. https://www.policyalternatives.ca/sites/default/files/uploads/publications/National%20Office/2017/09/Cost%20Savings%20From%20Pharmacare.pdf Office/2017/09/Cost_Savings_Resulting_from_Pharmacare.pdf.
39. Mackenzie H. Down the drain: how Canada has wasted $62 billion health care dollars without Pharmacare. 2017. https://nursesunions.ca/wp-content/uploads/2017/05/Down_The_Drain_Pharmacare_Report_December_2017.pdf.
40. Morgan SG, Law M, Daw JR, Abraham L, Martin D. Estimated cost of universal public coverage of prescription drugs in Canada. CMAJ. 2015;187(7):491–7. https://doi.org/10.1503/cmaj.150281.
41. Palmer WN, Nelson CA, Palmer NDL. Pharmacare Costing in Canada - Estimated Costs of Proposed National Pharmacare Programs.; 2016.
42. Gagnon M, Hebert G. The economic case for universal Pharmacare: costs and benefits of publicly funded drug coverage for all Canadians. Ottawa; 2010. http://old.nursesunions.ca/sites/default/files/universal-pharmacare-report-e.pdf.
43. Gagnon M-A. A roadmap to a rational Pharmacare policy in Canada. 1st ed. Canadian Federation of Nurses Unions: Ottawa; 2014.
44. Morgan SG, Law M, Daw JR, Abraham L, Martin D. Estimated cost of universal public coverage of prescription drugs in Canada. CMAJ. 2015;187(7):491–7. https://doi.org/10.1503/cmaj.141564.
45. Morgan SG, Martin D, Gagnon M-A, Mintzes B, Daw J, Lexchin J. Pharmacare 2020: the future of drug coverage in Canada. Vancouver; 2015. http://pharmacare2020.ca/
46. Morgan S, Hanley G, Raymond C, Blais R. Breadth, depth and agreement among provincial formularies in Canada. Healthc Policy. 2009;4(4):162–84.
47. Patented Medicine Prices Review Board. Alignment Among Public Formularies in Canada - Part 1: General Overview. Ottawa; 2017.
48. World Health Organization. WHO Model List of Essential Medicines - 19th List (April 2015). Essent Med. 2015;(April):1–45. http://www.who.int/medicines/publications/essentialmedicines/EML_2015_FINAL_amended_NOV2015.pdf.
49. Farkouh ME, Mphil AQ, Teoh H, Mbbs KAC, Leiter LA, Dphil JOF. Development of a preliminary essential medicines list for Canada. CMAJ Open. 2017;5(1):137–43. https://doi.org/10.9778/cmajo.20160058.
50. Morgan SG, Li W, Yau B, Persaud N. Estimated effects of adding universal public coverage of an essential medicines list to existing public drug plans in Canada. CMAJ. 2017;189(8):E295–302. https://doi.org/10.1503/cmaj.161082.
51. Canadian Agency for Drugs and Technology in Health. About CADTH. https://www.cadth.ca/about-cadth. Published 2018. Accessed 11 Mar 2018.
52. McMahon M, Morgan S, Mitton C. The common drug review: a NICE start for Canada? Health Policy (New York). 2006;77(3):339–51. https://doi.org/10.1016/j.healthpol.2005.08.006.
53. Forest P-G, Martin D. Fit for purpose: findings and recommendation of the external review of Pan-Canadian health organization - summary report: Government of Canada; 2018. https://www.canada.ca/content/dam/hc-sc/documents/services/health-care-system/reports-publications/health-care-system/findings-recommendations-external-review-pan-canadian-health-organization/findings-recommendations-external-review-pan-canadian-health-organization.pdf.
54. Government of Canada. Understand Permanent Resident Status. https://www.canada.ca/en/immigration-refugees-citizenship/services/new-immigrants/pr-card/understand-pr-status.html. Published 2017. Accessed 17 Sept 2018.
55. Government of Canada. Interim Federal Health Program – Information for individuals. https://www.canada.ca/en/immigration-refugees-citizenship/services/refugees/help-within-canada/health-care/interim-federal-health-program.html. Published 2017. Accessed 17 Sept 2018.
56. Government of Canada. Canada Health Act - Frequently Asked Questions - Canada.ca. https://www.canada.ca/en/health-canada/services/health-care-system/canada-health-care-system-medicare/canada-health-act-frequently-asked-questions.html#a12. Published 2018. Accessed 29 Jan 2018.
57. Parkin E. Briefing Paper - NHS Charges. 2018;(07227):1–22. http://researchbriefings.files.parliament.uk/documents/CBP-7227/CBP-7227.pdf.
58. Morgan SG, Daw JR, Law MR. Are income-based public drug benefit programs fit for an aging population? Montreal: Institute for Research on public policy; 2014. http://irpp.org/wp-content/uploads/2014/12/study-no50.pdf
59. Law MR, Kratzer J, Dhalla IA. The increasing inefficiency of private health insurance in Canada. CMAJ. 2014;186(12):470–4.
60. Flood CM, Thomas B, Moten A, Fafard P. Universal Pharmacare and Federalism. Montreal: Policy Options for Canada; 2018. http://irpp.org/wp-content/uploads/2018/09/Universal-Pharmacare-and-Federalism-Policy-Options-for-Canada.pdf
61. Canadian Doctors for Medicare. Rx : National Pharmacare. http://www.canadiandoctorsformedicare.ca/images/2013-07-21_CoF_Pharma_.pdf. Published 2011. Accessed 1 Mar 2018.
62. Canadian Medical Association. Health care transformation in Canada: change that works. Care that lasts; 2010. p. 48.
63. Canadian Federation of Nurses Unions. Canada's Nurses Serve up the Facts on Pharmacare to Premiers at Council of Federation 2016. http://nursesunions.ca/canadas-nurses-serve-up-the-facts-on-pharmacare-to-premiers-at-cof-2016/. Published 2016. Accessed 1 Mar 2018.
64. Canadian Federation of Nurses Unions. Pharmacare | Canada's Nurses. http://nursesunions.ca/campaigns/pharmacare/. Accessed 1 Mar 2018.
65. Registered Nurses Association of Ontario. Nurses Call for a National Pharmacare Program: RNAO Submission to the Standing Committee on Health; 2016.
66. Canadian Pharmacists Association. Position Statement - National Pharmacare Program. 2011:1. https://www.pharmacists.ca/advocacy/pharmacare-20/ Accessed 1 Mar 2018.
67. Canadian Pharmacists Association. Pharmacare 2.0 - Principles and Priorities. Ottawa; 2015. https://www.pharmacists.ca/advocacy/pharmacare-20/ Accessed 1 Mar 2018.
68. Canadian Pharmacists Association. Closing the Coverage Gap: Pan-Canadian Pharmacare. https://www.pharmacists.ca/advocacy/pharmacare-20/ Accessed 1 Mar 2018.
69. Canadian Pharmacists Association. *Rx* : PharmAccord - a Prescription for a Healthier Canada. Ottawa; 2017. https://www.pharmacists.ca/advocacy/pharmacare-20/ Accessed 1 Mar 2018.
70. Canadian Pharmacists Association. Submission to the Standing Committee on Finance for the Pre-Budget Consultations 2017 - Prescriptions for a Healthy and Prosperous Canada. Ottawa; 2017. https://www.pharmacists.ca/advocacy/pharmacare-20/ Accessed 1 Mar 2018.
71. Pomey MP, Forest PG, Palley HA, Martin E. Public/private partnerships for prescription drug coverage: policy formulation and outcomes in Quebec's universal drug insurance program, with comparisons to the medicare prescription drug program in the United States. Milbank Q. 2007;85(3):469–98. https://doi.org/10.1111/j.1468-0009.2007.00496.x.
72. Conference Board of Canada. Canadian Pharmacists Association. Ottawa: A Review of Pharmacy Services in Canada and the Health and Economic Evidence; 2016.
73. Canadian Society of Hospital Pharmacists. National Pharmacare : Position Statement. 2017:1–6. https://www.cshp.ca/sites/default/files/files/publications/Official%20Publications/Position%20Statements/National%20Pharmacare_Position%20Statement_2017_EN.pdf. Accessed 3 Mar 2018.
74. Health Charities Coalition of Canada. Position statement: access to medicines. 2016;(March):1–4. http://www.healthcharities.ca/media/30477/HCCC_PositionStatementATM_2016_EN.pdf. March 3, 2018.
75. Canada Health Coalition. Policy Conference on a National Public Drug Plan (2017). http://www.healthcoalition.ca/get-involved/international-conference-a-prescription-for-equity/. Published 2017. Accessed 3 Mar 2018.
76. White J, Canada Health Coalition. A National Public Drug Plan for All: Policy Brief. Ottawa; 2016. http://healthcoalition.ca/wp-content/uploads/2017/02/Policy-Brief-NPDP.pdf. Accessed 3 Mar 2018.
77. Canada Labour Congress. Pharmacare: A Plan for Everyone (Petition Campaign). http://www.aplanforeveryone.ca/. Published 2017. Accessed 3 Mar 2018.
78. CARP. Pharmacare Poll Highlights. http://www.carp.ca/2017/11/27/pharmacare-poll-highlights/. Published 2017. Accessed 19 July 2018.
79. Pharmacare2020. The Future Of Drug Coverage In Canada - Pharmacare 2020. http://pharmacare2020.ca/. Accessed 3 Mar 2018.
80. Angus Reid Institute. Prescription Drug Access and Affordability an Issue for Nearly a Quarter of All Canadian Households; 2015. http://angusreid.org/prescription-drugs-canada/.

81. Citizens' Reference Panel on Pharmacare in Canada. Necessary Medicines. Vancouver: Recommendations of the citizens ' reference panel on Pharmacare in Canada; 2016.
82. Canadian Organization for Rare Disorders. Should Rare Disease Patients Fear National Pharmacare? Press Release. https://www.raredisorders.ca/press-release/. Published 2018. Accessed 19 Sept 2018.
83. Graham J. National Pharmacare: prescription for restriction | Fraser Institute. Ottawa Citizen https://www.fraserinstitute.org/article/national-pharmacare-prescription-restriction. Accessed 19 July 2018.
84. Bateman J. Pharmacare 2020: the Canadian Tax Federation's Vision I Canadian Tax Federation. https://www.taxpayer.com/presentations/pharmacare-2020%2D%2Dthe-ctf-s-vision. Published 2013. Accessed 19 July 2018.
85. Innovative Medicines Canada. About - Innovative Medicines Canada represents Canada's innovative pharmaceutical industry. http://innovativemedicines.ca/about/. Accessed 11 March 2018.
86. Dion-Marquis S. Budget 2018: Innovative Medicines Canada welcomes new advisory council and renewed commitment to research and science. http://innovativemedicines.ca/budget-2018-innovative-medicines-canada-welcomes-new-advisory-council-renewed-commitment-research-science/. Accessed 4 Mar 2018.
87. Dion-Marquis S. Statement: Federal Cost of a National Pharmacare Program. http://innovativemedicines.ca/statement-costing-report-on-national-pharmacare/. Accessed 4 March 2018.
88. Canadian Life and Health Insurance Association. Letter to Minister of Health - Re: Facts about the cost implications of bringing prescription drugs into Medicare. 2015:1–7. https://www.clhia.ca/web/clhia_lp4w_lnd_webstation.nsf/page/5CEC3F8A27207E4E85257ED200643C4C/$file/Ltr%20to%20Min.%20Ambrose%20-%20costs%20of%20pharmacare.pdf to Min. Ambrose - costs of pharmacare.pdf.
89. Canadian Life and Health Insurance Association. News Release - Life and Health Insurance Industry Welcomes New National Advisory Council on Pharmacare. 2018. https://www.clhia.ca/web/clhia_lp4w_lnd_webstation.nsf/page/532F8A8F41087DE7852582B2005F06B0/$file/News%20Release%20-%20Advisory%20Council.pdf.
90. Canadian Life and Health Insurance Association. Letter to CFNU Regarding August 2014 Report on Pharmacare Policy. https://www.clhia.ca/web/clhia_lp4w_lnd_webstation.nsf/page/A48C50D2ED5C38DC85257D47006ABCD3/$file/Letter%20to%20Ms%20Silas%20re.%20Aug%202014%20report%20on%20pharmacare%20policy to Ms Silas re. Aug 2014 report on pharmacare policy.pdf. Published 2014. Accessed March 4, 2018.
91. Swedlove F. CLHIA Opening Remarks to the House of Commons Standing Committee on Health - Appearance on Pharmacare (Oct 19, 2017). https://www.clhia.ca/web/clhia_lp4w_lnd_webstation.nsf/page/E447014D8DFED32F852581C2004B2F7C/$file/CLHIA%20Opening%20Remarks%20on%20Pharmacare.pdf. Opening Remarks on Pharmacare.pdf. Published 2017. Accessed 4 Mar 2018.
92. Canadian Life and Health Insurance Association. Improving drug access and affordability: Can public and private payers do more, together? http://page.telushealth.com/rs/655-URY-133/images/perspectives_Can%20public%20and%20private%20payers%20do%20more%20together.PDF. Published 2017. Accessed 28 Feb 2018.
93. Canadian Institute for Health Information. National Prescription Drug Utilization Information System: Plan Information Document. Ottawa: CIHI; 2018. https://secure.cihi.ca/free_products/PlanInformation_1007_e1.pdf
94. Morgan S, Smolina K, Mooney D, Raymond C, Bowen M. Rx atlas. 3 Vancouver, BC: Centre for Health Services and Policy Research.; 2013. https://open.library.ubc.ca/clRcle/collections/facultyresearchandpublications/52383/items/1.0048514. Accessed 3 Mar 2018.

2

'Better medicines for children' within the Integrated Management of Childhood Illness framework

Xavier Nsabagasani[1*], Japer Ogwal-Okeng[2], Ebba Holme Hansen[3], Anthony Mbonye[4,5], Herbert Muyinda[1] and Freddie Ssengooba[6]

Abstract

Background: The Integrated Management of Childhood Illnesses is the main approach for treating children in more than 100 low income countries worldwide. In 2007, the World Health Assembly urged countries to integrate 'better medicines for children' into their essential medicines lists and treatment guidelines. WHO regularly provides generic algorithms for IMCI and publishes the Model Essential Medicines List with child-friendly medicines based on new evidence for member countries to adopt. However, the status of 'better medicines for children' within the Integrated Management of Childhood Illnesses approach in Uganda has not been studied.

Methods: Qualitative interviews were conducted with: two officials from the ministry of health; two district health officials and, 22 health workers from public health facilities. Interview transcripts were manually analyzed for manifest and latent content.

Results: Child-appropriate dosage formulations were not included in the package for the Integrated Management of Childhood Illnesses and ministry officials attributed this to resource constraints and lack of initial guidance from the World Health Organization. Underfunding reportedly undercut efforts to: orient health workers; do support supervision and update treatment guidelines to reflect 'better medicines for children'. Health workers reported difficulties in administering tablets and capsules to under-five children and that's why they preferred liquid oral dosage formulations, suppositories and injections.

Conclusions: The IMCI strategy in Uganda was not revised to reflect child-appropriate dosage formulations – a missed opportunity for improving the quality of management of childhood illnesses. Funding was an obstacle to the integration of child-appropriate dosage formulations. Ministry of health should prioritize funding for the Integrated Management of Childhood Illnesses and revising the Essential Medicines and Health Supplies List of Uganda, the Uganda Clinical Guidelines and, the Treatment Charts for the Integrated Management of Childhood Illnesses to reflect child-appropriate dosage formulations.

Keywords: IMCI, Better medicines for children, Dosage formulations and Uganda

* Correspondence: dianatim2001@yahoo.co.uk
[1]Child Health and Development Center, College of Health Sciences, Makerere University, Kampala, Uganda
Full list of author information is available at the end of the article

Background

Globally, an estimated 8.1 million children under-five die every year due to conditions that can be prevented or treated with evidence-based medicines [1]. In 1995, the World Health Organization (WHO) and United Nations Children's Emergency Fund (UNICEF) introduced the Integrated Management of Childhood Illnesses (IMCI) strategy to improve case management skills of health workers to diagnose and treat the major childhood illnesses. IMCI was meant to address three key elements. The first element was to develop and provide IMCI guidelines to enable health workers improve case management. Therefore, WHO regularly provides generic algorithms for IMCI to be adopted by countries following their epidemiological situation. WHO also supports countries in the selection of essential medicines for children by publishing the Model Essential Medicines List for children [2]. The second element was to build the capacity of health workers through training and support supervision to enable them use the provided IMCI algorithms to identify and treat illness. The third element was to strengthen the health systems so as to provide an environment and facilities conducive for managing children illnesses. This element covers ensuring that there is availability of priority medicines for children. Therefore, UNICEF recommends that governments should improve their health systems to ensure that the essential drugs are available [3]. Some studies have concluded that availability of medicines is a key condition for the success of IMCI [2–6].

In 2007, the 60th World Health Assembly made a resolution that urged member countries to include 'better medicines for children' in their essential medicines lists and clinical guidelines [4]. Following this resolution, later in 2007 WHO and partners launched the 'make medicines child size' campaign to create more awareness about child-appropriate dosage formulations [5]. Hence, it was sensible to integrate child-appropriate dosage formulations into IMCI, a strategy that is used to manage sick children in more than 100 countries worldwide. Uganda was among the first countries worldwide to adopt and scale up IMCI. According to personal communication with a ministry of health official, after piloting of the strategy in 1995, IMCI was adopted in 1997 as a national strategy for the management of the common childhood illnesses. The first phase of implementation of IMCI included adaptation of the globally recommended IMCI guidelines to the Ugandan setting and consequent training of the health workers in selected districts. With support from the United States Agency for International Development (USAID), the IMCI approach was first pilot tested in ten districts in 1996 and a 22 member national task force was established to coordinate the IMCI activities. In 1997, the IMCI approach was scaled up nationally.

According to the Uganda Government Heath Sector Strategic and Investment Plan III (HSSIP III), IMCI was recognized as the main approach for treating children in Uganda [6]. Despite that recognition, there are still gaps in policy provisions for child-appropriate dosage formulations and so far there has been no formal adoption of these formulations as a policy [7, 8]. Furthermore, there is still low availability and utilization of the WHO recommended lifesaving priority medicines for children in the public health facilities [9].

Despite these gaps, the perspectives: of administrators at the MoH; district health officials; and, health workers' practices and experiences of treating children within the IMCI approach using child-appropriate dosage formulations have not been explored. This paper is premised on the understanding that IMCI should be the vehicle for integrating child-appropriate dosage formulations in those countries where it is being implemented. It is therefore critical to assess the extent to which IMCI implementation at the facility level reflects the WHA resolution of 'better medicines for children'. This paper explores the perspectives of officials from MoH and the district health department about the integration of 'better medicines for children' into the IMCI approach. At the facility level, the paper explores health workers' knowledge and perspectives about child-appropriate dosage formulations, their practices and experiences in the management of childhood illnesses in Uganda using IMCI approach.

Methods

Study design

The study derives from the 60th WHA resolution of 'better medicines for children'. Therefore, the focus of the study was about the level of integration and application of the 'better medicines for children' concept into IMCI, the main framework for managing childhood illnesses in Uganda. The study design was also based on the premise that child-appropriate dosage formulations such as dispersible tablets, granules, sprinkles and pellets are the best for improving prescription, dispensing and administration of medicines to the under-five population [10]. In this paper, child-appropriate dosage formulations refer to medicines that are easily adjusted to reflect size, strengths, state of development, and condition of a child [10]. WHO recommended dispersible, scored tablets or the equivalent of the flexible solid oral dosage formulations as the most effective for children [1, 11]. This study applied these concepts as basis for the formulation of the analytical framework, the data collection methods and the tools that were used.

The analytical framework of the study draws from debates about policy processes and factors that influence success of implementation of policy and its sustainability [12–14]. Tansella &Thornicroft (2009) highlighted these factors in relation to how to accelerate the transfer of discoveries in health sciences into implementation of evidence based routine clinical practice. Tansella &Thornicroft articulated three phases of implementation of evidence based clinical practices: adoption in principle; early implementation and, persistence of implementation [12]. This framework helps to explain the process and context of IMCI adoption, implementation and its implication on the adoption of child-appropriate dosage formulations in a low income country Uganda. In this study, facilitators and barriers to the implementation of the IMCI program are considered. A multi-level analysis of perspectives is used and covers the national, district and facility levels.

Study setting

The study was conducted between July and August 2012 in Uganda, a landlocked low income country in the East African region. In Uganda, IMCI is the main approach for diagnosing, dispensing and administering medicines to treat childhood illnesses. Uganda was also among the first UN member states in sub-Saharan Africa to implement IMCI as a national program since 1995 [6]. An IMCI section was included into both the Uganda Clinical Guidelines 2010 and 2012 versions [15, 16].

In Uganda, procurement of medicines for public health facilities is under National Medical Stores (NMS) which distributes medicines provided in the Essential Medicines and Health Supplies List of Uganda (EMHSLU) using a push system. By the time of the study, the latest version of EMHSLU was that of 2012. Other medicine procurement and distribution channels included: the Joint Medical Stores (JMS)-an umbrella organization for the Uganda Catholic Medical Bureau (UCMB) and Uganda Protestant Medical Bureau and, a private sector procurement agent called Medicine Access Uganda Limited (MAUL). Some medicines are also accessed with direct support of donors and are channeled through some development partners: the Uganda Health Marketing Group (UHMG); partners funded by the President's Emergency Plan for AIDS Relief (PEPFAR); Malaria Consortium (MC) and, the United Nations (UN) agencies including UNICEF, the Joint United Nations Programme on HIV and AIDS (UNAIDS) and WHO.

The Ugandan public health care system is highly decentralized with districts and health sub-districts playing a key role in the administration of the delivery of health services. There is a hierarchy of public health facilities starting with the lowest service delivery point being at the village level now referred to as Health Center One (HCI) through to Health Center four (HCIV) at a county level. Above these there is , the district hospitals, regional and national referral hospitals at the top [6]. At HCI, services are provided by volunteers referred to as Village Health Team (VHTs) who do not have formal health training. In 2010, the VHTs were given an additional role of distributing medicines for the integrated community case management (ICCM) of childhood illnesses. The Health Center two (HCII) facilities are largely managed by Nursing Assistants who have minimal training in the medical field. In most of the rural facilities in Uganda, Nursing Assistants play a significant role in treating children. Health Center three (HCIII) facilities are supposed to be served by clinical officers, nurses, midwives and nursing assistants. In reality, due to staffing challenges at this level, Nursing Assistants still constitute the majority of the health workers. At Health Center Four (HCIV) level, in addition to the cadre of staff stated above, there should be at least a medical doctor. At the district hospital and above, there are both general doctors and specialists in addition to other cadres of health staff. In case of children, the specialists are pediatricians.

Study respondents

Qualitative in-depth interviews were held with: the Ministry of Health officials; the district health team and, health workers from the public health facilities. Health facilities included one national referral hospital and one regional referral hospital and sixteen lower level rural based health facilities in Jinja district. In Uganda, the concept of health workers refers to those people working in the health system with the qualifications recognized by government. Rural based health facilities were lower levels facilities in the rural areas of Jinja district. These included HCIIs, HCIIIs and HCIVs. Table 1 shows the categories of respondents and the themes included in the interview guide for each category.

At the Ministry of Health level, two officials from the child health division were interviewed. The child health division was behind the adaption and scaling up IMCI implementation in the country. The division also spearheaded the adaptation of the WHO IMCI algorithm, initial training and support supervision of health workers. Two health officials from Jinja district in eastern Uganda were purposively selected to participate in the study. The district health officials had been part of the early implementation of IMCI in the district.

At the facility level, five pediatricians were drawn from Mulago, the biggest national referral hospital located in the capital city Kampala. The national referral hospital is a teaching hospital for the Makerere College of Health Sciences. One pediatrician was drawn from Jinja hospital, the biggest eastern regional referral hospital located in Jinja town. Despite, the huge pediatric patient load in the regional referral hospital, there are only two pediatricians. Sixteen lower level health workers were drawn from 16 rural based health facilities in Jinja district.

All the respondents were purposively selected based on experiences and current responsibilities about the

Table 1 Respondents and the thematic areas covered

Respondent	Number	Main themes covered
MoH Program mangers officers)	2	• The historical context and the process of IMCI implementation • What worked and what did not work with IMCI and child-appropriate dosage formulation adoption • The level of integration of the child-appropriate dosage formulation into IMCI approach • Achievements and limitation of the integration
The district health team	2	• The historical context and the process of IMCI implementation • Perspective of the child-appropriate dosage formulations • Experiences of implementation of IMCI and child-appropriate dosage formulations under a decentralized arrangement • Financing, support supervision and refresher training
Pediatricians from Mulago hospital	5	• Practices about using child-appropriate dosage formulations to treat children under 5 years • Available information about child-appropriate dosage formulations • Coping mechanisms when there are no child-appropriate dosage formulations
Pediatrician from Jinja hospital	1	• Practices about using child-appropriate dosage formulations to treat children under 5 years • Available information about child-appropriate dosage formulations • coping mechanisms when there are no child-appropriate dosage formulations
Lower level rural based health workers	16	• Their perspectives and practices about using child-appropriate dosage formulations to treat children under 5 years within the IMCI framework • Available information about child-appropriate dosage formulations and the treatment protocols • Coping mechanisms when there are no child-appropriate dosage formulations

implementation of the IMCI strategy. At the facility level, those found treating children at the time of the visit were automatically selected for interviews. All interviews were held in privacy and in venues preferred by the respondents. Where it was felt that information saturation was realized we stopped interviewing more of that category of respondents. There were 16 health workers from the rural based health facilities. This number was high because we wanted to get information from the diverse categories (clinical officers, nurses, midwives and nursing assistants) who represented different levels of healthcare.

Jinja district has a population of more than 468,256 people and of these 299,109 (64 %) live in rural areas [17]. Administratively, the district is subdivided into seven rural sub-counties, one town council and three divisions in the municipality. Like the rest of the country, there is a hierarchy of health facilities ranging from Health Centre II to the regional referral hospital as described elsewhere [9]. Jinja district has a total of 69 health facilities, 49 of which are public, seventeen are run by NGOs and three are institutional (army, police and prisons). The major causes of child morbidity and mortality in the area include malaria (70 %), acute respiratory infections (16 %) and diarrheal diseases (32 %) [18]. Jinja is also a home of the neglected tropical disease of schistomiasis which affects both adults and children.

Data collection

Qualitative in-depth interviews were performed using an unstructured thematic interview guide. For each category of respondents, as earlier indicated, the key themes addressed are provided in Table 1. Data was collected by the first Author (a social scientist) and was assisted by a Research Assistant who is also a social scientist. All the interviews were conducted in English by the first author. On average the interviews lasted between 40 and 60 min.

Data analysis

Interviews were digitally recorded and later transcribed verbatim, printed and carefully read. The codes were then applied to the scripts. Data analysis was conducted manually using a thematic manifest and latent content analysis [19]. A coding sheet with the key themes was developed and later applied to the transcribed text. Deductive meanings that were theory guided were adopted from our pre-conceived abstractions and compared with the primary data. This was based on the understanding that category names and related codes can be generated from the already existing concepts, literature and the phrases used by the informants themselves [20].

Results

The study explored perspectives about the status of child-appropriate dosage formulations within the IMCI approach at three levels in Uganda: the central ministry level; the district level and the health facility level. The key themes that emerged were as follows:

- Lacking of funding cut across all the three levels and affected implementation of IMCI
- At the national level, the IMCI strategy had not been revised to include child-appropriate dosage formulations

- At the district level, the decentralized IMCI activities were not being implemented and this weakened the efforts to integrate the child-appropriate dosage formulation component. Ironically, re-centralization of medicine procurement and distribution to the National Medical Stores (NMS) reversed district's discretion to procure child-friendly medicines
- At the facility level, health workers' faced challenges of prescribing, dispensing and administering tablets and capsules to children. They remodeled ways to ensure that children received appropriate treatment. Lower level cadres of rural based health workers did not have sufficient information about the new treatment policies that might have included child-appropriate dosage formulations

Resource constraints

The predominant challenge to the integration of child-appropriate dosage formulations was the insufficient funding of IMCI activities at the national, district and facility levels. Table 2 shows that at the national level, resource constraints affected planning, development of relevant policy reforms and budgeting that in turn affected the integration of child-appropriate dosage formulations into the IMCI framework. This in turn had a spillover negative effect on the implementation of IMCI at the lower levels. MoH officials reported that due to lack of funding, it was not possible to revise the IMCI treatment charts to reflect child-appropriate dosage formulations. During the late implementation phase of IMCI, the project resources were already exhausted and when government took over, it failed to sustain most of the activities.

At the moment we do not have money for continuing some of the IMCI activities the way we are supposed to. Donors have shifted ICCM. We have adopted the IMCI approach as a routine but we do not have needed resources to sustain some of the core activities including revision of guidelines and refresher training (MoH, official).

MoH officials perceived some of the child-appropriate dosage formulations recommended by WHO such as dispersible tablets as a luxury for the already financially hard-pressed ministry. MoH officials were also aware of the fact that there were no funds for the decentralized IMCI activities. Districts were expected to use the Primary Health Care (PHC) grants to implement the decentralized IMCI activities and development partners were expected to supplement. However, the PHC grants were not enough to cater for all the decentralized IMCI activities and other already earmarked activities. Jinja district did not get support for IMCI from development partners.

As a ministry, we no longer handle IMCI refresher training. This function was decentralized to the districts that have to develop a budget to cater for the refresher training and support supervision. A few districts have been lucky and some partners like STRIDES are supporting IMCI. As of now we do not know what is going on in the districts except where the partners are operating now (Ministry of Health Official).

Table 2 The process of IMCI Development and implementation landmarks in Uganda

Levels	Implementation phases		
	Adoption phase	Early implementation	Situation at the time of the study
National	In 1995 IMCI selected as the main approach for Uganda. A 22- member working group was established for planning, training and adaptation. IMCI algorithm was adopted to fit the national health policy and treatment guidelines	By 1998 there was a national expansion plan with a pool of 250 trainers, 10 zonal teams to supervise IMCI implementation. Donors: World Bank, USAID, UNICEF and WHO put in resources for early implementation of IMCI. By 2003 all the districts in Uganda had been trained in IMCI	Budget constraints and lack of information about 'better medicnes for children' meant limited national level reflections about policies, plans, budgets and guidelines for child-appropriate dosage formulations. No resources for the sustainability of IMCI in terms of refresher trainings, revision of job aids and support supervision. The decentralization of IMCI to districts minimized the central MoH role both technically and financially.
Local (district)	Districts health officials were prepared in terms of training about IMCI.	Districts were prepared in terms of training about IMCI.	Resources were not available for the districts. Districts were getting minimal support from the ministry in form of PHC grants which covered a little on support supervision. Therefore, the districts were not prepared for training health workers on child-appropriate dosage formulations
Facility/ individual levels	Health workers were sensitized on the new approach of IMCI.	Health workers were trained on the new approach of IMCI for 3 weeks.	Health workers were no longer receiving refresher training and support supervision for IMCI related activities from the district health team because districts did not have the financial capacity to do so.

MoH was also aware of the human resource challenges especially understaffing and limited number of qualified health personnel especially in the rural areas. Such staff needed adequate refresher training and support supervision to acquaint them with new information about the global and national treatment policies for children.

Failure to revise the IMCI treatment charts

Despite of the fact that WHO consistently revises the IMCI algorithm to accommodate new evidence based medicine, MoH officials admitted that it has not been possible to adapt new WHO IMCI algorithms to the Ugandan setting due to funding challenges as already indicated. Other than the WHA recommendation of better medicines for children, there other national initiatives such as changes in malaria treatment policies which were not communicated to the lower cadre staff. All these were not reflected in the IMCI treatment charts and this resulted into confusion especially among the lower level rural based health workers who entirely depend on IMCI treatment charts to diagnose and prescribe medicine to children.

Lack of global and national level efforts to initiate the integration

Unlike the other initiatives such as malaria treatment policy, WHO did not initiate national discussions about child-appropriate dosage formulation and how they would be integrated into the IMCI framework. MoH expected external support especially from WHO and UNICEF to initiate and finance the integration of child-appropriate dosage formulations.

> *We did not see any justification for just introducing child-appropriate dosage formulations into the IMCI approach without any guidance from the World Health Organization. There were gaps in the information about the child-appropriate dosage formulations concept especially regarding where the medicines could be procured and at what prices. (Ministry of Health official).*

On the other hand, donors had stopped funding facility based IMCI by the time the resolution of 'better medicines for children' was made. The MoH officials recounted how they had advised donors to continue to support the facility based IMCI including procurement of medicines for which donors did not comply. The discussions about child-friendly medicines only gained momentum in 2012 after the UN declaration of life- saving priority medicines for children. Both government and donors agreed to include into the mainstream health service delivery system, lifesaving for children. This was a good opportunity since all the medicines in the list of priority lifesaving medicnes for children were recommended in child-appropriate dosage formulations. In spite of this new emphasis, MoH officials also confessed that it would take time before these medicines could be accessed as there would be need to revise the EMHSLU, UCG and IMCI treatment charts to reflect 'better medicines for children'.

Perspectives about child-appropriate dosage formulations

Table 3 highlights the context and explanations by the respondents at different levels about status quo of child-appropriate dosage formulations within the IMCI framework in Uganda. The table highlights the perspectives in the wider context of the three different levels (ministry, district and facility) and how this affected the integration of child-appropriate dosage formulations into the IMCI framework. Although there were some areas of convergence, the perspectives are presented according to the specific respondents: MoH officials, district health officials, pediatricians and lower level rural based health workers.

Perspectives from Ministry of Health

The concept of child-appropriate dosage formulations in Uganda centered on liquid oral dosage formulations (syrups) which were deleted from the EMHSLU 2012 and were for the interim replaced with tablets for adults that were extrapolated for children. The reasons for deleting syrups included high prices and handling challenges. The deleted syrups were no longer being supplied in the public health facilities.

> *We usually find a lot of problems with these syrups. They are messy, expensive, and difficult to handle during transportation. They are had to store especially in remote areas where there is no power for refrigeration (Ministry of Health official)*

When asked about other child-appropriate dosage formulations such as pellets, sprinkles and dispersible tablets, MoH officials stated that lack of market information and high cost of these formulations repulsed efforts to integrate them into the IMCI approach. MoH officials generally perceived some of these formulations to be expensive and this affected their efforts to integrate them into the EMHSLU.

Table 3 Perspectives of respondents about IMCI and child-appropriate dosage formulations

Actors	The context	The Point of view of the actors
MoH officials	• Budget constraints and lack of information about 'better medicines for children' meant limited national level reflections about policies, revision of guidelines, budgets and guidelines for child-appropriate dosage formulations • MoH decentralized refresher training and support supervision for IMCI for the districts and their development partners	• Lack of global initiatives to support the resolution of 'better medicines for children' at the national level and challenges of sustainable financing for IMCI implementation • When IMCI funding reduced and MoH could no longer provide oversight and refresher training for IMCI and these roles were left for local governments under decentralized services. However, MoH continues to acknowledge the fact that there were no sufficient resources for implementing IMCI under the decentralized arrangement • Concerns that donors and development partners had shifted their goals to fund the community based ICCM program completely leaving out support for IMCI at the facility level • Since the markets and prices for some of the child-appropriate dosage formulations such as sprinkles, pellets and dispersible tablet were not known. They were perceived to be expensive and therefore not affordable by the ministry. Other well-known child-friendly formulations such as syrups were too costly and moreover difficult to handle and store in a low income setting of Uganda. They were deleted from the EMHSLU 2012 due to these reasons.
The district health officials	• Underfunding of the decentralized responsibilities in the health sector • Donors had shifted interest to ICCM and abandoned IMCI	• Jinja district was not ready for the decentralized roles of conducting IMCI refresher training and support supervision due to financial constraints. They were concerned about lack of revised IMCI treatment charts. Centralization of medical supplies to NMS has deprived the district the opportunities to decide on the procurement of the right medicines for children
Pediatricians	• Pediatricians are limited and are only available in hospitals • Pediatricians are supposed to see children who are referred to them by the lower level health workers	• IMCI is a strategy to be used by the lower cadre staff. At the moment the approach is not robust enough to integrate new treatment changes • The IMCI strategy would benefit from improved IMCI guidelines that would address evidence based and child-appropriate dosage formulations • The Uganda Clinical Guidelines are insufficient and pediatricians were reportedly referring to other guidelines such as BNF and the internet to determine treatment. Prescribe some syrup such as amoxicillin syrup and other child-friendly syrups available in the private sector. Had an idea about dispersible tablets but did not use them because they were not available.
Lower cadre health workers (enrolled nurses and nursing assistants)	Cognitive Barriers, using outdated IMCI charts, limited interaction with the MoH officials in terms of support supervision	• Need refresher training on IMCI, updated guidelines and evidence based medicines • Need support supervision to enable them improve their skills • Some nursing assistants said that they did not know that the treatment policy for malaria had changed

The perspectives of the district health officials

The district officials' explanations of the failure to integrate child-appropriate dosage formulations were consistent with those of the MoH. Lack of funds purportedly affected implementation of the decentralized IMCI activities. While the district managers were aware of their decentralized roles in relation to IMCI training and support supervision of facilities, they were not capable of carrying out the responsibilities due to lack of resources as indicated in Table 3. Under the decentralized arrangement, there was a challenge of understaffing due to the failure of local government to attract qualified health workers especially in the rural health facilities. Consequently, the majority of health workers seeing children in these facilities were mainly nurses and nursing assistants. Due to their limited medical training and limited access to information, this category of staff need constant on- job training and job aids to help them understand new information. According to the district officials, this was not happening.

We are expected to carry out refresher training for different things including IMCI. The PHC grants that we receive are not enough for the many obligations. So we can only do a little in support supervision which also covers a wide range of other things. Refresher training for IMCI requires a lot of money which is not available. We are looking forward for some external support (District Health official, Jinja District).

District officials also underlined challenges of recentralizing procurement and distribution of medicine supplies to NMS which was supplying medicines that were not necessarily corresponding to the priorities of the district and health facilities. There was a general feeling that districts have no say about the medicines that are procured by NMS compared to before when the districts had the discretion to purchase the medicines they wanted. District official wondered why important medicines for children such as syrups were being left out by NMS.

We used to have important syrups to treat malaria and pneumonia especially among the under-five children and now there are no more because we depend on NMS for drug supplies. NMS no longer supplies syrups. They supply tablets instead. It is now difficult for our caregivers to administer tablets to children. There are so many associated problems, dividing the tablets affects dosing, children refuse to swallow the medicines and if they do so they can easily vomit (District Health Official, Jinja district).

Like the ministry, the district officials accentuated the limitation of unrevised IMCI treatment chart as a reference material especially for the nursing assistants who are not sufficiently medically trained but nevertheless were treating children in most of the low level rural based health facilities.

In most cases our health workers use guess work and hearsay from the private sector providers. For quite some time, despite the changes in treatment policies, the IMCI guidelines have not been revised. They are still using the initial IMCI treatment charts which still refer to chloroquine as the first line treatment for malaria. They are so outdated. Yet our nursing assistants have no other reference materials to treat children other that the unrevised IMCI treatment charts (District Health Official, Jinja District).

Due to resource constraints and limited opportunities to decide on procurement, the district officials argued that they did not control the provision of child–appropriate dosage formulations. They remain on the receiving end and accept whatever is distributed by NMS.

Perspectives from the health workers

Health workers who participated in the interviews were differentiated by their level of training. Level of training influenced the health workers' views about IMCI and child-appropriate dosage formulations. Health workers interviewed fall into two broad categories. The first includes pediatricians who are highly specialized health workers in diagnosing and treating children. Ideally pediatricians are supposed to handle referral cases from the lower level health workers from the outpatient department (in case of hospitals) and lower level health facilities. In the Ugandan public health facilities, pediatricians mainly work in hospitals where they are supposed to handle complicated cases. The second category included the rural based and less trained health workers who were mainly clinical officers, midwives, nurses and nursing assistants. Ideally, rural based health workers are supposed to treat less severe symptoms using IMCI and refer severe cases and any other complications to the pediatricians.

Pediatricians' perspectives and their practices

The general view from the pediatricians was that IMCI does not cater for child-friendly medicines due to lack of a conducive medicine policy environment. Pediatricians reported that they do not use IMCI approach because they are consultants for very sick children after their management using the IMCI has failed. It was therefore more practical to think of more advanced and international guidelines to diagnose complicated cases among children.

For us we are beyond IMCI. We handle problems where IMCI has failed. We are consultants who are supposed to read widely. We refer to the internet, the British National Formulary and for that matter, we read beyond the Uganda Clinical Guidelines. However, because the clinical guidelines are not followed (by some of the lower level health workers) we often handle children with ordinary conditions and this increases our patient load (Pediatrician, Jinja regional referral hospital).

Pediatrician supported provision of child-appropriate dosage formulations. From their own point of view, the best child-appropriate dosage formulations were mainly liquid oral dosage formulations (syrups). They were for example concerned about the government policy that phased out syrups that were being used for the treatment of pneumonia and malaria. They argued that some of the emerging complications and treatment failure were due to use of medicine formulations that were not appropriate for children.

Some of the children referred to us from the lower level health facilities will have received the right treatment in terms of the medicines. However, because most of these will have been given in formulations of tablets, caretakers usually report difficulties in administration of the medicines. These difficulties result into inaccurate dosing sometimes associated with vomiting of the medicines. Caretakers do not know what to do when the child vomits. Most of them stop giving the medicines. We have been hearing these complaints from the caretakers quite a lot (Pediatrician Jinja Regional Referral Hospital).

Pediatricians from the regional referral hospital and the national referral hospitals reported that the Uganda Clinical Guidelines (UCG) were insufficient for the management of the prevailing childhood illnesses. They therefore, did not necessarily prescribe medicines indicated in the UCG.

Pediatricians reported that they often prescribed medicines that were not in the public health facilities but were nevertheless considered to be child-appropriate by the pediatricians. When the medicines are not available, pediatricians said they referred caregivers to procure the medicines from the private pharmacies and private clinics where the medicines were available at a cost.

Perspectives and practices rural based health workers

Rural based health workers reported (it was also observed) that they were still using the outdated IMCI treatment charts of 2001. They had not been oriented on the new treatment policies for quite some time and support supervision had accordingly diminished. It was noted that child-appropriate dosage formulations such granules, sprinkles and dispersible tablets were not mentioned among the key dosage formulations that health workers used in their daily practice using IMCI. They were instead familiar with tablets, suppositories for malaria and, injectables for pneumonia and sepsis.

Some of the Nurses and Nursing Assistants who had been in service for some years said they were initially trained in IMCI. However, they had also spent a long time without attending IMCI related refresher courses and felt that refresher trainings would have informed them more about new medicines, changes in treatment regimens, new guidelines and any other new information about managing childhood illnesses.

We come to learn about these new medicines from our friends who work in private clinics. Some medicines are brought here for use when we have never heard about them. The IMCI charts you see hear are referring to very old medicines some of which have already been phased out. We are often confused by this (Nurse, rural based health facility).

Some of the midwives who were interviewed reported that they had been left out during the initial IMCI training perhaps because it was never anticipated that they would ever interface with children. However, due to staff shortages, midwives were found treating children. Midwives noted that their work of treating children would be enhanced if they were also trained on how to use IMCI charts to treat children.

Health workers reported information gaps due to failure to update IMCI treatment charts to reflect medicines recommended by the new treatment policies. Much as the UCG had been revised from the 2007 to 2010, then later in 2012, only the in-charges in the rural based facilities had access to the revised guidelines. Health workers reported experiencing challenges regarding new treatment policies that were by then not integrated into the IMCI treatment charts. This, according to some, undermined their confidence in relation to deciding on which medicines to give. The newly introduced medicines for malaria were not written anywhere on the IMCI treatment charts that they were using. For example, while Artemether Lumefantrine was the first line treatment for malaria recommended in the new national malaria treatment policy, the IMCI treatment charts referred to a combination of fancidar and chloroquine-medicines which had been phased out by the National Drug Authority. Their other source of confusion was that the fansidar-chloroquine combination was also being recommended in the UCG 2010. At the same time, there were other types of anti-malarial medicines such as artesunate suppository and artesunate injectable. Despite the artesunate rectal and injectable formulations not being widely available in the health facilities, health workers often came across them either in the private sector or the community. Some interfaced with them because they were being channeled through their health facility to the community for the ICCM program. Although they were advised by their supervisors to use Artemether lumefantrine for malaria, health workers had also informally heard about use of rectal artesunate from the community based health workers. Although rectal artesunate (both injectable and suppository) was up to date and considered appropriate for children, they were often out of stock and health workers did not know when to use these two formulations. Some health workers still knew that chloroquine was still the main medicine for malaria. One of the Nursing Assistants innocently asked why chloroquine was no longer being supplied in the health facilities.

The health workers' understanding of the new treatment protocols varied according to the level of training. Comparatively, senior health workers especially pediatricians were more conversant with the new treatment policies than the lower level health workers in the rural facilities who did not have sufficient information about new medicines for children. The missing interactions between the rural based health workers and their supervisors who included the district health teams and central level MoH staff partly explains the health workers' limited understanding of new treatment policies. Although medicine policies for key causes of morbidity among children had been changing, the transfer of information about new policies from the global through the national level to the facilities had not been effective. Besides that, most of the rural based health workers such as Nursing Assistants said they did not have access to the revised Uganda Clinical Guidelines of 2010. In most of the facilities, it was reported (and also observed) that the guidelines were locked in cupboards of their supervisors who were often absent. The few lower cadre health workers who had glanced at the Uganda Clinical Guidelines of 2010 indicated that the guidelines were too bulky for them to use in their daily work and for that reason they had put them aside.

> *These guidelines (Uganda Clinical Guidelines) are too big. You have to turn so many pages to get to the exact information about a disease. In addition to that, we have never been oriented on these guidelines. There are some technical terms which some of us cannot understand. We find the IMCI counseling and treatment charts easy to use. Unfortunately, these IMCI charts have outdated information where some of the medicines are no longer recommended (Nursing Aide rural based health facility Jinja district).*

On the other hand, the outdated IMCI treatment charts were visible with health workers who reported them to be more user friendly than the UCG. Some of the health workers wondered why medicines like the combination of chloroquine and SP which had already been phased out by the National Drug Authority were still appearing on the IMCI treatment charts. The same medicines were no longer being supplied by NMS and there were some health workers who did not know that chloroquine and SP had been phased out.

> *You hear that the treatment of malaria has changed from chloroquine and SP to ACTs. Our (IMCI treatment) charts continue to indicate chloroquine and fansidar for children. By the way we no longer get chloroquine among the medicines supplied here. What is happening? (A Nursing Assistant rural based health facility).*

Some of the health workers were not sure of the first line treatment for pneumonia. They wanted to know whether amoxicillin and cotrimoxazole should be prescribed interchangeably. They said they were using both septrine and amoxicillin (depending on what was available at the time of dispensing) as the first line treatment for pneumonia. The child-appropriate amoxicillin dispersible tablet was still limited in supply and was mainly delivered for the donor funded ICCM program. Dispersible amoxicillin tablets were often withdrawn from the village health team providers for use in the facilities to avoid expiry especially because fewer children were being seen by the community providers. Cotrimoxazole tablets were on a high demand because it was also being used for HIV/AIDS prophylaxis.

> *We are using both cotrimoxazole and amoxicillin as first line treatment for pneumonia depending on what is available in stock when the child is brought for treatment. In most cases, cotrimoxazole (septrine) is used because it is supplied more regularly. On the other hand, amoxicillin is rarely used because it is always out of stock. Much of what we see is a remnant of what was being taken to the community for ICCM. We even do not know the medicine which is recommended for pneumonia. We see some of the donors supplying amoxicillin to the community. On the other hand, government concentrates on the supply of cotrimoxazole. Sometimes we take the remainders of amoxicillin dispersible from because there are challenges of storing these medicines in the community for a long time. They can easily expire before use. In any case, we are seeing many more children here than they see in the community (Clinical officer, in-charge of a rural based health facility).*

Rural based health workers had limited knowledge about the globally recommended 'child size' medicines and child-appropriate dosage formulations concepts. There was a consistent affirmation by the health workers indicating that IMCI treatment charts and the clinical guidelines neither referred to 'child-appropriate' dosage formulations' nor the 'child size medicines'. In spite of this limitation, health workers presented informative viewpoints about the different dosage formulations they were using to treat children. Health workers in the rural areas highly commended IMCI as a suitable program for children but also hastened to add that the approach had flaws: lack of updated guidelines; missing support supervision and, lack of refresher trainings. They echoed lack of child-friendly medicines in the assortment of medicines supplied by NMS.

The rural based health-workers' viewed appropriateness of dosage formulations in terms of being easy to prescribe, dispense and administer. In their practice, they came across ordinary tablets and capsules, oral suspension powders and a few dispersible tablets. They also reported using injectables and suppositories to treat children under severe conditions. From the experiences they shared, formulations in tablet forms and capsules were a challenge for children to swallow. Yet tablets and capsules were the most supplied by government for children. Rural based health workers also expressed their opinions about formulations which they though were child-friendly. These were discussed with reference to the common diseases of malaria and pneumonia. For malaria, health workers maintained that coartem (Artemether lumefantrine) was child-appropriate in terms strengths. They do not have to split a tablet of coartem even for an infant. However, like any other tablet, Artemether lumefantrine has to be crushed before being administered to the child. Artemether lumefantrine they were using was not dispersible in water like the ones that were being provided in the community and hence this type was diffecult for children to swallow. Therefore, rural based health workers said they have often advised caregivers to crush the tablets in order to make them suitable for children. Even when broken into pieces, some health workers noted that tablets were still difficult for children to swallow especially when the tablets are bitter. Regarding pneumonia medicines, health workers complained about lack of septrine syrup in the health facilities. The most available was the adult size of 480 mg. As a result, health workers said they were breaking the big tablets of septrine into smaller pieces before administering them to children. Despite amoxicillin being the recommended first line medicine for pneumonia, the child-appropriate dispersible amoxicillin tablets which were available in only a few of the health facilities as remnants of what was used in the community. Some of the health workers admitted having limited understanding of what dispersible tablets were and how they are used. Some were concerned because they did not see dispersible tablets being mentioned anywhere in the Uganda Clinical Guidelines and the IMCI charts they were using.

We hear dispersible tablets being talked about, but we have not seen anywhere where they are written (Nursing Assistant, rural based health facility)

Perhaps due to limited knowledge and limited publicity, dispersible tablets were not considered as the most important as syrups, suppositories, injectables and ordinary tablets.

There were concerns that liquid oral formulations commonly referred to as syrups were missing and yet according to the health workers they are the best for children. The common "syrups" that the health workers had heard about were for septrine, amoxicillin and chloroquine. There were a few rural based health workers who were critical of syrups and said that they were problematic because they were too expensive and difficult to store and that was the reason why they were not being procured by government.

Sometimes there are some medicines whose consumption is low. In such cases, these are challenges of storage which makes the medicine susceptible to being damaged if they are syrups (Nurse, a rural based health facility).

The most commonly mentioned liquid oral formulations were metronidazole syrup used to treat diarrhea and nevirapine syrup for prevention of mother to child transmission. Metronidazole syrup was being supplied in all the health facilities. Health workers wondered why metronidazole syrup was regularly supplied in most of the health facilities and yet other important syrups for malaria and pneumonia were not provided. Although they had been deleted from the EMHSLU, syrups for septrine and amoxicillin were still perceived by health workers as critically needed for treating children and the concern was that the only available formulation for septrine was the tablet of 480 mg tablets meant for adults as earlier discussed. The available Amoxicillin capsules were perceived to be unsuitable for children.

Ok, I say syrups are expensive fine: but they should add in a few syrups especially antibiotics such as septrine and amoxicillin so that we can continue with them. We only have septrine tablets of 480 mg which are too big for these children. I think it can help if there is septrine syrup instead. The rest of the medicines can remain as tablets (a Nurse in a rural based health facility).

Injections were reported to be highly available and highly utilized for treating children especially for severe pneumonia conditions. Injections were rated as very important especially by the rural based health workers and were being used when 'syrups' were not available and were preferred for those children who vomit oral medicines.

For pneumonia, we always have problems with the medicines in stock. We mainly have septrine which is too big for the child to swallow. Septrine syrup would be ideal but currently syrups are not being provided by government and we do not know why. We also have amoxicillin capsules which are the most available but they are difficult for children to swallow and they are meant for adults. Therefore, for pneumonia, we often use injection of x-pen which is not allowed, we just need to use it for pre-referral treatment. We are forced to use it especially when the child is vomiting (Nursing Assistant in a rural based facility).

In a nutshell, rural based health workers persistently emphasized the fact that, the treatment guidelines and the IMCI treatment charts were not clear about child-appropriate formulations. Despite being the main approach used to diagnose and treat children, health workers rightly argued that IMCI had nothing to do with chid-appropriate dosage formulations. Only names of medicines were simply referred to as oral, injectable and suppository. Categories of oral medicines formulations which are child-friendly are not referred to in the guidelines.

Discussion

The overarching assumption for the WHA resolution of 'better medicine for children' was that beneficiary countries would adopt this recommendation into their policy and implementation frameworks. The study design was based on the premise that child-appropriate dosage formulations are the best option to improve prescription, dispensing and administration of medicines to the under-five population. Findings from the qualitative inquiry at the ministry; district and facility levels established that there has been no integration of child-appropriate dosage formulations into the IMCI approach in Uganda. From the perspectives of the respondents at the three levels, 3 related explanations for failure to integrate are apparent: (1) resource constraints that affected persistent implementation of the IMCI program (2) gaps in the global and national efforts to integrate child-appropriate dosage into the Ugandan essential medicines list (3) cognitive gaps and information distortions that have undermined health workers' confidence in prescribing, dispensing and administering medicines to children while using outdated IMCI treatment charts.

Resource constraints and persistent implementation of IMCI

Resource constraints were constantly referred to in the perspectives that were explored at the national, district and facility levels. Resource constraints question can be viewed in two dimensions. The first dimension was that whereas IMCI is the main approach used to manage childhood illnesses in Uganda, it has not been sufficiently funded to address ever-changing global policy prescriptions such as the integration of chid-appropriate dosage formulations. In reference to the theoretical framework, resource constraint barrier was highlighted as a barriers by Tansella &Thornicroft (2009) in their three phases of implementation model for evidence based clinical practices [12].

Due to resource constraints, MoH could not mutually adjust the health system to meet the new global demand of child-appropriate dosage formulations. Therefore, the recommendation for 'better medicines for children' came at a time when resources for supporting IMCI had already dwindled. Lack of sustainable funding for IMCI undermined its effectiveness in terms of the integration of child-appropriate dosage formulations.

The second dimension was that right from its inception, the recommendation for 'better medicines for children' later coined as 'child-appropriate dosage formulations', did not receive specific donor attention. Except for the Melinda Bill gates Foundation which facilitated piloting of the child size medicine in three countries of Ghana, India and Tanzania, there were no other global efforts to market the concepts of child-appropriate dosage formulations. The idea of child-appropriate formulations remained in the UN (UNICEF and WHO) circles for quite long and did not gain global prominence until the UN declaration of the 'essential commodities and lifesaving priority medicines for children'.

Dependence on external funding for critical programs such as IMCI has done a disservice in some aspects. Interestingly, bypassing the national systems, largely ignoring the existing policies and medicine supply systems, development partners in Uganda initiated and supported supply of child-appropriate dosage formulations to the community [7]. Although this marked the beginning of the era of child-appropriate dosage formulations in the country, failure to mainstream the support through IMCI the main approach for treating children and due to failure to revise policy provisions to reflect child-appropriate dosage formulations [8], the initiative from the development partners left a lot desired. The availability and utilization of child-appropriate lifesaving and priority medicines for children continued to remain low in public facilities [9]. In the same way, due to lack of funding, the sustainability of IMCI, which was initially a heavily donor funded program, became uncertain. The findings of this study support the argument of Tansella and Thornicroft that resources are critical even during the final phases of projects [12]. Similarly, Hogwood and Gunn (1984) argued that external circumstances to the implementing agency may impose crippling effects if there is no adequate time and resources for continuity [13].

At the time when resources were scarce MoH decentralized some of the key IMCI activities such as refresher training, support supervision to the district without decentralizing commensurate resources. It is not surprising therefore that these activities were not implemented by the district. According to Walt (1994), decentralization of responsibilities without the associated resource requirements may make local authorities vulnerable to policies which are not cost effective. On the other hand, decentralization of financial resources can help enforce the guidelines and other elements of the packages such as support supervision and refresher courses [14].

The success of the integration of child-appropriate dosage formulations will largely depend on the capacity of the health system to enforce compliance. Health system strengthening was anticipated as one of the fundamental elements of the IMCI strategy [21, 22]. This study supports the argument that dynamic and strong health systems would enable the system to achieve improved health outcomes [23]. In Uganda, there have been more investments in the ICCM with diminishing support for another equally important component, the facility based IMCI [7]. Notwithstanding the fact that the facility based IMCI and ICCM should be well integrated if it is to have an impact on mortality. In Uganda, as a result of this gap, the expected efficiency and effectiveness of the IMCI are not being much felt. While the community-based initiatives extend the delivery of interventions in remote areas where health services are hard to access, strengthening national health systems should be the long-term aim [24]. Health systems bottlenecks are a formidable challenge in the rural based health facilities in Uganda and this directly affects integrating child-appropriate dosage formulations. As a matter of fact, the health systems' gaps in Uganda who include lowly trained health personnel who have not been oriented about new medicines, whose IMCI treatment charts are outdated and in the context of limited supply of child-appropriate dosage formulations and challenges of referral explain the failure to easily integrate child-appropriate dosage formulations into IMCI. A study elsewhere shows a similar pattern regarding IMCI implementation whereby the workload, medicine supplies and poor supervisory mechanisms undermine the program [25].

Due to resource constraints, IMCI remains an unfinished business in the clinical practice in Uganda. Tansella & Thornicroft (2009) highlight the need for sustainable: advocacy, financial support, and continuous staff training and review of the information technology. This did not happen in the case of Uganda because IMCI was funded in the initial stages by the donors and this funding stopped later. Government was unable to sustain all the IMCI core activities that were initially supported by donors. In the end, the globally generated seeds of child-appropriate dosage formulations landed on the bare ground since IMCI as a key framework for treating children was not adequately funded. Tansella and Thornicroft (2009) in their framework about translation of evidence into practice have contended that the greatest impact of a policy is not adoption per se but rather from the long-term implementation of the practice where resources are key [12]. Hogwood and Gunn (1984) added that the combination of resources is a must for the implementation to take place [13].

Lack of global and national effort

MoH officials attributed lack of integration of child-appropriate dosage formulations to gaps in the global and national effort. Although the IMCI algorithm at the global was adjusted by WHO to take care of 'better medicines for children', this did not happen at the national level in Uganda. There were no official discussions involving recipient countries and WHO about how to introduce child size medicines in Uganda [7]. It has been reported that changes in Malaria treatment policies were largely influenced by WHO active involvement in financing and initiating local discussions about the new policies [26]. For the integration to take root, it would have been necessary at the national level to develop a policy framework for integrating these medicines into the essential medicines list and clinical guidelines. Macleod Stuart and colleagues (2013) argue that it is necessary to update clinical guidelines, train health workers accordingly about the need to integrate child-appropriate dosage formulations into the essential medicines lists and the standard treatment guidelines which would guarantee knowledge transfer and dissemination of the new medicine information [27]. The disarticulation between IMCI approach in Uganda and the global recommendations that emphasize child-appropriate medicine formulations [1, 11] was apparent. This disarticulation has been due to lack of specific policy focus on child-size medicines both in the essential medicines lists and the Uganda clinical guidelines (UCG) [8]. The Uganda government failed to formally adopt the global policy on child-appropriate dosage formulations [7]. Eventually this limited the avenues for IMCI to address the global requirement of integrating child-appropriate dosage formulations. For example, the Uganda Clinical Guidelines of 2010 and 2012 were silent about child-appropriate dosage formulations.

There was concern that quality and effective of treatment of children less than 6 years of age cannot be realized without integrating the child-appropriate dosage formulations into the essential medicines lists. World-wide essential medicines lists are considered vital for prioritizing medicines to procure. Holloway and Henry have shown that essential medicines along with training on standard treatment guidelines are associated with quality of medicine use in many countries [28]. In Uganda, child-appropriate dosage formulations are not among the essential medicines and worst still, health workers are not regularly oriented about the global changes in the medicines for children. Similarly, in South Africa health workers found training in IMCI informative and reportedly increased their skills for managing the sick children. Follow up visits would help encourage correct practice and motivate the newly trained IMCI practitioners [29].

The cognitive gap among health workers

Pediatricians were more confident about the Uganda national treatment policies of the key childhood illnesses and were also able to access state of art international standards for the management of childhood illnesses. However, pediatricians are very few and are mainly available in the hospitals. On the contrary, rural based lower cadre health workers such as Nursing Assistants did not have sufficient information about new treatment protocols. This information gap was associated with lack of revised guidelines, lack of refresher training and gaps in information mainstreaming when new treatment protocols are introduced through vertical programs such as the presidential malaria initiative. In this initiative, new medicines for treating malaria were recommended but were not reflected in the IMCI treatment charts and clinical guidelines. Medicines recommended in the clinical guidelines as first line treatment for malaria and pneumonia among under-five were outdated medicines which were also not even child-friendly [8]. At the same time, the new malaria treatment policies proposed through the vertical program of presidential malaria initiative were not effectively communicated to the lower cadre staff in rural based facilities. This is because of the limited integration of these vertical programs into the general health care delivery systems such as IMCI. Unless the issue of new knowledge is addressed in the IMCI approach to take care of evidence based medicines and new approaches to management of childhood illnesses, IMCI will eventually become irrelevant and will be taken over by vertical programs such as ICCM and malaria programs as has been the case before. Innovative solutions may be necessary to ensure that guidelines are updated to reflect child-appropriate medicines and at the same time health workers' skills should be updated and maintained [29].

Lack of information affects easy understanding of new developments about medicine policies. Okungu and Gilson (2014) argued that effective health policy communication is important for the uptake of new drug interventions and adherence to treatment regimens [30]. There was confusion about first line medicines due to information gap resulting from the failure to update the IMCI treatment guidelines, missing refresher courses and limited support supervision. It has been argued that development and implementation of (evidence-based) clinical practice guidelines is one of the promising and effective tools for improving the quality of care for children [31] especially when introduced in the context of rigorous evaluations and subsequent updates [32]. Some of the good attributes of clinical guidelines include an explicit description of the scientific evidence for which the recommendation is available; evidence that is straightforward and not conflicting; and when the evidence is based on relevant aspects of care in daily practice [33]. At the global level, the most recent version of IMCI guidelines was produced in 2014. Nevertheless, the new version is still vague about child-appropriate formulations. For example, in the UCG there are recommendations such as 'give oral amoxicillin for 5 days' on page 2 of the UCG or 'give first line oral antimalarial' on page 4 of UCG [34]. The IMCI treatment charts that were being used in all the rural based health facilities by the time of the study had not been updated since 2001. This explains the confusions and lack of confidence especially among the lower level rural based health workers.

Policy implications

According to the Health Sector Strategic and Investment Plan III, IMCI remains the main approach in the management of childhood illnesses in Uganda [6]. In reality, IMCI is the most appropriate approach for the rural based health facilities where children are treated by low cadre health workers. Therefore, IMCI should constantly receive adequate attention during the policy development, planning, budgeting and implementation processes. Without sufficient investments into the IMCI core activities, the expected gains from IMCI will not be achieved. Core investments should include regular adaptation of new generic guidelines from WHO, sufficient facilitation in terms of training, support supervision and regular to ensure that there is an environment in which health workers can apply their child care skills [35]. It also means that all the vertical programs such as the presidential malaria initiative and ICCM should be aligned with and integrated into the IMCI program whereby guidelines of these vertical programs are part and parcel of the IMCI treatment charts. Pediatricians continue to prescribe liquid oral formulation (syrups) which are not readily available in the public facilities and caretakers have to purchase them at high costs. The implication is that some of the caregivers who cannot afford the medicines might have to forego the treatment or procure under dose because they cannot afford. This infringes on the rights of the poor to health services.

Conclusion

The IMCI package for managing childhood illnesses in Uganda does not include the global recommendation of 'better medicines for children'. The poorly funded IMCI strategy has continued to stagnate due to lack of resources for updating the guidelines, procure evidence based medicines, conduct refresher training and support supervision for health workers. This stagnation continues to undermine appropriate and effective administration of medicines to children. The missing child-appropriate dosage formulations in the EMHSLU and UCG undermine low cadre rural based health workers efforts to appropriately treat children using the IMCI approach. There are still challenges in prescribing, dispensing and administration of tablets and capsules to children under-five. Depending on their level of medical training, health workers have come up with strategies for mitigating the challenges of administration of adult medicines to children. Lower cadre health workers prefer using injections and suppositories which they more appropriate for children who vomit. When revising the clinical guideline, it is important to seek the views of those providers managing children especially lower cadre staff who have narrow choices of medicines, have limited information about new medicnes and are also faced with challenges of medicine formulations that are inappropriate for children.

Recommendations

Both government and development partners should invest more into the IMCI strategy from a health systems approach to enable the systems to respond positively to the emerging global demands for child-appropriate dosage formulations. This would require more budget allocations to the child health division and other relevant departments. The IMCI treatment charts should be updated regularly to reflect child-appropriate dosage formulations. It will also necessitate revisiting the EMHSLU to reflect child-appropriate dosage formulations based on new evidence. There should be adequate budget provisions for refresher training and support supervision for the health workers on new evidence-based and national treatment policies for the common childhood ailments. More studies are needed to explore the experiences of the caregivers about access and use of child-appropriate dosage formulations.

Acknowledgements

This work was supported by the Danish Ministry of Foreign Affairs (DANIDA) [file number 09–100 KU] through the University of Copenhagen in collaboration with Makerere University, College of Health Sciences. We would like to thank the Jinja District Health Team and all the health workers who were our respondents for sparing time to participate in the study.

Authors' contributions

XN conceived the idea of the study. The study protocol was developed by XN with input from JOO, EHH, FS and AM. XN did the sampling, data collection and analysis. XN drafted the first version of the manuscript and revised it after critical comments from all the authors. All authors approved the final version of the manuscript.

Competing interests

The authors declare that they have no competing interests.

Author details

[1]Child Health and Development Center, College of Health Sciences, Makerere University, Kampala, Uganda. [2]Department of Pharmacology and Therapeutics, Gulu University, Gulu, Uganda. [3]Section for Social and Clinical Pharmacy, Department of Pharmacy, Faculty of Health and Medical Sciences, University of Copenhagen, Copenhagen, Denmark. [4]Department of Community Health, Ministry of Health Uganda, Kampala, Uganda. [5]Department of Health, Uganda Christian University, Mukono, Uganda. [6]School of Public Health, College of Health Sciences, Makerere University, Kampala, Uganda.

References

1. World Health Organization. Priority medicines for mothers and children, World Health Organization. Geneva: World Health Organization; 2011. available at: http://cdrwww.who.int/medicines/publications/A3prioritymedicines.pdf.
2. Hill S, Yang A, Bero L. Priority medicines for maternal and child health: a global survey of national essential medicines lists. PLoS One. 2012;7(5):e38055.
3. UNICEF. Integrated management of childhood illness. 2012. Available at: http://www.unicef.org/health/index_imcd.html. Accessed on 16 April 2015.
4. Gitanjali B. Essential medicines for children: should we focus on a priority list of medicines for the present? J Pharmacol Pharmacother. 2011;2(1):1–2.
5. World Health Organization, Make medicines child size 2010. Available at: http://www.who.int/childmedicines/en/. Accessed 19 March 2015.
6. Government of Uganda. Health sector strategic and investment plan 2010-2014/15: promoting People's health to enhance socio-economic development. Kampala: Ministry of Health; 2010.
7. Nsabagasani X et al. Explaining the slow transition of child-appropriate dosage formulations from the global to national level in the context of Uganda: a qualitative study. J Pharm Policy Pract. 2015;8(1):19.
8. Nsabagasani X et al. The "child size medicines" concept: policy provisions in Uganda. J Pharm Policy Pract. 2015;8(1):2.
9. Nsabagasani X et al. Availability and utilization of the WHO recommended priority lifesaving medicines for under five-year old children in public health facilities in Uganda: a cross-sectional survey. J Pharm Policy Pract. 2015;8(1):18.
10. Finny E. Children's medicines: a situation analysis in make medicines child size. 2011.
11. World Health Organization, Priority Life-saving Medicines for Women and Children 2012. Available at: http://www.who.int/reproductivehealth/publications/general/emp_mar2012.1/en/
12. Tansella M, Thornicroft G. Implementation science: understanding the translation of evidence into practice. Br J Psychiatry. 2009;195(4):283–5.
13. Hogwood BW, Gunn LA. Policy analysis for the real world. Oxford: Oxford University Press; 1984.
14. Walt G. Health policy : an introduction to PROCESS and POWER. London: Zed Books; 1994.
15. Government of Uganda. Uganda clinical guidelines: national guidelines for management of common conditions. Kampala: Ministry of Health Uganda; 2010.
16. Government of Uganda. Uganda clinical guidelines: national guidelines for management of common conditions. Kampala: Ministry of Health; 2012.
17. Republic of Uganda. National population and housing census: provisional results. Kampala: Uganda Bureau of Statistics; 2014.
18. Uganda Bureau of Statistics (UBOS) and ICF International Inc. Uganda Demographic and Health Survey 2011. Kampala, Uganda: UBOS and Calverton, Maryland: ICF International Inc.; 2012.
19. Graneheim U, Lundman B. Qualitative content analysis in nursing research: concepts, procedures and measures to achieve trustworthiness. Nurse Educ Today. 2004;24:105–12.
20. Marshall C, Rossman GB. Designing qualitative research. 4th ed. London: SAGE publications; 2006.
21. World Health Organization, Integrated Management of Chilhood Illnesses (IMCI) Implementation in the Western Pacific Region: IMCI and Health System Strengthening. Geneva: WHO; 2009. Accessed at www.wpro.who.int/child...health/.../info_package7.pdf?ua. Accessed 15th March 2016.
22. Patwari AK, Raina N. Integrated Management of Childhood Illness (IMCI): a robust strategy. Indian J Pediatr. 2002;69(1):41–8.
23. Travis P et al. Overcoming health-systems constraints to achieve the millennium development goals. Lancet. 2004;364(9437):900–6.

24. Bryce J et al. Reducing child mortality: can public health deliver? Lancet. 2003;362(9378):159–64.
25. Basaleem HO, Amin RM. Integrated management of childhood illness in Lahej, Yemen: a qualitative analysis from the perspective of health providers. East Mediterr Health J. 2011;17(2):101–8.
26. Nabyonga-Orem J, Ssengooba F, Macq J, Criel B. Malaria treatment policy change in Uganda: what role did evidence play? Malar J. 2014;13(1):345.
27. Macleod SM et al. Better drug therapy for the children of Africa: current impediments to success and potential strategies for improvement. Paediatr Drugs. 2013;15(4):259–69.
28. Holloway K, Henry D. WHO essential medicines policies and use in developing and transitional countries: an analysis of reported policy implementation and medicines use surveys. PLoS Med. 2014;11(9):e1001724.
29. Horwood C et al. Experiences of training and implementation of integrated management of childhood illness (IMCI) in South Africa: a qualitative evaluation of the IMCI case management training course. BMC Pediatr. 2009;9(1):62.
30. Okungu V, Gilson L. "...still waiting for chloroquine": the challenge of communicating changes in first-line treatment policy for uncomplicated malaria in a remote Kenyan district. Malar J. 2014;13:258.
31. Grol R. Successes and failures in the implementation of evidence-based guidelines for clinical practice. Med Care. 2001;39(8 Suppl 2):II46–54.
32. Grimshaw JM, Russell IT. Effect of clinical guidelines on medical practice: a systematic review of rigorous evaluations. Lancet. 1993;342(8883):1317–22.
33. Grol R et al. Attributes of clinical guidelines that influence use of guidelines in general practice: observational study. BMJ. 1998;317(7162):858–61.
34. World Health Organisation. Integrated Management of Childhood Illnesses. Geneva: WHO; 2014. available at: http://www.who.int/maternal_child_adolescent/topics/child/imci/en/.
35. Tulloch J. Integrated approach to child health in developing countries. Lancet. 1999;354 Suppl 2:SII16–20.

3

Prescription medicine sharing: exploring patients' beliefs and experiences

Kebede Beyene*, Trudi Aspden and Janie Sheridan

Abstract

Background: Prescription medicine sharing has been defined as the lending of medicines (giving prescription medicines to someone else) or borrowing of medicines (being given and using a medicine prescribed for another person). This qualitative study explored the views of patients, to elicit information regarding factors influencing medicine sharing behaviours, their experiences of the consequences of prescription medicine sharing, and their risk assessment strategies when deciding to share.

Methods: One-on-one, face-to-face, semi-structured interviews were carried out in Auckland, New Zealand between September 2013 and August 2014 with 17 patients, purposively sampled to provide information from different socio-demographic backgrounds. The interviews were audio recorded, transcribed verbatim and analysed using a general inductive approach. The study received ethical approval, and all interviewees provided written informed consent.

Results: Findings were captured within five overarching themes: types of shared medicines; perceived benefits of sharing medicines; negative experiences of sharing; factors influencing sharing behaviours; and risk assessment strategies. Participants reported that sharing helped them to avoid treatment costs and the inconvenience associated with medical visits such as booking appointments. Conversely, unanticipated side effects, allergies, and taking inappropriate medicines were the main adverse consequences of sharing. Altruism, limited access to medicines/health services, sociocultural factors, and having unused prescription medicines were factors influencing sharing behaviours. Participants reported assessing the safety of sharing a medicine primarily based on symptom matching, past illness experiences, and knowledge about the medicines.

Conclusions: This study enriches previous survey findings, by providing insight into patients' reasons for medicines sharing. Healthcare providers should consider asking their patients about any medicines they have shared and their future sharing intentions, in order to use the opportunity for discussing safer sharing practices, without promoting the behaviour. The findings are helpful for informing the development of potential interventions and targeted educational messages about safe medicine use for patients.

Keywords: Medicine sharing, Medicine borrowing, Medicine lending, Non-recreational sharing, Auckland

Background

Prescription medicine sharing has been defined as the lending of medicines (giving prescription medicines to someone else) or borrowing of medicines (being given and using a medicine prescribed for another person) [1]. Medicine sharing has two distinct types; these are recreational and non-recreational sharing. While recreational sharing can be defined as the sharing of abusable prescription medicines "to get high" or feel good, non-recreational sharing is the sharing of any prescription medicine for its intended therapeutic benefits. Although most forms of sharing are non-recreational in nature, [2] recreational sharing has received most of the research focus for the previous four decades [3–5]. Limited research evidence is available around non-recreational sharing; therefore, this study aimed to fill this gap.

While non-recreational sharing is not a new phenomenon, it has received increasing attention from researchers, due to its potential medical and public

* Correspondence: k.beyene@auckland.ac.nz
The School of Pharmacy, Faculty of Medical and Health Sciences, the University of Auckland, Private Bag 92019, Auckland 1142, New Zealand

health implications [1, 6–16]. Some of these implications are unmonitored adverse drug events, [6] drug resistance, [7] complications in clinical diagnosis, [6] and delay in care seeking [17]. Although borrowers are at higher risk than lenders, of unexpected side effects or allergies from shared medicines, [9] lenders could also deplete their own medicine supply and incur a risk of therapeutic failure. On the other hand, medicine borrowing may be beneficial in some instances, for example, in an emergency situation. For those who do not have easy access to health services or are dissatisfied with healthcare systems, sharing provides an alternative method for accessing prescription medicines [18–20]. Furthermore, in modern societies, medicines are often part of an individual's everyday life and might be shared to restore ill health or to facilitate social interactions [19].

A range of medicines has been reported to be shared [1, 8–11, 13, 20–26]; pain medications, allergy medications, and antibiotics were chief among them [1, 10, 23]. The sharing of asthma inhalers, [20] diabetes medications, [11] antihypertensives, [8, 10] corticosteroids, [21] acne medications, [21, 23] and antiretrovirals [25, 26] has also been reported to be common. Friends and family members were the main sources of shared medicines [1, 8, 23, 27]. Though medicine sharing is frequently reported amongst adults and adolescents, [9, 23] one study reported that the parental use of a child's prescribed medicine for another child also occurs [10]. While this form of sharing could help to alleviate a child's illness, administration of medicines not meant for a specific child could result in using inappropriate doses, hospital admission, or death [24].

Although there is no accepted, gold standard method for assessing medicine sharing, 5–66 % prevalence rates of sharing have been documented across studies [1, 8, 9, 11, 13–15, 21–23, 27, 28]. Females have been reported to be more likely than males to lend prescription medicines [1, 21, 23, 27]. In a representative national sample of 26,566 American adults, age was found to have more influence than gender on medicine lending or borrowing behaviour, with the prevalence of lending or borrowing behaviour increasing as age decreased [23]. Ethnicity and/or race appear to have less influence on medicine lending behaviour [29]. Lower income level, [27] unemployment, [10] larger household size, [10, 27] and having a chronic disease [21] have been found to be positive predictors of sharing behaviours, across studies. On the other hand, one study found that having health insurance, and a primary care provider who frequently asked about medicine usage were negatively associated with the borrowing behaviour of urban medical centre clients in New York [8].

Several factors have been reported to be reasons for medicine sharing behaviours. These include running out of previously prescribed medicine, [1, 10, 11, 23] inability to afford a medical visit or prescription charges, [8, 11, 13, 27, 30] emergency situations, [1] or convenience [8]. Being prescribed the same medicine or having the same health problem as the other person could also create opportunity for sharing medicines [1, 22]. Although several reasons contributing to medicine sharing were revealed by the above studies, many of these studies listed predetermined factors and asked participants to choose among them, [1, 9, 11, 14, 23, 27] and this process might limit the identification of a comprehensive range of motives for sharing from the patient perspective. Overall, little is known about the psychosocial, behavioural and cultural factors that influence medicine sharing. It is also unclear how patients assess the risk of sharing medicines and if, and how they assess risk in their decision making to lend/borrow medicines.

Further, previous research around sharing has tended to take a medical perspective and largely focussed on negative consequences of sharing behaviours [1, 6, 7, 17]. This approach may not provide a complete picture of sharing. People's decisions to share medicines might not differ from their decision to share other commodities, [31] and understanding the 'social context' of medicines could provide further insights into why people share medicines.

The majority of the evidence around adults' medicine sharing practices has been from cross-sectional surveys; limited qualitative studies are available describing non-recreational medicine sharing behaviours among adults [12]. A recent, extensive literature search by the research team has revealed only two qualitative studies that were specifically designed to assess medicine sharing behaviours [11, 31]. One of these studies explored older adults' sharing behaviours, [11] and the other was designed to determine people's willingness to share medicines in comparison with other sharable commodities and, as such did not provide details about sharing behaviours [31]. Our study has addressed this gap in the literature. The overall research process was guided by the central research questions: "Why do adults lend or borrow prescription medicines" and "How do they decide whether or not to do so?" These questions seek to understand sharing behaviours from medical and socio-cultural perspectives. The aims of the study were: (1) to understand adults' experiences of the consequences of prescription medicine sharing; (2) to identify factors influencing medicine sharing behaviours; and (3) to understand how patients decide if prescription medicines are safe to be shared. This study has provided new information regarding the types of shared medicines, factors contributing to and potential consequences of sharing and patients' medicine sharing risk assessment strategies. Therefore, the information may help healthcare providers to identify and address problems related to medicine sharing. The findings can also be used by patient support groups, medicine regulatory agencies, and other local and international organisations involved in promoting the safe use of medicines.

Methods

Design and sampling

A qualitative approach was adopted for this study. One-on-one, face-to-face, semi-structured interviews were conducted to explore adults' beliefs and experiences about prescription medicine sharing practices. In this type of research it is usual to recruit up to 30 participants or collect data until data saturation is reached, whichever comes first [32]. Participants were sampled purposively based on their age, gender, income, and employment status in order to gather a wide range of information from different socio-demographic backgrounds. English-speaking adults aged 18 years or older with experience or interest in medicine sharing were eligible to participate. Health-care professionals were excluded from participation. The interpretation of findings was guided by a 'harm reduction' philosophy focusing on minimising the risks/harms of sharing without necessarily considering it essential to eliminate sharing practices.

Study setting and recruitment

The study took place in Auckland, the largest city in New Zealand with a population of 1.4 million [http://www.statistics.govt.nz/Census/2013-census/profile-and-summary-reports/quickstats-about-a-place.aspx?request_value=13170&tabname=]. Participants were invited through local patient support group newsletter advertisements, pamphlet advertisements in a public library and a community pharmacy, and via email advertisements on university email lists. When participants approached the researchers, their eligibility was checked by the first author (K.B.) using a checklist developed for this purpose.

Data collection

To ensure consistency, all interviews were conducted by K.B. K.B. is a pharmacist, but not registered to practice in New Zealand, and this was made known to participants. An interview guide (see Additional file 1) was used to ensure broadly similar topics were covered with each participant whilst allowing them to introduce and expand upon individual experiences. The selection of topics was guided by the research team experience and a review of available literature [1, 8, 13, 16, 17, 23, 27]. The research proposal was also presented at School of Pharmacy, the University of Auckland, departmental seminars and feedback received from colleagues was used to refine the topics. The interview guide was piloted with two participants and the results discussed among the research team to further refine the guide. Pilot data were excluded from final analysis. The main topics explored in the final guide were: the types of medicines shared by participants, participants' beliefs and experiences about benefits and adverse consequences of medicine sharing, circumstances that lead to sharing medicines, participants' views regarding ways to minimise the potential harms of medicine sharing. After conducting the first four interviews, previously unforeseen topics were added to the interview guide. Participants also completed a short questionnaire describing their socio-demographic characteristics and medicine-taking habits.

Participants were interviewed at a time and location of their choice. With the exception of one participant (who preferred to be interviewed at home), all interviews were conducted at the University of Auckland. To ensure participants understood the purpose of the study, all participants were provided with a general definition of medicine sharing, and were instructed to focus on non-recreational prescription medicine sharing. With participants' consent, all interviews were audio recorded. At the end of each interview, the participant was given a document describing the potential risks of medicine sharing. Interviewing continued until data saturation was reached, which was considered to have occurred after 17 interviews (as no new themes were identified from the last three interviews). The mean duration of the interviews was 47 min (range: 30–72 min), and they were conducted between September 2013 and August 2014.

Data analysis

After each interview, the interviewer made field notes and this information was used to describe how each interview was conducted and to note issues or comments not sufficiently captured by audio recordings. This information aided interpretation of data. Interviews were transcribed verbatim by K.B. ($n = 6$) or an independent professional transcriber ($n = 11$), and the transcripts were checked against the audio recordings by K.B. All participants were offered an opportunity to edit their interview transcripts; however, with the exception of one participant, they did not read and edit them. To ensure anonymity, names, place of work, or any other identifying information was removed, and a unique code number was assigned to each transcript. The data were analysed using the general inductive approach (GIA) [33]. GIA is a thematic analysis approach with both deductive and inductive features. In GIA, while the general (or overarching) themes are derived from the research objectives (deductive feature), more specific categories/themes arise from the data (inductive feature) [33]. NVivo 10 software (QSR International) was used to support the analysis process. Before data coding began, the audio recordings, field notes, and the interview transcripts were repeatedly revisited by K.B. to identify salient topics in relation to the research objectives. The preliminary findings were also discussed amongst all authors at several meetings held during the course of the project. Initially, the authors met to agree on the coding procedure and a coding framework was developed to guide the process. Then, two of the authors (K.B. and T.A.) independently coded four, randomly selected interview transcripts, and then all authors met to resolve any coding discrepancies. The main discrepancy identified was an overlap between themes; for example, sharing medicines because of inability to pay for a medical visit was coded initially both under 'cost' and 'access' codes, but later a decision was made to code these data as 'cost.' Discrepancies and overlaps were remedied through mutual consensus among the research team. Afterwards, the codes from both coders were merged to create an initial codebook. Using the initial codebook, K.B. coded the remaining transcripts. The initial codebook was added to and adapted as the coding process progressed to incorporate emerging codes. Instead of line-by-line coding, the coder coded only sections of data meaningful to the research aims. Overall, two levels of coding were employed. The initial coding phase was used to reduce large tracts of unorganised data into a more manageable form based on the general research topic. The second phase involved more focused coding and was used to identify themes, patterns and relationships emerging across the data. The initial and second phase codes and their text segments were systematically organised to examine for any similarities or differences in order to draw conclusions. At this point, patterns and relationships started to emerge within and among major themes and sub-themes (see Table 1 for details). Information from each interview was compared with other interviews to elicit variation and to identify similarities and explain outlying data or negative cases. Mind maps and diagrams (drawn using Post-It notes and poster paper) were used to visualise the relationship between themes and sub-themes. After completion of coding, the data within each code were re-read and this process helped to identify and accurately re-code miscoded data into appropriate categories. The authors then met to discuss the main findings and to explore alternative interpretations of the findings. Overall, five overarching themes were identified. These were: types of shared medicines, perceived benefits of sharing, negative experiences from shared medicines, factors influencing sharing medicines, and risk assessment strategies.

Results

Participant characteristics

The sample comprised 12 females and five males, with a mean age of 41.2 years (Range: 23–69 years) and the majority of participants (n = 10) self-identified as New Zealand European (see Table 2 for detailed description of participants' characteristics). Twelve participants were recruited through email advertisements to the University of Auckland community, and two each through a public library and a patient support group. One participant was recruited from a community pharmacy.

Types of shared medicines

A range of medicines was reported to be shared (see Table 3). Although most of the sharing practice described was for medical purposes, sharing for non-medical purposes was also reported, for example, for cosmetic use (e.g., Botox®), to relax or to "get high" (e.g., strong pain medications), and for dietary supplementation (e.g., glucosamine). Participants also reported sharing homeopathic preparations which were sometimes recommended by their GP.

Perceived benefits of sharing medicines

Participants reported a range of benefits and these were categorised into two sub-themes.

Saves time and money

Participants stated that medicine sharing helped them to avoid doctors' fees and prescription charges, and reduced the burden associated with medical visits such as booking appointments, arranging transport, and the need to visit a pharmacy afterwards. Participants stated that visiting a doctor often requires taking time off work and can be costly in terms of income loss or the inconvenience it can create. Participants also reported sharing prescription medicines for conditions that require immediate treatment because of long waiting times at busy surgeries. Sharing also provided participants with easy access to medicines particularly when they considered themselves not sick enough to visit a doctor or when they only required a few doses of the medicine.

For those who were concerned about finances, sharing provided an opportunity to try the medicine before making a decision to pay for a doctor's appointment. When the shared medicine was found to be effective, some participants visited their doctor to inform them of their positive experience and obtain their own prescription.

> *I have psoriasis and I have some friends who have psoriasis. So if they said to me, "Oh my doctor gave me this [cream], and it was great." I might say, "Oh do you think I could try that a little bit?" I could see myself doing that. Maybe I'll see if it seems to work for me and I'll go to the doctor and get it myself.* (P07, 69-year-old female)

For some participants, medicine sharing was a way of preventing wastage of resources. Some considered discarding unused medicines to be wasteful, and was a

Table 1 Overview of codes, sub-themes and overarching themes

Codes (specific categories)	Code description	Sub-theme	Overarching theme
Pain, asthma and sleep medications, antibiotics, and so forth.	Classes of medicines shared by participants	NA	Types of shared medicines
Avoid doctor visit	Sharing avoids the need to visit a doctor	Saves time and money	Perceived benefits of sharing medicines
Avoid hidden costs	Sharing avoid taking time off work or avoid inconveniencing work – avoids hidden cost		
To avoid waste	To avoid buying a packet when only need one dose or might not work		
Convenience	Sharing is more convenient, the medicines are readily available, no need to visit a GP		
Emergency	Sharing when someone is in great need of the medication or during emergency		
To try the medicine	To see if the medicine works before obtaining a personal supply		
Misplacing medicines	Misplacing own medicines and temporarily sharing other's medicines		
Common minor condition	Sharing medicines when the patient perceives that the medical condition is minor		
Caring relationship	Sharing is a means of supporting each other during illness – caring relationship	Social support	
Inappropriate dose/wrong medicines	Person takes inappropriate doses or wrong medicines	Unsafe and ineffective treatment	Negative experience from shared medicines
Adverse drug events	Sharing might result in unanticipated side effects, drug interactions, allergy or contraindications		
Expired medicines might be shared	Expired medicines might be shared		
Risk of killing/harming	Sharing may have a risk of killing or harming a person		
Topical medicines are weaker than orally ingested medicines	Sharing topical medicines is not as risky as sharing pills – can be removed by washing		
Loss of medication instruction	Lack of information – e.g. borrower does not have information on risks, adverse outcomes, etc.		
Medical condition get worse	Sharing complicates simple medical conditions by delaying diagnosis and treatment		
Misdiagnosis	Sharing based on misdiagnosis could be dangerous		
Unhygienic	Sharing medicines (e.g., inhalers) is unhygienic	Public health risk	
Antimicrobial resistance	Sharing might increase drug resistance		
Spread infection	Sharing creams/ointments might spread the disease – cross infection		
Affects social relationship	Sharing addictive medicines may affect one's personal relationship with others	Risk of drug dependence	
Dependence	Sharing might result in drug dependence		
To help a friend or family	Sharing to help out others or to make someone feel better – caring relationship	Altruism	Factors influencing medicine sharing
Ran out	Ran out of previously prescribed medicines		
Cost	Sharing saves doctor's fee, prescription charges, or cost of unsubsidised medicines	Limited access to medicines/health services	
Access	Sharing when difficult to access medicines – for example prescription restriction and when pharmacy or doctors are inaccessible or where there is no nearby health facility		
Waiting times	Sharing medicines to avoid long appointment or waiting time at GP surgeries		
'After hours'	Sharing for pain occurring late at night or over the weekend – when a regular GP is not accessible		

Table 1 Overview of codes, sub-themes and overarching themes *(Continued)*

Traveling	Sharing medicine during family trip, holiday trips or when traveling overseas		
Forgetfulness	Someone forgets to carry around their own medicines		
Leftover medicines	Having leftovers/unused medicines creates opportunity for sharing	Leftover medicines	
Lack of information about safe disposal	Not knowing what to do with leftover or unused medicines		
HCPs not mentioning not to share	When patients do not receive information from health care providers about the risk of sharing		
Cultural influence	Cultural beliefs, family values and customs may influence medicine sharing	Sociocultural factors	
Embarrassment	Embarrassment about seeing a doctor or embarrassed to carry around own medicines		
Ads/Internet	TV ads or the Internet encourages self-diagnosis and sharing medicines		
Familiarity with the medical condition or the medicine	Familiarity with the medical condition or the medicine–facilitates sharing	Experience of, and knowledge about illness and its treatment	Risk assessment strategy
Complex medical condition	If the condition is complex – deterrent		
Uniqueness of medication for the person	Medicines meant for a specific condition are less likely to be shared		
Unaware of risk	Unaware of risk of sharing – facilitator		
Perception of efficacy	Assuming if the medicine worked for the lender it will do the same for the borrower		
Perceived danger of medicine	Concern about side effects – deterrent		
Borrower's responsibility	Borrower decides and accepts responsibility for consequences	Borrower's responsibility	
Same symptoms	Having the same symptoms facilitates sharing	Symptoms matching	
Same medicines	Attitude that taking similar medication as the other person might not have a negative effect on one's health		

NA not applicable

reason they were willing to share their unused medicines, as long as they believed them to be of benefit to someone else. During many of the interviews participants asked the interviewer if there was any way to return or donate unused medicines. Also of note, was that participants considered paying for medical visits to be a waste of money, when only a few doses of medicine are required.

Sometimes medicines were lost or misplaced and participants borrowed to avoid the inconvenience of getting a replacement prescription. Sharing also allowed some participants to avoid the fear of the consequence of missing a few doses of the medicines they were relying on (e.g. diabetes medications or asthma inhalers).

Sharing as a form of social support

Apart from cost reduction, medicine sharing had a positive impact on social interactions. During sharing, participants disclosed the nature of their illness to the other person, and this process helped them to share illness experiences and to sustain and nurture a social relationship. A university student described her boyfriend's positive experience as follows:

> *My boyfriend got a nasal spray* [for snoring] *from his friend, that really helped, that really worked, even brought them closer, because that's a very special experience.* (P08, 28-year-old female)

Negative experience from shared medicines

Participants described various risks and harms of medicine sharing and these were classified into three subthemes. While some participants revealed their own negative experiences from shared medicines, others provided hypothetical scenarios to explain the potential risks of sharing.

Unsafe and ineffective treatment

In an effort to help friends or relatives, participants engaged in "diagnosing" and "prescribing" which resulted in sharing their medicines with others. However, in so doing, some of the participants ended up giving inappropriate medicines to the other person. According to participants, it is often difficult for an untrained person to make the correct judgment regarding the dosage, potential contraindications, and side effects as this often requires technical knowledge

Table 2 Participant characteristics

Characteristics	Number ($N = 17$)
Gender	
Male	5
Female	12
Age in years[a] (Mean age = 41.2 years, Range: 23–69 years)	
20 - 30	6
31 - 40	2
41 - 50	3
51 - 60	2
60+	2
Ethnicity	
New Zealand European	10
Chinese	4
Others (Indian, Māori, Brazilian)	3
Highest level of education attended	
Tertiary education (college and above)	15
Secondary school	2
Working status	
Working full time	10
Working part time	1
Retired	2
Student	3
Unwaged	1
Monthly income (in NZD)[a]	
<1000	2
1001 – 2000	7
2001 – 4000	2
4001 – 6000	2
6000+	2
Have you been taking any prescription medicines in the past one year?	
Yes	16
No	1

[a]Data were not obtained from two participants

about medicines. Sharing can have life threatening consequences; one of the participants recounted the negative consequences occurring when her mother borrowed a medicine.

> *My mother, she was having pain. She had spondylitis so she was having severe pain and she was talking to her friend who is her next-door neighbour. So she said, "Oh you know what, I have this medicine and it worked fantastic for me" and she gave my mum, and she was given a CNS acting drug, she was given* [sic] *to take three tablets a day. My mum took the same dose and she went into coma that night.* (P10, 30-year-old female)

Table 3 Medicines shared by participants

Allergy medications (e.g., e.g., Zetop®, EpiPen®, hay fever medications)
Antibiotics (e.g., amoxicillin, Augmentin®)
Antidiarrhoeal medications
Antiemetic medications
Antihypertensives
Anti-inflammatory medications (e.g., diclofenac, naproxen)
Asthma inhalers (e.g., Ventolin®, Symbicort® inhaler)
Botox® (cosmetic use)
Cardiovascular medications (e.g., Cartia®, aspirin)
Cholesterol medications (e.g., simvastatin)
Constipation relief medications (e.g., VitoLax®)
Diabetes medications (e.g., metformin, glipizide)
Dietary supplements (e.g., glucosamine tablets)
Gastric/duodenal ulcer medications (e.g., omeprazole, Losec®)
Homeopathic medications
Hypnotics (e.g. nitrazepam, Valium®, melatonin)
Migraine medications (e.g., sumatriptan)
Muscle relaxants
Nasal spray to treat snoring
Nitrous oxide canister
Oral contraceptive pills
Pain medications (e.g. tramadol, morphine, codeine, pethidine)
Psoriasis medications
Topical antifungal/corticosteroids (e.g., Micreme H®, Betnovate®, eczema medications)

A few incidences of medicine sharing had resulted in allergic reactions. Most participants believed that the decision to share medicines often relies on symptom matching alone and that allergy histories might not be properly assessed. One participant described her negative experience as follows:

> *A long time ago my mum and I were in [country], we were living in a small town, we shared medicine once, after my mum took the medicine her eyes became swollen and she stopped the drug, and she went to the GP, and the GP actually told her that she is allergic to that kind of drug.* (P08, 28-year-old female)

Public health risk

Participants had different opinions regarding the risk of antibiotic sharing. Some of them had fewer concerns about sharing antibiotics particularly for common conditions; others were worried about treatment failure and antimicrobial resistance due to sharing and incomplete courses of antibiotics. Depleting one's own supply and ineffective treatment were other risks mentioned by those who had concerns about antibiotic sharing.

Sharing some forms of medicines (e.g. eye drops, asthma inhalers, creams or ointments) was considered by participants to be unhygienic and a way of spreading infections. Apart from the spread of infections, it appeared that participants had fewer concerns about the effects of some of these medicines. For instance, many participants were less concerned about the possible side effects or toxicity from shared creams or ointments, compared to pills. On the other hand, one participant warned that the likelihood of exacerbating skin conditions when using inappropriate creams could be high, and she explained the common misconceptions towards topical preparations amongst the public.

> *We think it's safer because we don't take it in and that's less chance of getting poisoned by it or something. It's probably not, that's what people think. If you eat it inside then people take more precautions. Whereas if it's topical like something on the skin, like if it's a cut or a burn or something then they just think it's less important than something that's happening inside.* (P16, 29-year-old female)

Risk of drug dependence

Participants also discussed about the impact of medicine sharing on drug dependence. Participants stated that although sharing by itself might not necessarily result in drug dependence, some medicines (e.g. strong pain medications) might be shared for thrill-seeking. Participants believed that this form of sharing could have a negative impact on social relationships. A participant who had been prescribed these medicines described strategies he uses to minimise the chance of being a source of abusable medicines, such as keeping social distance or concealing information from potential abusers.

> *If they [drug abusers] knew what I had [strong pain killers] they would be knocking at my door, "bro can I have a few of these, few of that?" So that's why I tell them nothing because I know what they use them for.* (P11, 50-year-old male)

Factors influencing medicine sharing

Participants reported many factors that could facilitate prescription medicine sharing practices; these were classified into four sub-themes.

Altruism

A desire to help others (i.e. altruism) was often the main motivator for those who reported sharing medicines. They shared their medicines for what they perceived to be a good reason, to help their loved ones when they were suffering from an illness. Participants' past illness experience could further encourage altruistic behaviour. This was described by one of them.

> *Just someone here at work had a terrible migraine and the person did not have access to medication, you know, and it's something that I suffer from migraine and I know how horrible it is so I just said look I have sumatriptan here, if you want I can give you.* (P12, 41-year-old male)

Although medicines were more often reported to be shared with family members, close friends, neighbours, or work mates, when it came to helping people in urgent need of medicine, social distance was less important.

> *Yes, one time actually, my boyfriend has asthma and I had his inhaler in my bag because I always carry around for him, and I was out in the pub and a guy had really bad asthma and his friend was running around and saying "Inhaler, inhaler", so I gave him, so yeah, I did do that, I am happy to do it, it was not like an emergency, but he definitely needed the inhaler.* (P09, 25-year-old, female)

Sometimes the lender used the sharing instance as an opportunity to establish a friendship with the borrower, although the main motivator, in doing so, was often altruism.

> *I get anxious so I take omeprazole or Losec®. ... And if somebody told me that their stomach was hurting and they needed one of those, I would do that* [share], *sure. I'm trying to be friendly and a bit of a socialist, you know (laughs), but I don't do it to save money.* (P07, 69-year-old female)

Limited access to medicines/health services

The cost of medical visits hindered participants with limited resources from seeking medical care and being prescribed their own medicines. Some of them revealed that their health insurance was limited and did not cover all their medical needs, for example, students and retired participants. Limited opening hours of local pharmacies and surgeries also influenced participants' sharing behaviours. For instance, participants reported sharing medicines for pain occurring late at night or at the weekend when local health facilities were not accessible. A university student associated her medicine sharing behaviour with the campus clinic opening hours as follows;

> *My health insurance is very limited, for example, it's only free if I go to the campus clinic, and the campus clinic you need to book and their opening hours is very short, I think they are closed at 3:00 PM or 4:00 PM. So*

it will be easier if I just get the medicine from someone I know and solve my problem. (P08, 28-year-old female)

Participants also reported sharing medicines while travelling when they could not access their regular doctor within a reasonable time.

Sociocultural factors

Social, cultural, and interpersonal interactions influencing participants' sharing behaviours were captured by this theme.

Although not nationally representative, participants were drawn from different communities, and it was noted that for some participants (e.g. those recently migrating to New Zealand) visiting a doctor and getting their own medicines was not an easy experience, partly because of cultural differences (e.g. communication barriers or differences in the health systems). Those participants considered medicine sharing to be a means of accessing prescription medicines without having to see a GP. It was also revealed that in some cultures sharing medicine and other commodities is a way of providing social support for others. One participant had lived in New Zealand for a number of years. He described the difference in perspectives about sharing medicines and the role of medicines, between people from his homeland and New Zealanders, as follows;

In New Zealand it's not culturally acceptable, you don't share someone else's drink whereas back home it is quite common so I guess that cultural difference may come into play.... [people from his homeland] are much more interventionist they will medicate people much more commonly than in New Zealand. So back home, I think there's much more medication sharing than in New Zealand. (P12, 41-year-old male)

Embarrassment was reported as a major reason why some patients do not visit their GP to obtain their own prescriptions. Participants also believed that younger patients might be embarrassed to carry around medicines they rely on and need to take in front of others (e.g., asthma inhalers) because doing so might be considered, by peers to be an indication of weakness.

Participants believed that advertising medicines on television might encourage people to self-diagnose and borrow medicines. It was noted by participants that when a prescription medicine is advertised on television it may lead the public into believing that the advertised medicine is safe to be shared, and might change their attitude towards the risks associated with sharing it. Younger participants appeared to be more influenced to share medicines by patient fora and various drug information sources on the Internet. One of the younger participants reported surfing the Internet to help her decide whether to take the medicine she had been offered by a friend.

I remember once I had a cat bite, the cat got some fungus infection and I got the infection on my skin as well. I talked to some friends who also had a cat and I asked whether they had this kind of problem as well, and yeah she said she had once a cat bite and she still have the ointment. So I Googled the drug and I thought that it suits my condition and I borrowed from her, and I just used it until the infection was gone, until I recovered. (P08, 28-year-old female)

Having leftover/unused prescription medicines

Participants were unsure what to do with unused medicines and many of them mentioned passing their unused medicines on to others. Most of the participants revealed that they received little information from healthcare providers about the safe disposal of leftover medicines. Some participants criticised their doctors for failing to understand their actual need and for supplying them surplus pills. A retired woman with back pain was among those who were unhappy with their doctor's prescribing behaviour.

Sometimes I have a really bad back problem and so for a little while I went to a back person [doctor] *and I think they're very negligent. He gave me a million tramadol, you know, it was like so much and they just give you these giant prescriptions and so I don't think I would share that tramadol. To me I would put that into a more serious; it's not like an aspirin.* (P07, 69-years-old female)

Although the above participant did not share her tramadol this was not the case for all participants. Some of them reported sharing their spare medicines (e.g. antibiotics), and they believed that having an oversupply of medicines motivated them to do so.

Risk assessment strategies

Participants reported different strategies that helped them to assess whether it was safe for them to share medicines and these were classified into three sub-themes.

Experience of, and knowledge about illness and its treatment

Their own experience with the medicine also helped participants to assess risks of sharing. If participants had been taking the medicine and if they knew what it was for and were confident that it could help the other person, they were more likely to share the medicine. On the other hand, if participants thought that their medicines were specific to their condition, if they were unfamiliar with the medicine or when they were not confident enough about the borrower's medical condition they were less likely to share.

Knowledge about illness and its treatment could also play a significant role in decisionmaking. For example, those who were aware of the risk of misdiagnosis of bacterial infections, risk of allergy and/or antimicrobial resistance firmly opposed sharing oral antibiotics. However, most participants were unaware of the potential risks of topical antimicrobials and were willing to share them. Although the meaning of 'complicated condition' was different among participants, they were also generally uncomfortable with sharing medicines which are meant for conditions such as cancer, diabetes, heart problems, or hypertension.

Friends' positive experiences with a medicine and obtaining the medicine from a trusted person (i.e., a person with good knowledge of medicine or who used it for long time) also had an influence on participants' decisions to borrow medicines.

Borrower's responsibility

Some participants were not concerned about assessing risks when lending medicines. They believed that they were not qualified to diagnose the borrower's condition or to assess the risk of the medicine. Further, they stated that it is up to borrowers to decide if the medicine suits their condition and/or to check allergic reactions.

> *I assumed that he didn't have any sort of particular allergies or something towards the chemical but I think it's not up to the person who's offering the medicine to diagnose the other person and give him the right drugs. It's just I have this, maybe you want to try it, maybe you don't – I don't really care.* (P14, 23-year-old female)

Symptoms matching

Symptoms matching was another strategy used by participants to assess the possible risks of sharing medicines. Participants believed that if someone had similar symptoms to the other person then the medicine would most probably work for him/her and be safe. Participants also frequently reported that they would be willing to try a medicine which worked for their friends with a similar condition to see if it would also work for their condition.

Discussion

This research explored the positive and negative consequences of, and factors influencing non-recreational medicine sharing practices of adults. Furthermore, the study examined factors considered by patients when deciding to share a medicine. These findings advance our understanding of non-recreational medicine sharing and provide further insights into the social, cultural, economic, and therapeutic aspects of medicine sharing. Although the potential risks of medicine sharing are well known to researchers [21, 22, 27] and regulatory authorities, [http://www.fda.gov/RegulatoryInformation/Legislation/FederalFoodDrugandCosmeticActFDCAct/] the non-medical aspects of sharing have been largely unexplored. From the medical perspective, medicine sharing is often considered to be undesirable behaviour [6, 17]. However, patients often see their sharing practices as positive and the study indicates that they often have sound justifications for doing so, as described in our findings.

In line with other research, a wide range of medicines were reported to be shared [1, 8–11, 13, 14, 21–23]. A number of previously unreported medicines were also reported; these include melatonin, muscle relaxants, Botox®, homeopathic preparations, and migraine medications.

With the rising cost of health-care, it has been noted that patients with lower incomes may adopt different cost-coping strategies such as intentional non-adherence, increasing debt burden, or cutting back (or economising) on necessities such as clothes and food [34]. Our findings suggest that medicine sharing may be another coping strategy. This finding is also in line with earlier studies reporting financial hardship as a reason for medicine sharing and underutilisation of available health-care services [19, 20, 30]. Also of note, in some developing countries the prevalence rates of medicine sharing are high (55–66 %) [14, 28] when compared with reports from developed countries (5–27 %) [1, 8, 10, 11, 23].

For most participants, medicine sharing was not a major concern. Some participants did not perceive their medicine sharing to be risky. Instead, they weighed up the risks and benefits of sharing particular medicines primarily based on their previous illness experiences and symptoms matching. In most instances, participants did not disclose the medicines they have shared or their sharing intention to healthcare providers; one possible explanation for this could be a fear of upsetting their healthcare providers. Overall, participants described a multifaceted system for determining the safety of the medicines they had shared. It appears that medicine sharing practices described in this study sample often involved a thoughtful decision making process rather than irresponsible behaviour or ignorance. However, although sharing medicines had many benefits for participants, we are concerned by some forms of sharing. For instance, opioid painkiller effectiveness for non-cancer chronic pain is controversial, [35] and its continuous use may diminish pain threshold levels or lead to substance use disorders [36]. Antibiotic sharing practices might result in therapeutic failure and may contribute to the emergence of antimicrobial resistance [1].

Van der Geest et al., in their anthropological study of pharmaceuticals, pointed out that medicines can be exchanged between individuals to facilitate social interactions [37]. The authors further noted that medicines are representations of ideologies and lifestyle. Our study findings support this; we found that "prescribing" for others and medicine sharing were common practices, and these practices had a positive impact on participants' social relationships. Many of the participants had been offered medicines by friends or relatives for free, and the sharing decision appeared to be influenced by altruistic reasons rather than the expectation of a reward. Therefore, any efforts to design interventions need to consider sharing behaviours within the context of wider social interactions.

Inconvenience, and embarrassment about seeing a doctor were other reasons why some participants shared medicines. This may be a coping strategy by patients in response to a healthcare system that does not address their needs and expectations. Language, cultural barriers and a lack of information about the healthcare system were reported to be contributing factors to poor access to health services and medicine sharing practices amongst immigrants in New Zealand [38] and elsewhere [39]. Similarly, immigrants in this study reported challenges they have faced in accessing medicines or health services (such as limited health insurance, an inability to pay doctors' fees, and language barriers), particularly upon their arrival in New Zealand, and the contribution of those challenges towards medicine sharing practices. Providing more information for migrants on the healthcare system and using translators in healthcare facilities were suggested as strategies to reduce some of the problems mentioned [38].

This study also revealed that some participants initially try to self-medicate their problems with borrowed medicines before visiting their doctor. This behaviour might lead to a delay in clinical diagnosis and an increase in complications from simple conditions [6]. Moreover, if patients do not inform their prescribers they might be unaware of the patient's sharing practices, and as a result they may prescribe medicines that should not be taken with the medicine the patient has borrowed [8]. Sharing unused/leftover medicines is also concerning. Some of these medicines might have passed their expiry date and/or their active ingredient might have deteriorated due to unfavourable storage conditions. Providing systems/pathways for unused/unwanted medicines to be safely disposed of (e.g. promoting collection of unused medicines by pharmacies) and prescribing medicine in quantities tailored to the actual need of the patient is more likely to reduce the amount of leftovers and associated sharing practices. Some of the adverse reactions reported by participants are potentially life threatening. However, no study to date has tracked the extent and severity of adverse drug reactions occurring as a result of shared medicines, and this is an important area for future research.

Overall, the findings indicate that some individuals are sharing 'high risk' medicines and this suggests the importance of incorporating questions assessing medicine sharing behaviours into prescribing, dispensing and medicine reconciliation activities. Available electronic medication records can assist in the process of identifying individuals sharing medicines. Posters and leaflets which show the potential risks of sharing medicines could be used to increase risk awareness. In addition, non-compliance with medication regimens is likely to increase the amount of leftover medicines, thus adherence counselling is crucial to reduce the opportunity for sharing.

This study is not without limitations and the findings should be interpreted in the light of these. Participants were not a representative sample of New Zealand adults, and thus their views may not be generalisable, although care was taken to recruit a sample from a broad range of backgrounds. This could potentially limit the transferability of findings. Those who could not speak English were excluded from the study. These individuals are more likely to have different cultural backgrounds and they might have unique concerns and expectations regarding their health and medicine sharing, particularly as language and communication barriers are more likely to increase medicine sharing.

As the professional qualification of the interviewer was made known to all participants, and it is possible that such information could have potentially influenced participants' responses. For example, some participants might believe that sharing medicines is not condoned by some health professionals and may not have wanted to disclose the nature of some of their sharing practices to the interviewer. To minimise the potential for such social desirability bias, all interviewees were informed of the general purpose of the research and the measures taken to ensure confidentiality of information. They were further informed that there was no right or wrong answer to any of the questions. This appeared to put participants at ease. In some interviews the interviewer was challenged by participants to give his opinion on topics such as the possibility of sharing medicines in some instances and legal issues related to medicine sharing. However, such opinions were not supplied, except in instances where further explanation was sought relating to the intention of the interview questions. The study authors are pharmacists, and despite acknowledging both the benefits and harms of this practice, this could have influenced the study design and data interpretation. However, attention was paid to providing balanced perspectives. Lastly, the fear of punishment from a previous 'bad' experience about medicine sharing may have exclude some individuals from participation.

Limitations aside, this study revealed that medicine sharing is a behaviour more complex than some previous quantitative studies suggest. Accordingly, the findings have important implications for healthcare providers who regularly engage in patient consultations about the safe use of medicines and for future research on medicine use behaviours. A cross-sectional survey among larger cohorts is currently being conducted by the authors to examine the extent to which each identified factor influences patients' medicine sharing decisions, and the relationships between these factors.

Generally, as noted by Shoemaker and Ramalho de Oliveria, understanding medicine use behaviours requires carefully analysis of patients' perspectives and should not rely only on health professionals' perspectives [40]. Thus, taking into account how patients understand medicine sharing is critical in designing effective interventions to reduce harms from this practice.

Conclusions

This study enriches previous survey findings, by providing insight into patients' reasons for medicines sharing. For example, altruism, forgetfulness, cost of GP visits, illness denial and embarrassment, lack of awareness regarding the risk of sharing, which have received little attention in previous surveys, were identified as important factors influencing sharing behaviours. Health care providers need to be aware that the sharing of prescription medicines is not uncommon. The authors suggest that healthcare providers consider engaging patients in discussions which may provide further insights into factors influencing sharing behaviours for particular individuals. Overall, it might be impractical to stop people from sharing their prescribed medicines (and even undesirable under some circumstances), and minimising the potential risks/harms of sharing should, therefore, be a priority whilst also acknowledging the meaning such behaviours have for patients, and their reasons for sharing. Quantitative research is required to examine the extent to which the identified factors related to sharing influence patients' decisions to share.

Acknowledgement

We would like to acknowledge our research project funders, New Zealand Pharmacy Education and Research Foundation (Grant Number - 244) and the University of Auckland. We thank all individuals and organisations who took part in the study. We are also grateful to Gregory Duncan, Eastern Health Clinical School, Monash University, for reviewing the draft manuscript and providing useful suggestions.

Authors' contributions

KB designed the study protocol and instruments, carried out data collection and analysis, and drafted the first manuscript. TA and JS were involved in all aspects of the study – developing and revising the study protocol and instruments, analysing data, interpreting results and revising the manuscript for publication. All authors read and approved the final manuscript.

Competing interests

The authors declare that they have no competing interests.

References

1. Goldsworthy RC, Schwartz N, Mayhorn CB. Beyond Abuse and Exposure: Framing the Impact of Prescription-Medication Sharing. Am J Public Health. 2008;98(6):1115–21.
2. Goldsworthy RC. Recreational Versus Nonrecreational Prescription Borrowing: Time for an Expanded Conceptualization? J Adolesc Health. 2010;46(4):402.
3. McCabe SE, West BT, Teter CJ, Ross-Durow P, Young A, Boyd CJ. Characteristics associated with the diversion of controlled medications among adolescents. Drug Alcohol Depend. 2011;118(2–3):452–8.
4. Cooper JR, Czechowicz DJ, Petersen RC, Molinari SP. Prescription drug diversion control and medical practice. JAMA. 1992;268(10):1306–10.
5. Garnier LM, Arria AM, Caldeira KM, Vincent KB, O'Grady KE, Wish ED. Sharing and selling of prescription medications in a college student sample. J Clin Psychiatry. 2010;71(3):262–9.
6. Makowka A, Zawiasa A, Nowicki M. Prescription-medication sharing among family members: an unrecognized cause of a serious drug adverse event in a patient with impaired renal function. Clin Nephrol. 2014;83(3):196–200.
7. Dimitrov D, Boily M, Mâsse B, Brown E. Impact of Pill Sharing on Drug Resistance Due to a Wide-Scale Oral Prep Intervention in Generalized Epidemics. J AIDS Clin Res. 2012;5(4):S5–004.
8. Ward L, Patel NM, Hanlon A, Eldakar-Hein S, Sherlinski K, Ward SH. Prescription Medication Borrowing among Adult Patients at an Urban Medical Center. J Urban Health. 2011;88(6):997–1014.
9. Goldsworthy RC, Mayhorn CB. Prescription Medication Sharing Among Adolescents: Prevalence, Risks, and Outcomes. J Adolesc Health. 2009;45(6):634–7.
10. Gascoyne A, Beyene K, Stewart J, Aspden T, Sheridan J. Sharing prescription medicines: results of a survey of community pharmacy clients in Auckland, New Zealand. Int J Clin Pharm. 2014;36(6):1268–76.
11. Ellis JC, Mullan J, Worsley T. Prescription medication hoarding and borrowing or sharing behaviours in older residents in the Illawarra, New South Wales, Australia. Australas J Ageing. 2011;30(3):119–23.
12. Beyene KA, Sheridan J, Aspden T. Prescription Medication Sharing: A Systematic Review of the Literature. Am J Public Health. 2014;104(4):e15–26.
13. Goulding E, Murphy M, Di Blasi Z. Sharing and borrowing prescription medication: a survey of Irish college students. Ir J Med Sci. 2011;180(3):687–90.
14. Auta A, Banwat SB, Francis RA. Prevalence of prescription medication sharing behaviour among students. Int J Pharm Life Sci. 2011;2(4):651–4.
15. Goebel JR, Compton P, Zubkoff L, Lanto A, Asch SM, Sherbourne CD, Shugarman L, Lorenz KA. Prescription sharing, alcohol use, and street drug use to manage pain among veterans. J Pain Symptom Manage. 2011;41(5):848–58.
16. Ellis JC, Mullan J. Prescription medication borrowing and sharing: risk factors and management. Aust Fam Physician. 2009;38(10):816–9.
17. Mayhorn CB, Goldsworthy RC. Borrowing prescription medication: Implications for healthcare warnings and communications. Proceedings of the Human Factors and Ergonomics Society Annual Meeting. 2009;53(20): 1608-1611.
18. Kamutingondo S, Groot S, Hodgetts D, Nikora LW. Understandings and social practices of medications for Zimbabwean households in New Zealand. MAI Review. 2011;3:1–17.

19. Hodgetts D, Nikora LW, Rua M. Maori men and the indirect procurement and sharing of prescription medications. AlterNative: Int J Indigenous Peoples. 2011;7(2):152–62.
20. Pai S, Boutin-Foster C, Mancuso CA, Loganathan R, Basir R, Kanna B. "Looking out for each other": a qualitative study on the role of social network interactions in asthma management among adult Latino patients presenting to an emergency department. J Asthma. 2014;51(7):714–9.
21. Hogan DJ, Moreland A, Lane P, Lal S. Exchange of prescription medications by dermatology outpatients. J Am Acad Dermatol. 1990;23(5):953.
22. Thompson S, Stewart K. Prescription medication use practices among non-institutionalised older persons. Int J Pharm Pract. 2001;9(3):141–51.
23. Petersen EE, Rasmussen SA, Daniel KL, Yazdy MM, Honein MA. Prescription medication borrowing and sharing among women of reproductive age. J Womens Health. 2008;17(7):1073–80.
24. Schillie SF, Shehab N, Thomas KE, Budnitz DS. Medication overdoses leading to emergency department visits among children. Am J Prev Med. 2009; 37(3):181–7.
25. Kurtz SP, Buttram ME, Surratt HL. Vulnerable infected populations and street markets for ARVs: potential implications for PrEP rollout in the USA. AIDS Care. 2014;26(4):411–5.
26. Kiarie JN, Kreiss JK, Richardson BA, John-Stewart GC. Compliance with antiretroviral regimens to prevent perinatal HIV-1 transmission in Kenya. AIDS. 2003;17(1):65–71.
27. Daniel K, Honein M, Moore C. Sharing prescription medication among teenage girls: Potential danger to unplanned/undiagnosed pregnancies. Pediatrics. 2003;111(5):1167–70.
28. Audet CM, Baptista A, Groh K, Moon TD, Sidat M, Vergara A, Vermund SH. Barriers to antiretroviral therapy adherence in rural Mozambique. BMC Public Health. 2011;11:650.
29. Caviness CM, Anderson BJ, de Dios MA, Kurth M, Stein M. Prescription medication exchange patterns among methadone maintenance patients. Drug Alcohol Depend. 2013;127(1):232–8.
30. Anglin MK, White JC. Poverty, health care, and problems of prescription medication: a case study. Subst Use Misuse. 1999;34(14):2073–93.
31. Dohn MN, Pilkington H. Sharing Medicine: The Candidacy of Medicines and Other Household Items for Sharing, Dominican Republic. PLoS One. 2014; 9(6):e101007.
32. Creswell J. Qualitative inquiry and research design: Choosing among five approaches. 2nd ed. Sage Publications, Inc: Thousand Oaks; 2007.
33. Thomas DR. A general inductive approach for analyzing qualitative evaluation data. Am J Eval. 2006;27(2):237–46.
34. Heisler M, Wagner TH, Piette JD. Patient strategies to cope with high prescription medication costs: who is cutting back on necessities, increasing debt, or underusing medications? J Behav Med. 2005;28(1):43–51.
35. Martell BA, O'Connor PG, Kerns RD, Becker WC, Morales KH, Kosten TR, Fiellin DA. Systematic review: opioid treatment for chronic back pain: prevalence, efficacy, and association with addiction. Ann Intern Med. 2007; 146(2):116–27.
36. Compton P, Charuvastra V, Ling W. Pain intolerance in opioid-maintained former opiate addicts: effect of long-acting maintenance agent. Drug Alcohol Depend. 2001;63(2):139–46.
37. Van der Geest S, Whyte SR, Hardon A. The anthropology of pharmaceuticals: a biographical approach. Annu Rev Anthropol. 1996;25(1996):153–78.
38. Babar Z, Pengelly K, Scahill SL, Garg S, Shaw J. Migrant health in New Zealand: exploring issues concerning medicines access and use. J Pharm Health Serv Res. 2013;4(1):41–9.
39. Derose KP, Bahney BW, Lurie N, Escarce JJ. Review: immigrants and health care access, quality, and cost. Med Care Res Rev. 2009;66(4):355–408.
40. Shoemaker SJ, Ramalho de Oliveira D. Understanding the meaning of medications for patients: the medication experience. Pharm World Sci. 2008;30(1):86–91.

4

Assessment of WHO/INRUD core drug use indicators in two tertiary care hospitals of Bahawalpur, Punjab, Pakistan

Muhammad Atif[1*], Muhammad Rehan Sarwar[1], Muhammad Azeem[1*], Danial Umer[1], Abdul Rauf[1], Arslan Rasool[1], Muhammad Ahsan[1] and Shane Scahill[2]

Abstract

Background: Medicines are a main therapeutic intervention provided within hospitals and their proper use in the outpatient setting is important for patients and the community. The objective of this study was to evaluate drug use patterns in the outpatient departments (OPDs) of two tertiary care hospitals (Bahawal Victoria Hospital and Civil Hospital) in the Bahawalpur district of the Punjab province of Pakistan by employing the standard World Health Organization/International Network of Rational Use of Drugs (WHO/INRUD) drug use indicators.

Methods: A descriptive, cross-sectional study design was employed. For assessing the prescribing indicators a sample of 2400 prescriptions were systematically reviewed out of a total of 1,560,000 prescriptions written from 1st April 2014 to 31st March 2015. A total of 600 randomly selected patients and all pharmacy personnel were observed and interviewed to investigate the patient-care and facility-specific indicators. We used the published ideal standards for each of the WHO/INRUD indicators for comparison purposes.

Results: Among the prescribing indicators, the average number of drugs per prescription was 2.8 (SD = 1.3), the drugs prescribed by generic name were 56.6 %, the encounters with an antibiotic prescribed were 51.5 %, no injections were prescribed and 98.8 % of the drugs prescribed were from the Essential Drugs List (EDL). Among the patient-care indicators, the average consultation time was 1.2 min (SD = 0.8), the average dispensing time was 8.7 s (SD = 4.9), the percentage of drugs actually dispensed was 97.3 %, the percentage of drugs adequately labeled was 100 % and the patients' knowledge of correct dosage schedule was 61.6 %. Among the facility-specific indicators, all OPDs had a copy of the EDL and 72.4 % of the key drugs were available in stock.

Conclusion: Irrational use of drugs was observed in both OPDs. Polypharmacy, brand prescribing, over-prescribing of antibiotics, short consultation and dispensing times, lack of patients' knowledge about prescribed medicines and unavailability of all key drugs in stock were the major issues that need attention of the healthcare authorities. This study necessitates the requirement to implement the relevant WHO recommended core interventions to promote rational use of medicines in these hospital-based OPDs.

Keywords: Rational, Use of drugs, Prescribing pattern, Patient-care, Facility-specific

* Correspondence: pharmacist_atif@yahoo.com; azeem634@hotmail.com
[1]Department of Pharmacy, The Islamia University of Bahawalpur, Bahawalpur, Pakistan
Full list of author information is available at the end of the article

Background

The World Health Organization (WHO) defines rational use of medicines as "patients receive medications appropriate to their clinical needs, in doses that meet their own individual requirements, for an adequate period of time, and at the lowest cost to them and their community" [1]. According to the WHO, more than 50 % of all medicines are prescribed, dispensed or sold inappropriately [2]. As a result, patients are unable to follow their treatment plan correctly. One of the consequences of irrational use of medicines is lack of patients' confidence in the healthcare system. In the developing countries, for example Pakistan, the problem is exacerbated by limited resources and inadequate drug policy [3].

The most common causes of inappropriate use of medicines are; self-medication, polypharmacy, inappropriate use of antibiotics, overuse of injectable medicines and prescribing of medicines outside of usual clinical practice guidelines [2]. Some other causes of irrational use of medicines include knowledge, attitudes and practices of patients and practitioners, the working environment, the drug supply system, legal regulations, information and misinformation about the medicines and profit intentions of the pharmaceutical companies [4–8]. Unsafe and ineffective treatment, prolongation of disease state, harm and distress to the patients, increased cost of treatment, aggravation of chronic conditions for example diabetes, hypertension, epilepsy and neurological disorders, and antibiotic resistance are some of the consequences of the irrational use of medicines [9].

The fundamental steps to limit the irrational use of medicines is to identify the types, extent and reasons of their irrational use [2]. In the 1990′s, WHO in collaboration with the International Network of Rational Use of Drugs (INRUD) developed standard indicators to evaluate drug use practices at healthcare centers [10]. Though originally developed to assess drug use patterns in primary healthcare centers, these indicators have been used at tertiary healthcare facilities for similar purposes [11–13]. The indicators called "core drug use indicators" are classified into prescribing, patient-care and facility-specific indicators (Table 1).

The purpose of this study was to investigate the drug use patterns at ten outpatient departments (OPDs) in each of the two tertiary care hospitals in the Bahawalpur district of Southern Punjab, Pakistan. The findings are able to be used as a benchmark for the healthcare facilities and as a basis for further follow-up of quality of drug use. In the context of Pakistan, the findings of this study will further help policymakers to take necessary measures to stimulate appropriate use of medicines.

Table 1 Core drug use indicators and their optimal values

Core drug use indicators	Optimal values
Prescribing Indicators	
Average number of drugs prescribed per patient encounter	1.6–1.8
Percent medicines prescribed by generic name	100
Percent encounters with an antibiotic prescribed	20.0–26.8
Percent encounters with an injection prescribed	13.4–24.1
Percent medicines prescribed from essential medicines list or formulary	100
Patient-Care Indicators	
Average consultation time (minutes)	≥10
Average dispensing time (seconds)	≥90
Percent medicines actually dispensed	100
Percent medicines adequately labeled	100
Percent patients with knowledge of correct doses	100
Facility-Specific Indicators	
Availability of essential medicines list or formulary to practitioners	100
Percent key medicines available	100

Note: Core drug use indicators are obtained from World Health Organization source [2, 10]

Methods

Study setting

The study was conducted in the Bahawal Victoria Hospital (BVH) and the Civil Hospital of Bahawalpur district of the Punjab province of Pakistan. Ten OPDs from each of the two hospitals were included. The BVH, located in the central part of the city, is a 1600-bed tertiary care hospital with all standard medical and surgical facilities. The Civil Hospital is newly established 400-bed tertiary care hospital.

Study design and outcome measures

This descriptive, cross-sectional study was conducted to evaluate the performance of the selected OPDs in three general areas related to rational drug use; prescribing, patient-care and facility. The optimal values for the prescribing [11], patient-care and facility-specific indicators [9, 14] were adopted from previous studies. For this study, the optimal values for the consultation and dispensing times were set as ≥10 min and ≥90 s, respectively (Table 1).

Zhang and Zhi developed an index system to gauge the performance of a healthcare system in terms of drug utilization [14, 15]. For the calculation of non-polypharmacy, rational antibiotic and injection safety indices, the following formula was used;

$$Index = \frac{\text{Optimal value}}{\text{Observed value}}$$

All other indices (index of generic name, index of Essential Drugs List (EDL), consultation time index, dispensing time index, index of drugs actually dispensed, index of labelling of drugs, index of patients' knowledge, index of EDL availability and index of key drugs availability in stock) were calculated by the following formula;

$$Index = \frac{\text{Observed value}}{\text{Optimal value}}$$

The optimal index for all indicators was set as 1. The values closer to 1 indicated rational drug use and vice versa. The Index of Rational Drug Prescribing (IRDP) was calculated for all OPDs by adding the index values of all prescribing indicators. Based on the IRDP values, the OPDs were ranked from 1 to 10 (rank 1 for the higher IRDP value and rank 10 for the lower IRDP). In a similar fashion, the Index of Rational Patient-Care Drug Use (IRPCDU) and the Index of Rational Facility-Specific Drug Use (IRFSDU) were calculated. Finally, the Index of Rational Drug Use (IRDU) was calculated for all OPDs by adding up the total of IRDP, IRPCDU and IRFSDU. Subsequently, OPDs were ranked based on the IRDU indices. The OPD with higher IRDU value was considered the best performing OPD in terms of rational drug use, and was given the first rank.

Data collection

The standard core drug use indicator forms were used to collect the data [10]. The WHO guidelines and methods were observed to ensure data reliability [10]. The data was collected during the period 1st December 2014 to 31st March 2015.

Prescribing indicators

Trained data collectors retrospectively selected 2,400 prescriptions (120 prescriptions per OPD) out of the total 1,560,000 prescriptions written during the 1 year period (i.e., 1st April 2014 to 31st March 2015). A systematic random sampling technique was used to collect the data and the sampling unit was the patient encounters at each of the OPDs [11]. To minimize the sampling bias (seasonal alterations or supply cycle of medicines), the encounters per year were uniformly divided into four quarters and 30 prescriptions were randomly selected from each quarter, irrespective of acute or chronic illnesses, including a mixture of health conditions and a range of patient ages.

Patient-care indicators

Patients visiting the OPDs, between 1st December 2014 and 31st March 2015 for diagnosis and treatment of health problems were invited to participate in the study. A total of 600 patients (30 patients per OPD) were randomly selected during the OPD hours. Trained data collectors explained the purpose of the study to the respondents and obtained their consent before data collection began. The consented patients were observed and interviewed to obtain the required information [10].

Facility-specific indicators

For the facility-specific indicators, all available pharmacy personnel were invited to participate in the study and the consented participants were interviewed to obtain the required information [10].

Data analysis

Statistical Package for Social Sciences (IBM, SPSS Statistics for Windows, version 21.0. Armonk, NY: IBM Corp.) was used for data analysis. Descriptive statistics such as frequencies, percentages, average/mean, and standard deviation were used to present the data.

Results

Prescribing indicators

The average number of drugs per encounter was 2.82 (SD = 1.3) and percentage of drugs prescribed by the generic name was 56.6 % (SD = 1.2). Over half (51.5 %, SD = 0.5) of the prescriptions had an antibiotic prescribed. There was no injection encounter recorded. The percentage of drugs prescribed from the EDL was 98.8 % (SD = 1.3) (Table 2).

Patient-care and facility-specific indicators

The average consultation time was 1.2 (SD = 0.8) minutes and the average dispensing time was 8.7 (SD = 4.9) seconds. 97.3 % (SD = 1.3) of drugs on the prescriptions were actually dispensed. All dispensed drugs were adequately labelled. Over two-thirds (61.6 %, SD = 0.6) of patients had the correct knowledge about the dosage of the medications they had been prescribed (knowledge about when and in what quantity the medicine should be taken). A copy of the EDL was available 100 % (SD = 0.0) of the time. Nearly three-quarters (72.4 %, SD = 0.4) of key drugs were available in stock (Table 3).

The IRDP values show that the gynecology OPD was performing well in the BVH and the pulmonology OPD was the leading department in the Civil Hospital. Similarly, the IRPCDU values indicated that the surgery OPDs in both hospitals showed better results compared with all other OPDs. The gynecology, ENT and pediatrics OPDs in the BVH and the ophthalmology OPD in the Civil Hospital showed relatively better results with regard to facility-specific indicators. Overall, the IRDU values showed that the gynecology OPD in the BVH and the pulmonology OPD in the Civil Hospital were the best performing OPDs (Table 4) in terms of core drug indicators.

Table 2 WHO/INRUD prescribing indicators in two tertiary care hospitals of Bahawalpur (*N* = 2400)

OPD wards	Prescribing indicators									
	Average drugs/ encounter		% drugs prescribed by generic name		% encounters with an antibiotic prescribed		% encounters with an injection prescribed		% drugs prescribed from EDL/formulary	
	BVH	Civil	BVH	Civil	BVH	Civil	BVH	Civil	BVH	Civil
Gynecology	3.1	2.8	66.0	51.3	38.0	43.3	0.0	0.0	100	87.1
Ophthalmology	1.2	1.6	28.2	84.1	48.0	71.6	0.0	0.0	100	99.4
Dermatology	2.2	2.8	44.2	54.4	48.0	35.0	0.0	0.0	100	98.8
ENT	3.2	2.8	72.5	62.2	80.0	55.8	0.0	0.0	100	100
Surgery	3.2	2.7	62.5	55.7	86.0	28.3	0.0	0.0	100	99.3
Pulmonology	3.7	2.0	55.6	56.0	54.1	6.6	0.0	0.0	100	98.3
Dental	2.8	2.5	45.1	39.3	95.0	95.0	0.0	0.0	100	99.7
Cardiology	4.6	4.1	52.8	67.0	0.0	10.0	0.0	0.0	100	95.5
Pediatrics	2.5	3.0	57.4	53.5	65.0	84.1	0.0	0.0	100	98.9
Medical	3.2	2.5	65.1	58.6	39.0	47.5	0.0	0.0	100	100
Mean	3.0	2.7	54.9	58.2	55.3	47.7	0.0	0.0	100	97.7
MEAN (SD)[a]	2.8 (1.3)		56.6 (1.2)		51.5 (0.5)		0.0 (0.0)		98.8 (1.3)	

[a]Calculated based on the total sample size, *OPD* outpatient department, *EDL* essential drugs list, *BVH* Bahawal Victoria Hospital, *ENT*, ear, nose & throat

Discussion

This study set out to assess drug use practices through analysis of the core indicators of the WHO/INRUD across a range of OPDs in two tertiary care hospitals in Pakistan. Though irrational prescribing practices exist all over the world [9], the gravity of the problem is high in low and middle income countries and so Pakistan makes for a sensible context in which to explore this issue. Our study reports: a higher number of drugs prescribed per prescription, over-use of antibiotics, low rate of prescribing by generic name and short dispensing and consulting times. Key drugs were available less than three-quarters (72.4 %) of the time. Patient knowledge of correct doses was found to be lower than like studies in other developing countries. On the positive side, the EDL was always available in these OPDs and 98.8 % of drugs prescribed were from the list. The implications of these findings are discussed in terms of previous studies and future policy, practice and research.

Prescribing indicators

Our findings suggest the average number of drugs per prescription was higher than the admissible range and there was considerable over-prescribing of antibiotics.

Table 3 WHO/INRUD patient-care and facility-specific indicators in two tertiary care hospitals of Bahawalpur (*N* = 600)

OPD wards	Patient-care and facility-specific indicators													
	Average consultation time (minutes)		Average dispensing time (seconds)		% drugs dispensed		% drugs adequately labeled		% patients knowledgeable		% copy of EDL		% key drugs in the stock	
	BVH	Civil	BVH	Civil	BVH	Civil	BVH	Civil	BVH	Civil	BVH	Civil	BVH	Civil
Gynecology	2.2	0.9	7.8	6.7	100	100	100	100	47.0	73.0	100	100	100	80
Ophthalmology	0.7	0.6	4.8	5.9	100	100	100	100	87.0	67.0	100	100	43.0	86
Dermatology	1.1	0.7	9.0	5.1	67.6	100	100	100	73.0	70.0	100	100	50.0	75
ENT	0.9	0.7	7.5	6.3	94.9	100	100	100	27.0	50.0	100	100	100	71
Surgery	1.1	2.1	17.2	6.8	100	100	100	100	100	67.0	100	100	50.0	75
Pulmonology	1.3	2.1	7.6	8.0	96.7	100	100	100	70.0	47.0	100	100	71.0	71
Dental	1.7	0.7	8.0	6.2	100	100	100	100	40.0	60.0	100	100	75.0	50
Cardiology	1.6	2.4	18.6	8.6	100	100	100	100	67.0	50.0	100	100	75.0	75
Pediatrics	1.4	0.7	6.1	7.4	86.0	100	100	100	47.0	60.0	100	100	100	67
Medical	1.1	0.7	18	7.4	100	100	100	100	67.0	63.0	100	100	75.0	58
Mean	1.3	1.1	10.5	6.8	94.5	100	100	100	62.5	60.7	100	100	73.9	70.8
MEAN (SD)[a]	1.2 (0.8)		8.7 (4.9)		97.3 (1.3)		100 (0.0)		61.6 (0.6)		100 (0.0)		72.4 (0.4)	

[a]Calculated based on the total sample size, *OPD* outpatient department, *EDL* essential drugs list, *BVH* Bahawal Victoria Hospital, *ENT* ear, nose & throat

Table 4 Index of rational drug use in two tertiary care hospitals of Bahawalpur

IRDU		OPDs									
		Gynecology	Ophthalmology	Dermatology	ENT	Surgery	Pulmonology	Dental	Cardiology	Pediatrics	Medical
Prescribing Indicators											
Non-polypharmacy index	BVH	0.58	1.00	0.82	0.56	0.56	0.49	0.64	0.40	0.72	0.56
	Civil	0.64	1.00	0.64	0.64	0.67	0.90	0.72	0.44	0.60	0.72
Generic name index	BVH	0.66	0.28	0.44	0.72	0.62	0.56	0.45	0.53	0.57	0.65
	Civil	0.51	0.84	0.54	0.62	0.56	0.56	0.39	0.67	0.53	0.59
Rational antibiotic index	BVH	0.71	0.56	0.56	0.34	0.31	0.49	0.28	1.00	0.41	0.69
	Civil	0.62	0.37	0.76	0.48	0.95	1.00	0.28	1.00	0.32	0.56
Injection safety index	BVH	1.00	1.00	1.00	1.00	1.00	1.00	1.00	1.00	1.00	1.00
	Civil	1.00	1.00	1.00	1.00	1.00	1.00	1.00	1.00	1.00	1.00
Essential drugs list index	BVH	1.00	1.00	1.00	1.00	1.00	1.00	1.00	1.00	1.00	1.00
	Civil	0.87	0.99	0.99	1.00	0.99	0.98	0.99	0.95	0.99	1.00
IRDP	BVH	3.95	3.84	3.82	3.62	3.49	3.54	3.37	3.93	3.70	3.90
	Civil	3.64	4.20	3.93	3.74	4.17	4.44	3.38	4.06	3.44	3.87
Rank	BVH	1	4	5	7	9	8	10	2	6	3
	Civil	8	2	5	7	3	1	10	4	9	6
Patient-Care Indicators											
Consultation time index	BVH	0.22	0.07	0.11	0.09	0.11	0.13	0.17	0.16	0.14	0.11
	Civil	0.09	0.06	0.07	0.07	0.21	0.21	0.07	0.24	0.07	0.07
Dispensing time index	BVH	0.09	0.05	0.10	0.08	0.19	0.08	0.09	0.21	0.07	0.20
	Civil	0.07	0.06	0.06	0.07	0.08	0.09	0.07	0.10	0.08	0.08
Dispensed drugs index	BVH	1.00	1.00	0.67	0.94	1.00	0.97	1.00	1.00	0.86	1.00
	Civil	1.00	1.00	1.00	1.00	1.00	1.00	1.00	1.00	1.00	1.00
Labeled drugs index	BVH	1.00	1.00	1.00	1.00	1.00	1.00	1.00	1.00	1.00	1.00
	Civil	1.00	1.00	1.00	1.00	1.00	1.00	1.00	1.00	1.00	1.00
Patients' knowledge index	BVH	0.47	0.87	0.73	0.27	1.00	0.70	0.40	0.67	0.47	0.67
	Civil	0.73	0.67	0.70	0.50	0.67	0.47	0.60	0.50	0.60	0.63
IRPCDU	BVH	2.78	2.99	2.61	2.38	3.30	2.88	2.66	3.04	2.54	2.98
	Civil	2.89	2.79	2.83	2.64	2.96	2.77	2.74	2.84	2.75	2.78
Rank	BVH	6	3	8	10	1	5	7	2	9	4
	Civil	2	5	4	10	1	7	9	3	8	6
Facility-Specific Indicators											
Index of EDL	BVH	1.00	1.00	1.00	1.00	1.00	1.00	1.00	1.00	1.00	1.00
	Civil	1.00	1.00	1.00	1.00	1.00	1.00	1.00	1.00	1.00	1.00
Index of key drugs in stock	BVH	1.00	0.43	0.50	1.00	0.50	0.71	0.75	0.75	1.00	0.75
	Civil	0.80	0.86	0.75	0.71	0.75	0.71	0.50	0.75	0.67	0.58
IRFSDU	BVH	2.00	1.43	1.50	2.00	1.5	1.71	1.75	1.75	2.00	1.75
	Civil	1.80	1.86	1.75	1.71	1.75	1.71	1.50	1.75	1.67	1.58
Rank	BVH	1	5	4	1	4	3	2	2	1	2
	Civil	2	1	3	4	3	4	7	3	5	6
Grand Total											
IRDU	BVH	8.73	8.26	7.93	8.00	8.29	8.13	7.78	8.72	8.24	8.63
	Civil	8.33	8.85	8.51	8.09	8.88	8.92	7.62	8.65	7.86	8.23

Table 4 Index of rational drug use in two tertiary care hospitals of Bahawalpur *(Continued)*

Rank	BVH	1	5	9	8	4	6	10	2	7	3
	Civil	6	3	5	8	2	1	10	4	9	7

OPD outpatient department, *EDL* essential drugs list, *BVH* Bahawal Victoria Hospital, *ENT*, ear, nose & throat, *IRDP* index of rational drug prescribing, *IRPCDU*, index of rational patient-care drug use, *IRFSDU* index of rational facility-specific drug use, *IRDU* index of rational drug use

We also found that just over half (56.6 %) of drugs were prescribed by the generic name whilst the aim is for 100 % prescribing by generic. These findings are alarming for a number of reasons. Polypharmacy can adversely influence treatment outcomes in a way that patients are at a higher risk of adverse events [16]. Similarly, unnecessarily prescribed medicines and those prescribed by brand names can put extra financial pressure on patients as well as healthcare budgets [2]. According to the WHO, it is the aim that generic prescribing takes precedent over originator brand prescribing because it helps with improved communication and clarity amongst healthcare providers. Moreover, generic medicines are less expensive than originator branded medicines [17]. The over-use of antibiotics is occurring internationally and leads to increase in adverse drug reactions and hospitalization, but also contributes significantly to an increase in antibiotic resistance and Pakistan appears no different [18].

In our study, we found that injectable medicines were not prescribed and the EDL was followed in 98.8 % of the prescriptions. It is likely that injectable medicines were not prescribed because in Pakistan they are more commonly reserved for emergency cases, and in the context of this study, such patients would be managed in Accident and Emergency (A&E) departments, and A&E departments were not included in our study.

We have summarized the findings of closely related studies, irrespective of country of origin, to facilitate comparisons (Table 5). With regard to prescribing indicators, our findings are closely related to earlier studies in this field. For example, studies from Afghanistan (3.9) [19], India (5.6) [20], Ghana (4.8) [21] and Nigeria (5.2) [22] showed higher numbers of drugs per prescription. Similarly, in studies from Andorra (6 %) [23], Palestine (5.5 %) [24], Lebanon (2.9 %) [25] and India (11.5 %) [3], generics were less commonly prescribed than was seen in this study. In contrast to this, studies from Cambodia (99.8 %) [26], Timor-Leste (92 %) [27] and Ethiopia (98.7 %) [11] showed higher levels of generic prescribing, which might be the consequence of more effective and better enforced drug policies in these countries; or simply a lack of very expensive originator branded drugs.

Patient-care indicators

The results of the current study demonstrate that the average consultation and dispensing times were 1.2 min and 8.7 s, respectively (dispensing time = time when a patient reaches and leaves the pharmacy counter. Waiting time not included). This is much less than the proposed optimal norms. The shorter consultation and dispensing times reported in our study could be a result of the large number of patients attending the OPDs in these two tertiary care hospitals. Insufficient consultation time leads to inappropriate patient examination and history taking and poor physician–patient interactions [9]. On the other hand, shorter dispensing time is insufficient to provide complete

Table 5 Summary of core drug use indicator studies from developed and developing countries

Indicators	Study reference									
	Developed countries					Developing countries				
	[14, 35]	[38]	[39]	[40]	[41]	[9]	[42]	[26]	[22]	[43]
Average no. of drugs per encounter	2.4	0.7	2.9	2.6	2.2	2.5	2.2	2.4	3.0	2.2
% Generic	61.2	——	17.7	14.3	4.4	95.4	74	99.8	63.1	99
% Antibiotic	32.2	10.4	39.1	26.2	13.5	39.2	37	66	54.2	43
% Injection	2	0.0	9.1	8.3	1.6	9.9	11	2.4	38.0	18
% drugs EDL	99.2	——	——	19.8	——	95.4	78	99.7	75.6	98.8
Average consultation time (minutes)	7.3	22.5	2.8	——	——	7.1	5.8	4.4	6.1	3.7
Average dispensing time (seconds)	100	——	54.6	——	——	47.4	17	234	18.1	37
% Drugs dispensed	99.6	——	97.9	——	——	95.9	66	100	99.1	84.5
% Drugs labeled	10	——	66.9	——	——	0.0	63	0.0	55.9	86.2
% Patient knowledge	79.3	70	26.9	——	——	94	54	55	86.5	81.7
% EDL availability	90	——	———	——	——	80	50	100	100	100
% Drugs in stock	59.2	———	————	——	——	78.3	55	86.6	91.7	86.5

Saudi Arabia [14, 35]; Sweden [38]; Kuwait [39]; Bahrain [40]; United Arab Emirates [41]; Egypt [9]; Brazil [42]; Cambodia [26]; Swaziland [22]; Mozambique [43]

drug related information to the patients. Several studies from various under-developed countries reported almost similar findings [22, 28, 29]. However, studies from Nigeria [30], Nepal [31] and Ethiopia [32] showed better results probably because of adequate patient-to-healthcare worker ratio. According to our findings, 61.6 % of the patients had knowledge of correct dosage schedule for all prescribed drugs. This is much lesser than the optimal value of 100 %. It was higher than that reported in Tanzania (37.9 %) [33] and Malawi (27 %) [34] but much lower than high achieving nations such as Nigeria (93 %) [30] and Egypt (94 %) [9]. Patient's knowledge about correct dosage is highly significant to avoid over use and abuse of drugs, and could prevent adverse events that ultimately affect patients' health and quality of life.

In contrast to dispensing time, consultation time, and patients' knowledge of correct dosage, the percentage of drugs actually dispensed and the drug labelling practices were close to the optimal values. This may be due to the fact that the medical professionals were aware of the drugs available in the hospital and followed appropriate guidelines with regards EDL use.

Facility-specific indicators

The study revealed that all OPDs had a copy of the EDL which is in line with the proposed norm. However, only 72.4 % of key drugs were available in on hand in these OPDs. Shortage of any essential drugs in the hospital is disadvantageous for patients in that doctors may not be able to prescribe the correct drugs or they are limited to prescribing out-of-stock medicines which may pose extra fiscal burden on the patients' through "out of pocket" expense. Similar to our findings, studies from Saudi Arabia (59.2 %) [35], Nigeria (62 %) [36], Malawi (67 %) [34] and Ethiopia (65 %) [32] showed lower values for availability of key drugs in the stock. In contrast, Tanzania (100 %) [37], Swaziland (91.7 %) [22], Nigeria (90.9 %) [22] and Nepal (90 %) [31] appear to report better results.

Implications

In addition to the implications for literature (outlined previously) there are also considerations for policy, practice and future research. Our findings will benefit policy makers who have an interest in process improvement and service delivery performance. The finding that only 72.4 % of key drugs were available throughout the study warrants consideration by policy-makers, who may need to put incentives or legislation in place to ensure better access to these essential drugs. There are also areas of practice which could be improved on particularly around the potential over-use of antibiotics and the prescribing of drugs by generic name. The two hospitals would benefit from having guidelines in place for the optimal and responsible use of antibiotics which could be monitored and feedback provided on a regular basis to prescribers. An awareness campaign and incentives could also be put in place to increase the prescribing of drugs by generic name. This intervention could be set up as a program evaluation and add to the current research agenda in this area. One approach could be to implement and evaluate WHO recommended core interventions on a pilot scale to devise policies to achieve improved performance and the long-term benefits associated with this.

Conclusion

Polypharmacy, brand prescribing, over-prescribing of antibiotics, short consultation and dispensing times, lack of patients' knowledge about prescribed medicines and unavailability of all key drugs in stock were the major issues that need attention of the healthcare authorities. WHO recommended core interventions could be implemented on pilot scale to devise policies to achieve long-term benefits.

Limitations

As with any study there are limitations which need to be considered.. First, our findings could not be generalized for the whole of Pakistan and should not be extrapolated to the international environment. The findings do however add to a growing literature, particularly around medicines use and pharmaceutical health systems in developing countries. It is also important to consider that a uniform healthcare policy is implemented throughout Pakistan and medical graduates from various institutions are working in the Bahawalpur district. It is expected that the practices would be similar to other tertiary care hospitals in Pakistan. Second, different OPDs in each of the tertiary care hospitals demonstrate varying degrees of optimal drug use and systems to support these. To address this bias, the mean values were calculated for each of the OPD, separately. Third, very limited data on core drug use indicators is available in tertiary care settings and we compare our findings with international data based on primary healthcare settings.

Abbreviations

EDL, essential drugs list; INRUD, International Network for the Rational Use of Drugs; IRDP, index of rational drug prescribing; IRDU, index of rational drug use; IRFSDU, index of rational facility-specific drug use; IRPCDU, index of rational patient-care drug use; SPSS, statistical package for social sciences; WHO, World Health Organization

Acknowledgements

The authors would like to thank the record officers at the BVH and Civil for their help in data retrieving. No funding was involved in the preparation of this article or in the decision to submit it for publication.

Authors' contributions

MAT conceptualized and designed the study. SS also participated in design of the study. MRS, MAZ, DU, AR, ARS and MA collected, analyzed and interpreted the data. MRS, MAZ and MAT drafted the manuscript. SS and MAT critically revised the manuscript. All authors read and approved final version of the manuscript.

Competing interests

The authors declare that they have no competing interests.

Author details

[1]Department of Pharmacy, The Islamia University of Bahawalpur, Bahawalpur, Pakistan. [2]School of Management, Massey University, Auckland, New Zealand.

References

1. World Health Organization. The Rational use of drugs: report of the conference of experts, Nairobi, 25–29 November 1985. 1987. http://apps.who.int/medicinedocs/en/d/Js17054e/. Accessed October 18 2015
2. World Health Organization. Promoting rational use of medicines: core components - WHO policy perspectives on medicines. 2002. http://apps.who.int/medicinedocs/en/d/Jh3011e/. Accessed October 18 2015
3. Kshirsagar M, Langade D, Patil S, Patki P. Prescribing patterns among medical practitioners in Pune, India. Bull World Health Organ. 1998;76(3):271–5.
4. World Health Organization. The use of essential drugs: sixth report of the WHO Expert Committee. 1995. http://apps.who.int/iris/handle/10665/37340. Accessed October 18 2015
5. Geest S, Hardon A, Whyte S. Planning for essential drugs: are we missing the cultural dimension. Health Policy Plan. 1991;5(2):182–5.
6. Hogerzeil HV. Promoting rational prescribing: an international perspective. Br J Clin Pharmacol. 1995;39(1):1–6.
7. Sachs L, Tomson G. Medicines and culture–a double perspective on drug utilization in a developing country. Soc Sci Med. 1992;34(3):307–15.
8. Abdo-Rabbo A, Haaijer-Ruskamp F, Basharahil K. Baseline prescribing and health facility indicators in Yemen. J Fac Med Baghdad. 2000;42(4):824–9.
9. Akl OA, El Mahalli AA, Elkahky AA, Salem AM. WHO/INRUD drug use indicators at primary healthcare centers in Alexandria, Egypt. J Taibah Univers Med Sci. 2014;9(1):54–64.
10. World Health Organization. How to investigate drug use in health facilities: selected drug use indicators. 1993. http://apps.who.int/medicinedocs/en/d/Js2289e/. Accessed October 18 2015
11. Desalegn AA. Assessment of drug use pattern using WHO prescribing indicators at Hawassa University teaching and referral hospital, south Ethiopia: a cross-sectional study. BMC Health Serv Res. 2013;13:170.
12. Malangu N. Indicators in a Zaire hospital. INRUD News. 1992;3(1):2.
13. Isah A, Ohaju-Obodo J, Isah E, Ozemoya O. Drug use profile in a Nigerian city hospital. Pharmacoepidemiol Drug Saf. 1997;6(5):319–24.
14. El Mahalli A. WHO/INRUD drug prescribing indicators at primary health care centres in Eastern province, Saudi Arabia. East Mediterr Health J. 2012;18(11):1091–6.
15. Zhang Y, Zhi M. Index system, appraising method for comprehensive appraisal. J North Jiaotong Univer. 1995;19:393–400.
16. Hohl CM, Dankoff J, Colacone A, Afilalo M. Polypharmacy, adverse drug-related events, and potential adverse drug interactions in elderly patients presenting to an emergency department. Ann Emerg Med. 2001;38(6):666–71. doi:10.1067/mem.2001.119456.
17. Atif M, Azeem M, Sarwar MR. Potential problems and recommendations regarding substitution of generic antiepileptic drugs: a systematic review of literature. SpringerPlus. 2016;5:182.
18. World Health Organization. Antimicorbial resistance. 2015. http://www.who.int/mediacentre/factsheets/fs194/en/. Accessed June 19 2016
19. Ahmad F, Danish AS, Rahmani MR. Prescribing practice at private clinics in jalalabad, Afghanistan. INRUD News. 1995;5(2):21
20. Akhtar M, Vohora D, Pillai K, Dubey K, Roy M, Najmi A, et al. Drug prescribing practices in paediatric department of a north indian university teaching hospital. Asian J Pharm Clin Res. 2012;5(1):146–9.
21. Bosu W, Ofori-Adjei D. An audit of prescribing practices in health care facilities of the Wassa West district of Ghana. West Afr J Med. 1999;19(4):298–303.
22. S.O.N. Uzoma AL, Eva Ombaka. Drug Use studies in Church Facilities in Africa. INRUD News. 1995;5(1):20.
23. Vallano A, Montane E, Arnau JM, Vidal X, Pallares C, Coll M, et al. Medical speciality and pattern of medicines prescription. Eur J Clin Pharmacol. 2004; 60(10):725–30. doi:10.1007/s00228-004-0802-8.
24. Fattouh R, Abu HB. Impact of using essential drug list: analysis of drug use indicators in Gaza Strip. East Mediterr Health J. 2010;16(08):886–92.
25. Hamadeh GN, Dickerson LM, Saab BR, Major SC. Common prescriptions in ambulatory care in Lebanon. Ann Pharmacother. 2001;35(5):636–40.
26. Chareonkul C, Khun VL, Boonshuyar C. Rational drug use in Cambodia: study of three pilot health centers in Kampong Thom Province. Southeast Asian J Trop Med Public Health. 2002;33(2):418–24.
27. Stanley Chindove AX. Nelson Martins. Medicines prescribing patterns for the treatment of common diseases at community health centres in 3 districts of Timor-leste. Int J Pharm. 2012;2(3):439–44.
28. Chattopadhyay A, Mondal T, Saha TK, Dey I, Sahu BK, Bhattacharya J. An audit of prescribing practices in CGHS dispensaries of Kolkata, India. IOSR J Dent Med Sci. 2013;8(01):32–7.
29. Hogerzeil H, Ross-Degnan D, Laing R, Ofori-Adjei D, Santoso B, Chowdhury AA, et al. Field tests for rational drug use in twelve developing countries. Lancet. 1993;342(8884):1408–10.
30. Henry CN, Ogaji IJ, Sariem CN. Drug use pattern with standard indicators in Jos University Teaching Hospital Nigeria. West Afr J Pharm. 2013;24(1):88–93.
31. Kafle K. INRUD drug use indicators in Nepal: Practice patterns in health posts in four districts. INRUD News. 1992;3(1):15.
32. Angamo MT, Wabe NT, Raju N. Assessment of patterns of drug use by using World Health Organization's prescribing, patient care and health facility indicators in selected health facilities in Southwest Ethiopia. J App Pharm Sci. 2011;01(07):62–6.
33. Nsimba SED. Assessing prescribing and patient care indicator for children under five years old with malaria and other disease conditions in public primary health care facilities. Southeast Asian J Trop Med Public Health. 2006;37(1):206–14.
34. Gelders S, World Health Organization. Drug use indicator survey, 1991-Malawi Essential Drugs Programme.1992. http://apps.who.int/medicinedocs/en/d/Js21679en/. Accessed October 18 2015
35. El Mahalli A, Akl O, Al-Dawood S, Al-Nehab A, Al-Kubaish H, Al-Saeed S, et al. WHO/INRUD patient care and facility-specific drug use indicators at primary health care centres in Eastern province, Saudi Arabia. East Mediterr Health J. 2012;18(11):1086–90.
36. Bimo D. Report on Nigerian field test. INRUD news. 1992;3:9–10.
37. Massele AY, Nsimba SE, Rimoy G. Prescribing habits in church-owned primary health care facilities in Dar Es Salaam and other Tanzanian coast regions. East Afr Med J. 2001;78(10):510–4.
38. Tomson G. Pilot study of drug use indicators in Sweden. Inrud News. 1992;3(1):3.
39. Awad A, Al-Saffar N. Evaluation of drug use practices at primary healthcare centers of Kuwait. Eur J Clin Pharmacol. 2010;66(12):1247–55.
40. Naseeb TA, Nasser MA. Drug prescribing indicators in primary health care centers in Bahrain. Saudi Med J. 2005;26(9):1436–8.
41. Sharif S, Al-Shaqra M, Hajjar H, Shamout A, Wess L. Patterns of drug prescribing in a hospital in dubai, United arab emirates. Libyan J Med. 2008; 3(1):10–2. doi:10.4176/070928.
42. Lopes A, Teixeira A, Gurgel M, Miranda M, Oliveira M, Oliveira M, et al. Drug use of evaluation in health services in Fortaleza, Brasil. INRUD News. 1996;6:17.
43. Folkedal SF G, Banqueiro EG. Rational Drug Use Field Tests: Experience from Mozambique. INRUD News. 1994;4(2):21.

5

Impact of pharmacists as immunizers on influenza vaccination coverage in the community-setting in Nova Scotia, Canada

Jennifer E. Isenor[1,2,3*], Jessica L. Killen[1], Beverly A. Billard[4], Shelly A. McNeil[2,3], Donna MacDougall[2,5], Beth A. Halperin[2,6], Kathryn L. Slayter[2,7] and Susan K. Bowles[1,2,3,8]

Abstract

Background: Annual immunization is the most effective way to prevent influenza and its associated complications. However, optimal immunization rates are not being met in Nova Scotia, Canada. Additional providers, such as pharmacists, may improve access and convenience to receive vaccines. Pharmacists began immunizing patients 5 years of age and older within the publicly funded universal influenza vaccination program during the 2013-2014 influenza season. The objective of this study was to evaluate influenza immunization coverage rates before and after pharmacists in Nova Scotia gained authority to immunize as part of the publicly funded universal influenza vaccination program.

Methods: Influenza immunization data was obtained from the Department of Health and Wellness from 2010 to 2015. Data included billing data from physicians and pharmacists, and local public health data. Vaccination coverage was calculated as proportion of vaccinations received in comparison to the total population.

Results: Prior to pharmacists immunizing, overall vaccination coverage for Nova Scotia residents 6 months of age and older was 35.8 % in 2012-2013, increasing to 41.8 % coverage in 2013-2014 the year pharmacists began immunizing. A decrease of 1.9 to 39.9 % was observed in 2014-2015. In patients 65 years of age and older living in the community, coverage has increased from 61.8 % in 2012-2013 to 71.6 % in 2013-2014, and again to 73.3 % in 2014-2015 with the addition of pharmacists immunizing. Prior to pharmacists immunizing the highest coverage noted for this portion of the population was 61.8 %.

Conclusions: The addition of pharmacists as immunizers within a publicly funded universal influenza vaccination program was found to increase overall vaccination coverage in the first year and to maintain higher coverage rates in the second year than those observed before pharmacists began immunizing. Increases in coverage in both years were observed in the elderly. Future research will be required to determine the ongoing impact of the addition of pharmacists as immunizers and other strategies to improve vaccination coverage.

Keywords: Pharmacist, Immunization, Influenza vaccination, Pharmaceutical services, Vaccine coverage, Canada

* Correspondence: Jennifer.Isenor@Dal.ca
[1]College of Pharmacy, Dalhousie University, 5968 College Street, PO Box 15000, Halifax, Nova Scotia B3H 4R2, Canada
[2]Canadian Center for Vaccinology, IWK Health Centre and Nova Scotia Health Authority, Dalhousie University, 5850/5980 University Ave, Halifax, Nova Scotia B3K 6R8, Canada
Full list of author information is available at the end of the article

Background

Receiving the seasonal influenza vaccine each year is the most effective way for an individual to protect themselves from influenza [1, 2]. Globally, influenza rates are estimated between 5 to 10 % for adults and 20 to 30 % among children. Worldwide, this translates to an approximate three to five million cases of severe influenza per year, with an estimated 250,000 to 500,000 deaths attributed to influenza [3]. Influenza is of greatest concern to those who are at high risk of complications, such as the elderly, pregnant women, or those with co-morbidities [1, 4].

Annual influenza immunization is the most effective way to reduce the risk of influenza-related complications. As such, several jurisdictions have identified goals for vaccine coverage rates [5–7], for example, the Office of Disease Prevention and Health Promotion in the United States has set annual influenza vaccine targets at 80 % for noninstitutionalized individuals aged 18 to 64 years, and 90 % for anyone aged 18 years and older who is institutionalized and for health care personnel [6]. In Canada, the National Advisory Committee on Immunization (NACI) has set vaccine coverage goals of 80 % for people 65 years of age or older, those younger than 65 years of age with high risk comorbidities, and health care workers; 95 % for residents of long term care; and 100 % coverage for vaccinators [7]. There are many challenges to reaching these goals, including accessibility and convenience of obtaining vaccinations. In Canada, pharmacists are viewed as highly trusted health care providers with the potential to decrease these barriers and improve vaccination coverage [8, 9]. In 2013, legislation was introduced in Nova Scotia (NS), Canada that allowed pharmacists, with appropriate certification, the authority to immunize adults and children 5 years of age and older [8]. Currently, pharmacists are able to administer the influenza vaccine in 9 of 10 provinces in Canada [10]. In 2013-2014, pharmacists in NS were able to provide influenza vaccines as part of the publicly funded universal vaccination program, which had been implemented in 2010 [11]. Although data from the United States, where pharmacists have been providing immunization services since 1995, demonstrate increased uptake of influenza immunization with the addition of pharmacist immunizers, little is known about the impact of pharmacist immunizers in Canada [12–15]. In British Columbia, pharmacy vaccination clinics were introduced and immunization rates in older people increased [13]. Our evaluation of the first year that pharmacists provided immunization services within the publicly funded universal influenza program showed an increase in overall vaccination rates, despite a decrease in vaccinations administered by physicians and public health [12].

This study expands on the previous NS data and compares NS influenza immunization rates prior to the addition of pharmacists as immunizers, with the 2 years following introduction of immunization services by pharmacists within the publicly funded universal influenza vaccination program [12].

Aim of the study

The aim of this study was to compare estimated influenza vaccination coverage in Nova Scotia, Canada in the 3 years prior to the expansion of pharmacist scope of practice to include administration of vaccinations with the 2 years in which pharmacists were permitted to administer influenza vaccines.

Methods

Census data and aggregate immunization data, which included physician and pharmacist billings and local public health data, were obtained from the Nova Scotia Department of Health and Wellness (DHW). Data was provided as number of vaccinations per district in the health authority by each type of care provider—physicians, pharmacists and public health/other (which included occupational health employees and home care nurses), and by year (end-August one year, to end-August the following year). For the purposes of comparison 2010-2011, 2011-2012 and 2012-2013 were defined as the pre-pharmacist involvement influenza seasons; 2013-2014 and 2014-2015 were considered the post-pharmacist involvement seasons. Vaccination coverage by provider was defined as the percentage of Nova Scotia residents vaccinated by each provider type, in relation to the entire population of Nova Scotia. Although pharmacists can only provide immunizations to those 5 years of age and older, data for those 6 months and older was used when comparing coverage between providers due to missing age related data necessary for alternate comparisons.

Data analysis

Estimated vaccination coverage and 95 % confidence intervals for influenza immunization were constructed for each year using the number of influenza immunizations administered as the numerator, and the census data most proximal to the year of interest as the denominator (2010-2011and 2011-2012 used 2006 census data; 2012-2013 and 2013-2014 used 2011 census data and 2014-2015 used 2013 census data). Coverage was calculated using total populations and estimates grouped by age and sex, and compared between vaccination provider groups. Comparisons between the proportions of the immunized populations each year were made using Chi-Square with Bonferronni correction for multiple comparisons. All data analysis was completed using EXCEL XLSTAT version 2015.

Results

In 2013-2014, 430 pharmacists in NS were licensed to immunize, and in 2014-2015, 293 additional pharmacists were licensed to vaccinate, bringing the total to 723.

In 2014-2015, overall vaccination coverage for all Nova Scotia residents 6 months of age or older decreased by 1.9 % (95 % CI, 1.76–2.04) from 41.8 % (95 % CI, 41.68–41.88) in 2013-2014 to 39.9 % (95 % CI, 39.78–39.98) (Fig. 1). The highest vaccination coverage achieved before pharmacists began immunizing was 38 % (95 % CI, 37.93–38.13) in 2010-2011. In 2011-2012 and 2012-2013 vaccination coverage was between 35 % and 36 %. Comparison of immunization rates by gender did not show any differences between years, with a ratio of approximately 55 % of vaccine recipients being female and 45 % being male.

The vaccination coverage provided by pharmacists increased between 2013-2014 and 2014-2015 from 8.4 to 10.2 % (Fig. 2). The vaccination coverage provided by physicians to patients 6 months of age or older decreased from 27.2 % in 2013-2014 to 24.5 % in 2014-2015 (Fig. 2). Likewise, the coverage provided by public health also decreased from 6.2 to 5.2 % between 2013-2014 and 2014-2015 (Fig. 2).

For individuals 65 years of age and older, overall vaccination coverage increased by 9.8 % (95 % CI, 9.5–10.2) to 71.6 % (95 % CI, 71.4–71.8) in the first year that pharmacists began immunizing, and increased by another 1.7 % (95 % CI, 1.4–2.0) in the second year, resulting in overall coverage of 73.3 % (95 % CI, 73.1–73.5) in 2014-2015 (Fig. 3). Physicians remained the primary providers of immunizations in this age group (Fig. 3). Prior to pharmacists immunizing, overall coverage rates in this population were 61.8 % (95 % CI, 61.5–62.0) in 2012-2013. The data were unavailable for years prior to 2012. A decrease in immunization coverage was noted for children 6 to 59 months from 45.4 % coverage in 2013-2014 to 40.6 % in 2014-2015, an age group that pharmacists are not permitted to immunize.

The vaccination coverage provided by pharmacists to the age groups 18–23 years and 24–64 years remained relatively unchanged from the 2013-2014 influenza vaccination season to the 2014-2015 season. There was a decrease in the coverage provided to 5–17 year olds compared to 2013-2014 data (12.5 to 9.9 %), whereas there was an increase in the coverage provided to those 65 years and older (27.4 to 33.1 %).

Discussion

Our data demonstrate that the increase observed in influenza immunization rates immediately following implementation of pharmacist-provided immunization services within the universal influenza program was sustained in the second year of the program. Although a 1.9 % (95 % CI, 1.76–2.04) reduction in overall rates was observed between the first and second year of pharmacists in the immunizer role, immunization rates remained higher than those observed prior to the introduction of pharmacist immunizers in NS. Of note, immunization coverage declined in 2014-2015 in those 6 to 59 months of age, whom pharmacists are not permitted to immunize, and therefore contributed to the overall decline in rates, independent of pharmacists' ability to immunize. Furthermore, immunization rates continued to increase among those 65 years of age and older, an age group that pharmacists are permitted to immunize.

Limitations of this study include potential errors related to secondary use of health claims aggregate data, such as errors in age-related coding, gender coding or

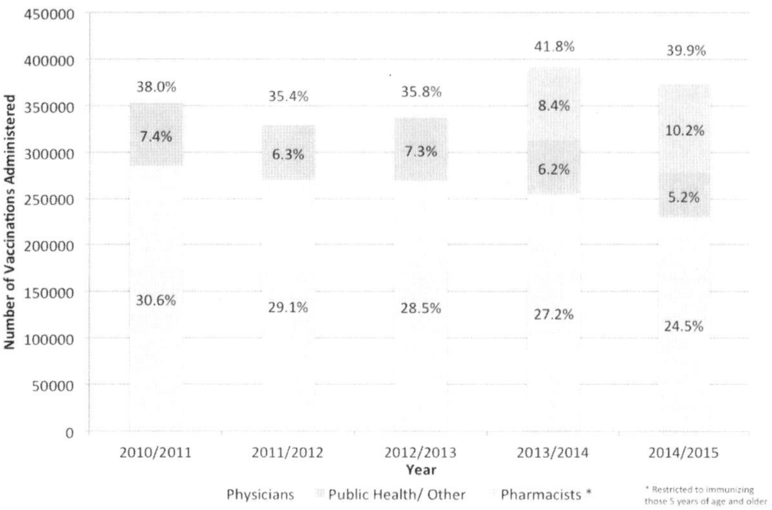

Fig. 1 Number of vaccinations administered and vaccination coverage by year and provider type represented as coverage of total population (%) for Nova Scotia residents 6 months of age or older

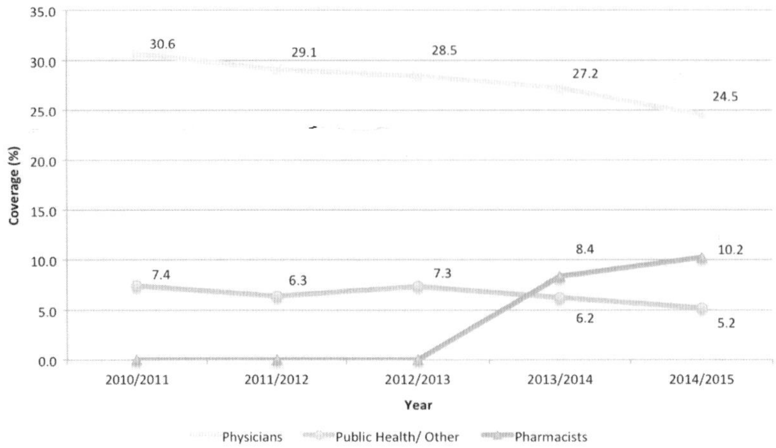

Fig. 2 Trends in influenza vaccination coverage by provider type for patients 6 months of age or older

improper reporting and billing. Missing age related data in 2012-2013 prevented complete comparisons for the age range that pharmacists can provide immunizations (5 years of age and older). In assessing vaccinations for patients less than 9 years of age, it is not possible to assess the proportion of patients who received two doses of influenza vaccine as recommended in the first year vaccinated against influenza, an important consideration given the lack of efficacy of a single dose in this group [11]. However, over-reporting should be consistent in all years evaluated and by all providers. In addition, the number of children between 5 and 9 years of age who were immunized by pharmacists was small; therefore the overall impact on results would be expected to be minimal. Other potential confounders that may have resulted in an increase or decrease in coverage over the years studied include the 2009 H1N1 pandemic and potential residual effects on coverage in 2010-2011, and a perceived vaccine shortage in 2013-2014 related to a distribution delay [16, 17]. Decreased public confidence due to widespread media coverage regarding poor vaccine effectiveness secondary to a mismatch with the predominant circulating

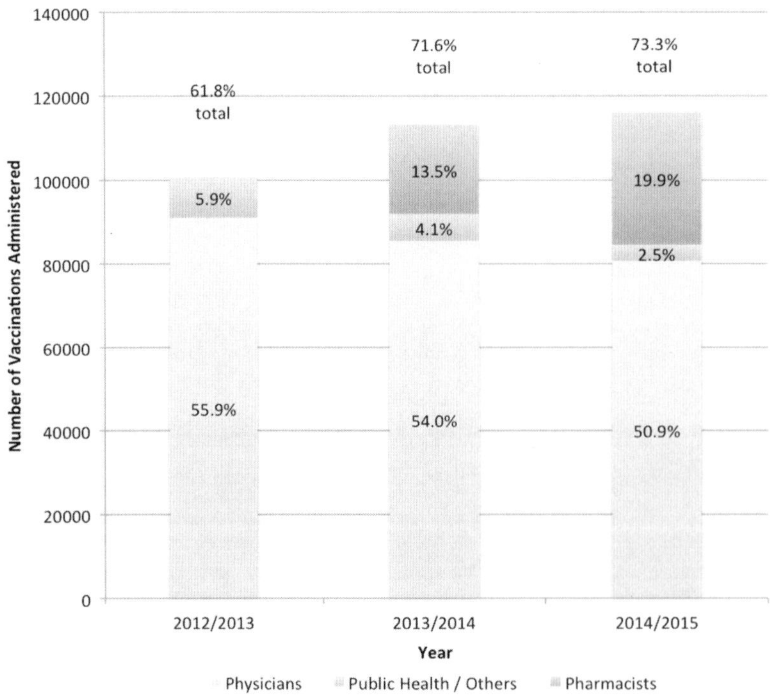

Fig. 3 Vaccination coverage by provider group and total population coverage for Nova Scotia residents 65 years of age and older, excluding those in long term care

strain in 2014-2015 is an additional confounder, which may have resulted in decreased vaccine uptake that year [11].

Higher rates for vaccination coverage noted in 2010-2011 may have been associated with the first year of the universally funded influenza vaccination program, or the residual impact of the pandemic H1N1 seen in 2009-2010 [16]. There is no apparent reason why coverage decreased from 2011 to 2013. The highest vaccine coverage in the years studied was observed in the 2 years that included pharmacist involvement in the program with the first year being the highest, possibly in part due to additional advertisements from pharmacies and increased media attention and news reports on the addition of pharmacists to the influenza vaccination campaign in the province. The slight decrease in vaccination coverage observed in 2014-2015 could be related to the reduced vaccine effectiveness observed in the 2013-2014 season during which the vaccine match to the dominant circulating H3N2 strain was poor [18].

These data lend further support to the benefit of pharmacist involvement in influenza vaccination programs in Canada or countries with similar health systems. Data from 2013-2014, the first year that pharmacists provided immunization services in NS, demonstrated an overall increase in vaccination coverage with the addition of pharmacists as immunizers and not merely a shift, although there is some, of vaccinations from other providers to pharmacists [12]. This is consistent with data from the United States that showed the benefit of pharmacists in increasing overall influenza immunization rates, which showed that those over 18 years of age were more likely to become vaccinated when the vaccine was provided at their community pharmacy [14].

With respect to NS data, a steady decline in the number of vaccinations provided by physicians each year was observed, leading to the question of whether immunization services previously provided by physicians are now being substituted by pharmacists. Arguing against this is that the rate of decline began prior to pharmacists providing influenza vaccination (Fig. 2). The reasons for the decrease in the proportion of vaccinations administered by physicians are likely complex, involving both practitioner and patient factors. Possible explanations include increased responsibility for physicians, leading to time constraints and longer wait times for each patient, and shorter patient-physician interactions resulting in less time to provide immunizations [19, 20]. In NS and other parts of Canada, perceived shortages and concerns around distribution of family physicians may be a barrier to patient access, which could directly lead to fewer vaccinations administered by physicians [21, 22].

Vaccination coverage by public health, while varying from year to year, has remained relatively steady between 5 and 8 % annually. The decrease in vaccinations administered by public health in 2013-2014 and 2014-2015 was expected because fewer public health clinics were offered as a conscious effort to allow public health practitioners to focus on other activities since pharmacists were authorized to also provide influenza vaccination.

By the end of the second year of pharmacist-provided immunization, there was an increase in coverage from 71.6 to 73.3 % in those individuals greater than 65 years of age, approaching the national goal of 80 % coverage for community dwelling seniors [2]. The overall increase in coverage in this population was not observed across all immunization provider groups. While pharmacists and public health saw an increase in the number of elderly being vaccinated, the number of older adults immunized by physicians continued to decline. Between 2013-2014 and 2014-2015, the demographics of the population being vaccinated by pharmacists changed, with an increase in the proportion being administered to the elderly, and a decreasing proportion being administered to all other age groups. This could indicate that people 65 years of age and older are an important demographic for pharmacists to engage or that this age group is most readily accessed by pharmacists. In general, older adults visit their pharmacy more frequently than younger people because they have more chronic conditions, providing more opportunity for pharmacists to make vaccination recommendations to this population [23]. As elderly are also at higher risk of complications, pharmacists may make greater effort to ensure vaccination in this population than in younger people presenting to their pharmacy. It may also relate to the confidence that older individuals have in pharmacists such that they are more willing to be vaccinated by a pharmacist than younger individuals. Our findings are consistent with both US and Canadian data that also observed patients 65 years of age and older were more likely to become immunized with the addition of pharmacists as immunizers [13, 14].

With regards to gender, there have been no significant changes in coverage noted with the addition of pharmacists as immunizers, however each year there is a significant difference between more females than males receiving their influenza vaccination. This could be associated with the fact that women see their physician more regularly than men, or visit their pharmacy more often than men to pick up prescriptions, allowing physicians and pharmacists to make a recommendation for vaccinations [24]. This difference was also observed in 2001 by Grabenstein et al., noting that 60 % of patients receiving immunizations from 21 pharmacies in the US were female [25].

Conclusions

The addition of pharmacists as immunizers has resulted in an increase in influenza vaccine coverage rates in

Nova Scotia, Canada. The impact appears to be greatest among adults who are 65 years of age or older and was sustained over the first 2 years in which pharmacists vaccinated. Future studies should address the impact of the addition of pharmacists over a longer time period and explore the potential for targeted interventions by pharmacists to increase vaccine coverage among other at-risk populations.

Acknowledgements
The authors would like to thank Elaine Holmes and Tania Alia for their initial assistance in study design and ongoing input and Beth O'Reilly for her assistance in manuscript preparation.

Funding
This study was funded by a grant from the Drug Evaluation Alliance of Nova Scotia (DEANS).

Authors' contributions
JI and SB conceived and designed the study, led the data analysis and drafting of the manuscript. JK assisted in data collection, analysis and drafting of the manuscript. BB assisted in study design, data collection, data analysis and drafting of the manuscript. DM, BA, and KS assisted in study design, data analysis and drafting of the manuscript. All authors read and approved the final manuscript.

Competing interests
SM has received research funding from GSK, Pfizer, Novartis, Sanofi Pasteur, and Merck unrelated to the conduct of this study. DM and BH have received research funding from GSK and Sanofi, unrelated to the conduct of this study. JI has received research funding from GSK, unrelated to the conduct of this study.

Author details
[1]College of Pharmacy, Dalhousie University, 5968 College Street, PO Box 15000, Halifax, Nova Scotia B3H 4R2, Canada. [2]Canadian Center for Vaccinology, IWK Health Centre and Nova Scotia Health Authority, Dalhousie University, 5850/5980 University Ave, Halifax, Nova Scotia B3K 6R8, Canada. [3]Faculty of Medicine, Dalhousie University, 1459 Oxford St, Halifax, Nova Scotia B3H 4R2, Canada. [4]Nova Scotia Department of Health and Wellness, PO Box 488, Halifax, Nova Scotia B3J 2R8, Canada. [5]School of Nursing, St. Francis Xavier University, PO Box 5000, Antigonish, Nova Scotia B2G 2W5, Canada. [6]School of Nursing, Dalhousie University, 5869 University Avenue, PO Box 15000, Halifax, Nova Scotia B3H 4R2, Canada. [7]IWK Health Centre, 5850/5980 University Avenue, Halifax, Nova Scotia B3K 6R8, Canada. [8]Department of Pharmacy, 1796 Summer St, Nova Scotia Health Authority- Central Zone, Halifax, Nova Scotia B3H 3A6, Canada.

References

1. National Advisory Committee on Immunization (NACI). Statement on seasonal influenza vaccine for 2014-2015. http://www.phac-aspc.gc.ca/naci-ccni/flu-grippe-eng.php (2014). Accessed 05 Aug 2015.
2. Public Health Agency of Canada. Vaccine coverage amongst adult Canadians: Results from the 2012 adult National Immunization Coverage (aNIC) survey. http://www.phac-aspc.gc.ca/im/nics-enva/vcac-cvac-eng.php. (2014). Accessed 06 Jun 2015.
3. World Health Organization. Influenza (seasonal) fact sheet #211. http://www.who.int/mediacentre/factsheets/fs211/en/ (2014). Accessed 21 Feb 2016.
4. Bowles S, Strang R. Infectious diseases: influenza. In: Jovaisas B, editor. Compendium of therapeutic choices. Ottawa: Academic; 2014. p. 1403–13.
5. NHS England Department of Health. The national flu immunisation programme 2015/16. https://www.gov.uk/government/uploads/system/uploads/attachment_data/file/418428/Annual_flu_letter_24_03_15__FINALv3_para9.pdf (2015). Accessed 16 May 2016.
6. Office of Disease Prevention and Health Promotion. Immunization and infectious diseases. https://www.healthypeople.gov/2020/topics-objectives/topic/immunization-and-infectious-diseases/objectives (2016). Accessed 16 May 2016.
7. Public Health Agency of Canada. Final report of outcomes from the national consensus conference for vaccine-preventable diseases in Canada. CCDR. 2007;33S3:1–56.
8. Canadian Pharmacists Association. Environmental scan: pharmacy practice legislation and policy changes across Canada. blueprintforpharmacy.ca/docs/kt- tools/environmental-scan—pharmacy-practice-legislation-and-policy-changes-may-2014.pdf (2014). Access 06 Jun 2015.
9. Kimmel SR, Burns IT, Wolfe RM, Zimmerman RK. Addressing immunization barriers, benefits, and risks. J Fam Pract. 2007;56(2 Suppl Vaccines):S61–9.
10. Canadian Pharmacists Association. Pharmacists' expanded scope of practice. http://www.pharmacists.ca/pharmacy-in-canada/scope-of-practice-canada/ (2016). Accessed 21 Feb 2016.
11. Public Health Agency of Canada. Statement on seasonal influenza vaccine for 2015-2016. http://www.phac-aspc.gc.ca/naci-ccni/flu-2015-grippe-eng.php (2016). Accessed 12 May 2016.
12. Isenor JE, Alia TA, Killen JL, Billard BA, Halperin BA, Slayter KL, McNeil SA, MacDougall D, Bowles SK. Impact of pharmacists as immunizers on influenza vaccination coverage in Nova Scotia, Canada. Hum Vaccin Immunother. 2016;12(5):1225–8.
13. Marra F, Kaczorowski J, Gastonguay L, Lynd LD, Kendall P. Pharmacy-based immunization in rural communities strategy (PhICS): A community cluster-randomized trial. Can Pharm J. 2014;147(1):33–44.
14. Steyer TE, Ragucci KR, Pearson WS, Mainous AG. The role of pharmacists in the delivery of influenza vaccinations. Vaccine. 2004;22(8):1001–6.
15. Grabenstein JD, Guess HA, Hartzema AG, Konrad TR. Effect of vaccination by community pharmacists among adult prescription recipients. Med Care. 2001;39(4):340.
16. Centers for Disease Control and Prevention.The 2009 H1N1 pandemic: summary highlights. http://www.cdc.gov/h1n1flu/cdcresponse.htm (2010). Accessed 16 Jan 2016.
17. CBC News. Flu shots across Nova Scotia in high demand. http://www.cbc.ca/news/canada/nova-scotia/flu-shots-across-nova-scotia-in-high-demand-1.2490598 (2014). Accessed 16 Jan 2016.
18. Centers for Disease Control and Prevention. Morbidity and mortality weekly report (MMWR): Influenza activity- United States, 2014-15 season and composition of the 2015-16 influenza vaccine. http://www.cdc.gov/mmwr/preview/mmwrhtml/mm6421a5.htm (2015). Accessed 10 Jan 2016.
19. Braddock 3rd CH, Snyder L. The doctor will see you shortly. The ethical significance of time for the patient-physician relationship. J Gen Intern Med. 2005;20(11):1057–62.
20. Dugdale DC, Epstein R, Pantilat SZ. Time and patient-physician relationship. J Gen Intern Med. 1999;14(1):34.
21. CBC News. Nova Scotia doctor shortage needs action, ex-medical dean says. http://www.cbc.ca/news/canada/nova-scotia/nova-scotia-doctor-shortage-needs-action-ex-medical-dean-says-1.3137431 (2015). Accessed 16 Jan 2016.
22. DesRoches J. Myth: Canada needs more doctors. http://www.cfhi-fcass.ca/SearchResultsNews/12-05-29/80fe1ee3-444d-4114-b9ee-d9da20439293.aspx (2012). Accessed 26 May 2016.
23. Canadian Association of Chain Drug Stores. 9000 points of care: improving access to affordable health care. http://9000pointsofcare.ca (2014). Accessed 26 Aug 2015.
24. Centers for Disease Control and Prevention. New study profiles women's use of health care. http://www.cdc.gov/nchs/pressroom/01news/newstudy.htm (2010). Accessed 06 Jan 2016.
25. Grabenstein JD, Guess HA, Hartzema AG. People vaccinated by pharmacists: Descriptive epidemiology. J Am Pharm Assoc. 2001;41(1):46.

6

Interaction and medical inducement between pharmaceutical representatives and physicians

Shahrzad Salmasi[1], Long Chiau Ming[2] and Tahir Mehmood Khan[3,4*]

Abstract

Background: It has been proven that the interaction between pharmaceutical representatives and physicians can directly influence the latter's prescribing behaviour. This meta-synthesis aims to explore the available studies regarding the nature of the interaction that takes place between pharmaceutical representatives and physicians. It highlights the different aspects of that interaction by investigating the reasons why these meetings happen in the first place, their benefits and drawbacks and their impact on patients' health and, ultimately, the health of the public.

Methods: A search for published articles was conducted in April 2015. Three databases (PubMed, Ovid Medline, and ProQuest) were searched for articles published between January 2000 and April 2015. Authors worked autonomously and in pairs to select eligible articles. In this case, the meta-synthesis approach was used to develop a fuller understanding and to facilitate new knowledge by bringing together qualitative findings on physician-PR interaction. 'Meta-synthesis' is the process of amalgamation of a group of similar studies with the aim of developing an explanation for their findings (Walsh and Downe, J Advanc Nurs 50: 204–211, 2005). A thematic content analysis was conducted on the 15 included full text articles (qualitative and quantitative studies) whereby the original authors' understanding of key concepts in each study was identified and listed in a summary form in the data extraction sheet under "key findings" column. These findings were then juxtaposed to identify homogeneity and dissonance (Walsh and Downe, J Advanc Nurs 50: 204–211, 2005). Homogenous findings were then coded together on a different data extraction table to form a theme.

Results: A total of 15 articles met the inclusion criteria and were included in this meta-synthesis;six from the United States, two from Libya, and one each from Turkey, Peru, India, Germany, the United Kingdom, Yemen, and Japan. Six main themes were derived from the included articles: 1-the frequency of pharmaceutical representatives' visits, 2-the perceived ethical acceptability of the interactions between pharmaceutical representatives and physicians, 3-the attitudes held by physicians towards visits by pharmaceutical representatives, 4-their perception of the effect of such visits on prescription patterns, 5-reasons to accept or reject pharmaceutical representatives, and lastly, 6-guidelines.

Conclusions: The physicians referred to pharmaceutical representatives as efficient and convenient information resources and were willing to meet them and accept their gifts. It was also evident that most physicians believed that their prescribing would not be influenced by pharmaceutical representatives.

Keywords: Inducement, Motivation, Health care quality, Pharmaceutical marketing, Prescription behavior, Marketing ethics, Pharmaceutical representatives

* Correspondence: tahir.mehmood@monash.edu
[3]School of Pharmacy, Monash University, Sunway City, Selangor, Malaysia
[4]Department of Pharmacy, Abasyn University, Peshawar, Pakistan
Full list of author information is available at the end of the article

Background

The pharmaceutical industry significantly influences the economy and healthcare system of a country. According to The World Health Organization(WHO), by 2017,the global pharmaceuticals market will be worth approximately US$400billion with one third of thesales revenue of pharmaceutical companies spent on marketing their products [1]. Physicians are the prime target of pharmaceutical marketing teams, in which pharmaceutical representatives (PRs) play a crucial role [1]. The job of the PRs is to visit physicians to promote their company's products [2, 3]. In addition, free physician samples, gifts, company supported conferences, workshops and events are also brought to the notice of physicians through PRs. Among all the promotional expenses, detailing is the largest category; estimated US$20.4 billion has been used for this purpose in United States (US) in 2015 [4, 5].

Given the above, PR-physician interactions have the potential to result in a conflict of interest whereby physicians might fail to abide by their moral, legal and professional obligations for personal gain [6, 7]. Research has shown that the interaction between PRs and the physicians can directly influence the latter's prescribing behaviour; it has been observed that the rate of prescriptions increases after physicians see a PR or accept free samples [8]. This has led to increasing concern over irrational and inappropriate prescribing practices [9] which could jeopardize patient care, harm the patients, promote the misuse of drugs, increase costs to the healthcare system, distort public opinion of the healthcare industry and erode the trust of the patients in the integrity of medical decision making [8, 10].

Wazana et al., published a review in 2000 that identified the extent of and attitudes toward the interplay of relationship and its impact between physicians towards the PR [11]. Wazana's review received a mixed response from the health care communities because he proposed that the extent of physician-PR interactions could potentially affect prescribing and professional behaviour [12–18]. Ten years later, Spurling et al. who performed a systematic review on 58 articles, reported that exposure to information from pharmaceutical companies was associated with either lower prescribing quality or increase in prescribing frequency or no association was detected. Finally, with only one exception among the 58 studies included in the review by Spurling et al.; exposure to information from PRs was associated with an increase in prescribing costs or no association was detected. They reported that interaction of physicians with PRs does not negatively affect prescribing [3]. This is the first meta-synthesis that fills the literature gap on the interaction between PRs and physician. The purpose of this meta-synthesis, therefore, is to explore the available studies regarding PR-physician interactions especially to highlight the detailing aspects of such interactions from the physician's point of view.

Methods

A systematic literature search of computerized databases was conducted in April 2015 using PubMed, Ovid Medline and ProQuest. A meta-synthesis approach was used to integrate results from various studies in order to give a comprehensive overview of the interaction that takes place between pharmaceutical representatives and physicians [19]. Research papers published between January 2000 and April 2015 which presented evidence concerning such interactions, were included. The search strings used can be found in Supporting Information Additional file 1: Table S1.

The search strings used were very specific. This is because we were not interested in marketing methods other than detailing. Our purpose was to focus on the interaction that takes place between PRs (and not any other promoter/ representatives from other industries who might meet with physicians) and physicians (and not any other prescriber such as prescribing nurses, dentists, etc.). Hence the search strings were chosen carefully to retrieve the most relevant studies. To ensure all relevant papers were included, we searched the references of the studies that were included. Furthermore, Monash integrated search panel for Science Citation Index were also used to screen the relevant citations of the included studies.

A total of 218 papers were identified using the search strings outlined in Additional file 1: Table S1. Duplicates and articles published before the year 2000 were excluded. The title and abstract of the 72 remaining papers were assessed for eligibility against the inclusion criteria. This was performed independently by two reviewers, who classified the papers into three groups of "to include", "to exclude" and "unclear". Both reviewers (SS and TMK) met to compare their independent reviews. A paper would be included or excluded once agreed by both reviewers. In the case of disagreement, or when either reviewer was unsure, the opinion of a third person (LCM) was sought.

The inclusion criteria were articles focusing on detailing and physician interaction with PRs. Studies related to marketing methods other than detailing, such as direct to consumer advertising and ghost writing were excluded. Papers written in languages other than English were excluded as we did not have the necessary skills to interpret them. We also excluded studies focused on prescribers other than physicians, such as prescribing nurses. Opinion papers and interventional studies were also excluded.

The full text of 25 papers was read by the first author. A number of studies were identified at this stage as not being written in English (i.e. their title and abstract were written in English but the full-text was not) and these were therefore excluded, along with a number of others that were found to be irrelevant. This left 15 papers. Details about the number of the included and excluded articles are shown in Fig. 1. The Preferred Reporting Items for Systematic Reviews and Meta-Analyses (PRISMA) checklist is presented in Additional file 2: Table S2.

Analysis and theme synthesis

'Qualitative meta-synthesis' is the process of amalgamation of a group of similar qualitative studies with the aim of developing an explanation for their findings [20]. In this case, the meta-synthesis approach was used to develop a fuller understanding and to facilitate new knowledge by bringing together qualitative findings on physician-PR interaction. The 15 included papers were subjected to data extraction using a pre-designed data-extraction Excel worksheet on Microsoft Office® 2014. A thematic content analysis was conducted on the15 included full text articles whereby the original authors' understanding of key concepts in each study was identified and listed in a summary form in the data extraction sheet under "key findings" column. These findings were then juxtaposed to identify homogeneity and dissonance [20]. Homogenous findings were then coded together on a different data extraction table to form a theme. Six broad themes were formulated for the results section; 1-The frequency of pharmaceutical representatives' visits, 2-The perceived ethical acceptability of the PR-physician interactions, 3-Physicians' attitudes towards PR visits, 4-Physicians'perceptions of the effect of PR visits on prescription patterns, 5-Reasons to accept/reject PRs and 6-Guidelines. Findings were scrutinized under each theme to see if further sub-categories were warranted. The arguments for and against PR interaction with physicians were very rich. We were hence unable to take account of all the arguments, in great detail. Moreover, while all the included studies presented information about PR-physician interactions, they reported different aspects of such interactions since they examined the interaction from different angles, hence a thematic analysis was chosen to classify and summarize the findings in a systematic, easy to understand manner. Through the six themes formulated, we hope to provide an overview of the main aspects of the PR-physician interactions identified.

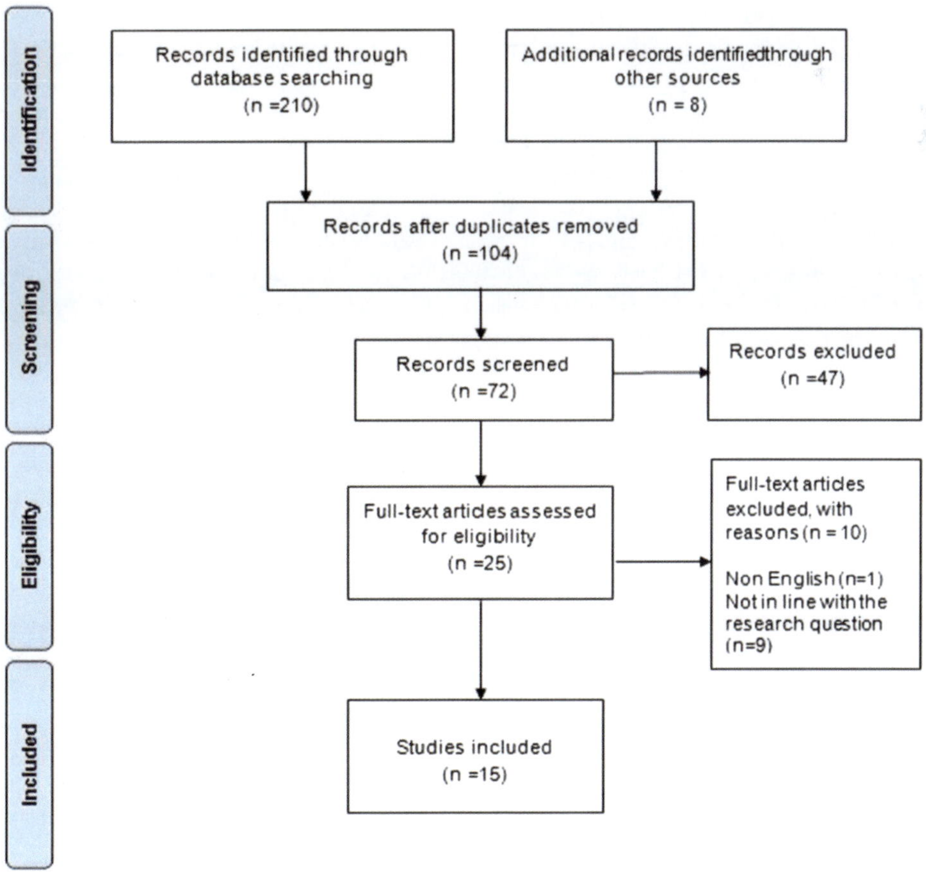

Fig. 1 PRISMA diagram demonstrating the search strategy and its results

Results

A total of 15 publications were included in the study covering studies undertaken in a range of countries; six from the US, two from Libya, one each from Turkey, Peru, India, Germany, the United Kingdom (UK), Yemen and Japan. Eight of these articles focused on physicians' attitudes and views regarding physician-PR interactions [9, 21–27]; four focused on the nature of the interaction [26, 28–30]; two concentrated on the frequency of these interactions [31, 32]; and two focused on the reasons behind such interactions [33, 34]. The detailed themes and extracted text is presented in Additional file 3. Study and participants' characteristics can be found in Table 1.

Theme 1.0: The Frequency of PRs visits

The first step in investigating and understanding the interaction between the PRs and the prescribers is to determine how frequent such interactions are, and if they are significant enough.

Research has shown that frequency of PR visits to physicians- skilled health-care professionals trained and licensed to practice medicine- is considered to be a good indicator of an active relationship between physicians and the pharmaceutical industry. Lieb et al. reported that 77.0% (n = 160) of German respondents met with PRs at least once a week, and 19.0% (n = 39) were visited by PRs on a daily basis [29]. Other studies also reported that PRs visit physicians regularly in order to promote their products [9, 21, 22, 26, 29, 32]. De Ferrari et al. studied the relationship between the specialty of the prescriber and the frequency of PR visits [9]. Physicians involved in teaching and those practicing paediatric medicine, were reported to receive more frequent visits, while anaesthetists were found to be least frequently visited by PRs [9]. Two studies reported that PRs visited physicians working in a private setting more frequently, while physicians working in community and university hospitals experienced less frequent visits [22, 23].

Theme 2.0: Perceived ethical acceptability of the PR-physician interactions

The job of PRs is to introduce and market their company's products. PRs ensure that physicians are informed of the benefits of the products and are therefore willing to prescribe them to their patients. The interaction between PRs and physicians entails a number of marketing methods such as gifts, sponsorships, free drug samples and free lunches. Moreover, in recent years, simple brand reminders such as stationery with the company's logo and product name on them have increasingly been replaced by gifts of greater value, ranging from jewellery to iPads [30]. According to policymakers, such gifts have the potential to act as an ethical inducement and negatively impact prescribing behaviour and, ultimately, patient health [11, 30]. Brett et al., for example, conducted a survey in South Carolina where physicians were asked to rate 18 scenarios of interactions between physicians and PRs from the most ethically appropriate (score = 0) to the least ethically appropriate (score = 5). Results showed that physicians made distinctions about the ethical appropriateness of gifts of different value and different type; recreational gifts were rated to be significantly less ethically appropriate than educational gifts, as were the more expensive gifts [23]. According to De Ferrari et al., activities perceived to be most ethical were the provision of medical samples (81.8%) and continuing medical education (68.9%) [9, 25]. Roy et al. further added that, in India, some physicians justify gifts as compensation for the time spent listening to the PR, time which could have been spent on a patient [30].

> *"PRs never try to bribe to sell their drug. (Gifts) are just a gesture to say thanks for the time the doctor gives. Let's say a doctor sees three patients in 15 minutes, the PR us costing him those three patients in his 15-minute talk. So the PR tries to compensate with gifts since obviously he can't compensate in cash"* [30].

In contrast, there were others who felt that air conditioners, washing machines, microwaves, cameras, televisions and expensive crystals were acceptable gifts [30].

Theme 3.0: Physicians' attitudes towards PR visits

The physician's attitude is what determines whether they would be inclined to believe the information provided by the PR. Qualitative data demonstrating the attitude of physicians are presented in Additional file 4: Table S3.

3.1 Perceived legitimacy of the PR

Legitimacy refers to the accuracy and accountability of the PRs as a source of information. According to Prosser et al., a relationship has been observed between the frequency of visits and the perceived legitimacy of the information provided: the more frequently visited physicians were more likely to consider the information provided to be of "high quality" [33].

Physicians have been reported, in a number of studies, to consider the information provided by the PRs as *"not trustworthy"*, *"very variable"* and *"depending on which PR you see"*; they also disclosed that the PRs usually choose the promotion of their company's product over the actual benefits for the patient by hardly ever mentioning the drug interactions and the side-effects [9, 21, 29, 30, 33].

On the other hand, some physicians from a number of different studies recognized the professional authority of

Table 1 Characteristics of the included studies

Study	Participant's Specialty (N)	Gender M/F	Years of Practice (N)	Practice Setting	Country
Morgan et al. 2006 [25]	Gynecologists (397)	125/92	NA	Obstetrics-gynaecology partnership or group (44.2%) Solo practice (27%) Multispecialty group (14.9%) University full-time faculty and practice (10.7%) Health maintenance organisation (3.3%)	US
Anderson et al. 2009 [28]	Gynecologists (251)	143/108	Mean (SD): 22 (11)	Private practice (178) Community hospital (25) University hospital (30) Other (16)	US
Wang et al. 2009 [27]	Ophthalmology trainees (122): 1st year residents (32) 2nd year residents (44) 3rd year residents (28) Fellows (17) Unknown (1)	NA	NA	NA	US
Misra et al. 2010 [24]	Psychiatry trainees (17): Residents (12) Fellow trainee (5) Psychiatry faculty (58): Assistant professor (21) Associate professor (6) Professors (13)	NA	NA	Academic medical centre	US
Fischer et al. 2009 [34]	Internal medicine (29) Family medicine (17) Pediatric medicine (2) Geriatric medicine (3)	23/38	15	Academic affiliation (21) Community-based practice (24) Academic affiliation & community-based practice (8) Other (8)	US
Brett et al. 2003 [23]	Residents (39) Faculty physicians (37)	49/27	NA	Medical school	US
Sarikaya et al. 2009 [32]	Medical students 2nd year students (280) 3rd year medical students (308)	168/140	NA	Marmara University School of Medicine (MUSM) Ege University School of Medicine (EUSM)	Turkey
Saito et al. 2010 [26]	Internal medicine (214) General surgery (181) Orthopedic surgery (177) Pediatrics (221) Obstetrics (210) Psychiatry (197) Ophthalmology (209)	1084/326	<10 (339) 11–20 (488) 21–30 (428) >31 (155)	Office (822) Hospital (588)	Japan
Roy et al. 2003	Senior executives in drug companies (15) PRs (36) Physicians (25) Chemists (25)				India
Alssageer et al. 2013 [31]	General Practitioner (GP) (274) Surgeon (99) Resident MO (41) Anesthesiologist (61) Specialist (91) Others (42)	371/237	1-3 (288) 4–6 (82) 7–9 (45) >10 (193)	Public (512) Private (34) Both (62)	Libya
Alssageer et al. 2012 [22]	GP (274) Surgeon (99) Resident MO (41) Anesthesiologist (61) Specialist (91) Others (42)	371/237	1-3 (288) 4–6 (82) 7–9 (45) >10 (193)	Public (512) Private (34) Both (62)	Libya

Table 1 Characteristics of the included studies *(Continued)*

Prosser et al. 2003 [33]	GP (107)	76/31	<10 (6) 11–20 (55) >20 (46)	Health authorities in the North West of England (107)	UK
Al-Areef et al. 2013 [21]	Physicians (32) (interns, GPs/medical officers, residents and specialists)	4/28	NA	NA	Yemen
Lieb et al. 2010 [29]	Neurologists/psychiatrists (83) Primary care physicians (76) cardiologist (49)	104/98 Unknown gender (6)	NA	NA	Germany
De Ferrari et al. 2014 [9]	Internal medicine (59) General surgery (32) Pediatrics (28) Anesthesiologist (13) Obstetrics (16)	96/52	NA	Peruvian public general hospital.	Peru

Abbreviations: *GP* General Practitioner, *NA* not applicable/available, *UK* United Kingdom, *US* United States of America, *MO* Medical Officer, *SD* Standard deviation

PRs as information providers and expressed satisfaction with the information provided. Just under half of all the participants (47.6%) in a study in Peru, for example, stated that the information provided by PRs helps them "learn about new products" and "stay up-to-date". Similarly, Roy et al. reports that physicians were satisfied with the information provided despite the fact that side-effects were hardly ever mentioned [30]. De Ferrari et al. also reported that 24% of faculty (n = 10) and 18% of psychiatry residents (n = 3) believed that PRs provide useful and accurate information on new drugs [9].

Overall, while opinions on this matter differ among physicians, it can be concluded that physicians consider the information provided by PRs, factual but, to an extent, biased.

3.2 Perceived benefits of the interaction with PRs

The perceived benefits of the interaction are the reason why physicians continue to see PRs, despite knowing that the information provided by them may, in some cases, be biased. These perceived benefits are explained below.

3.2.1 Easy access to information Research indicates that physicians considered the convenience of acquiring information from PRs, regarding both old and new drugs, to be the main benefit of meeting with them, This is true regardless of the country the physicians practiced in [21, 23, 24, 26, 29, 33, 34].

Physicians also reported that PRs are useful for obtaining research papers and journal off-prints. Physicians' busy schedules leave them no time to look for evidence. Thus, representatives are seen as 'short-cuts' and "valuable sources of information", simplifying the acquisition and evaluation of new product information [33].

"I'm sure you could manage if you didn't see another drug rep and I'm sure you could get the information if you wanted to, it's just that it's not that accessible, and it's also whether you would have the time to actually sit and read it" [33].

"Although you try and keep up with journals and such like that, some things go by, you do miss things. So I feel like I'm keeping up to date a little bit. If I didn't see reps I feel that I would be slightly disadvantaged in terms of my awareness of medications coming through" [33].
"[It is positive] that they can inform us about new products [...] being launched in the market for the first time. Secondly, we can [hear about] alternatives from other companies that have the same effectiveness, low cost and less side effects" [21].

The user-friendly and face-to-face nature of the interactions permits physicians to ask questions, and get instant answers;

" I think the answer is it's user friendly, it's very user friendly and its easy listening, you know, with your coffee listening to what they've got to say" [33].

Furthermore, according to Prosser et al. [33], several physicians have commented that they remember the information better when communicated verbally;

" I can remember the information better after having talked to them" [33].
"Seeing a representative face to face tends to make a more lasting impression than reading" [33].

3.2.2 Free gifts and drug samples The other perceived benefit of meeting PRs is the gifts and free samples provided by them. Such gifts can range from materials that are supposed to directly help the patients (blood sugar diaries, educational materials) to personalized gifts for the doctor; from cheap stationery to expensive so-called gifts that act as inducements [21, 34]. According to

Alssageer et al.(n = 423) 86% of respondents reported to have received printed material (n = 480; 79%), simple gifts (stationery, n = 442; 73%) or drug samples (n = 418; 69%) at least once during the last twelve months [31].

> *"Sometimes we need representatives in providing some medicines that we need it, some books or bulletin. Really, they help us in getting books, CDs and lectures from abroad that provided by some companies. They support us on this side a lot"* [21].

Free medication samples are the most frequently accepted gifts in the US and Germany. Physicians consider these gifts to be the most ethically acceptable and a great advantage of meeting with PRs [9, 29, 34].

Physicians and PRs justify such gifts on the grounds that free medications can be used to help patients who are unable to afford medications due to financial constraints. Free samples can also be used to determine the dose and side-effects before the patient has to invest in them [34, 36].

> *"We want to make people happy and you make people happy often when you give them a sample"* [34].

Morgan et al. reported that the main reason for which the free drug samples are distributed is patients' financial needs, followed by patients' convenience and to build a good relationship with the patient, but less than two-thirds of physicians distributed free samples with a good basis of knowledge as to the efficacy of the sample product [25].

3.2.3 Social aspects of the interaction Some physicians liked the casual, friendly aspect of the interaction and thought of the representatives as more of their friend than a promoter;

> *"Going out to dinner as a group....That's why we do it, more of a social setting outside of the wards"* [34].

3.3 Perceived drawbacks of the interaction with PRs

Despite the above-mentioned positive attitudes towards PRs, the prescribers do admit that there are certain drawbacks to seeing PRs. These drawbacks, in their opinion, are:

3.3.1 Negative impact on the patient Some physicians believe that PRs take up a proportion of the doctor's time, which could have been spent attending to patients [29, 30].

> *"Doctors always perceive MRs' visits as an intrusion. Every minute taken up by the MR is time which could have been spent seeing patients and making money in the clinic. Often, MRs queue up early in the morning for doctors who allow only the first three MRs to see them"* [30].

Al-Areefi et al. reported that some physicians hate the fact that PRs interrupt their patient care process, especially those working in the emergency departments with a high workload and a large number of patients to attend to. These physicians have absolutely no time to listen to PRs and even refer to them as "time wasters" [21].

Some other physicians reported discomfort with or dislike of the interactions, and this appeared to be rooted in their perception that PRs harm the ethical reputation of the profession and adversely affect patients [21, 34].

> *"My rule is I [listen but] don't believe anything they're saying"* [34].

3.3.2 Pressure from PRs Studies suggest that drugs often complain about the "pushy" behaviour of PRs that puts them under pressure to prescribe a certain product from a certain company. They have been reported to have experienced aggressive sale techniques, which they defined as: asking physicians to justify their current prescribing and even direct requests using emotional appeals to the physicians to prescribe a certain medicine as a favour to the PR. Such aggressive marketing methods are criticized by physicians [29, 30, 33].

> *"Such approaches could discourage prescribing a representative's product or seeing a particular representative again. What we don't like is a drug rep coming in and questioning us, because I don't think that's their role or asking us what we do prescribe, and then why. We don't like that. Some of them can be quite pushy"* [33].

> *"In some cases, the representative imposes on the physician to prescribe a certain product. We can prescribe it in rare cases for some diseases. Some representatives say: I have certain amount of medicine in your pharmacy and it's not dispensing, prescribe, just one or two'. This forced us to refuse to meet him again, because he imposes [on] me to prescribe his product for any patient without any reason"* [21].

Studies also indicate that physicians feel obliged to the PR because of previous service they may have provided. Although this is not a direct pressure from the PR, it can still pressure the prescribers indirectly and affect their prescription patterns, which they dislike [21].

Both direct and indirect pressure from PRs are disliked by physicians and can result in the physician deciding to stop seeing that particular PR [29, 30, 33].

Theme 4.0: Physicians' perceptions of the effect of PR visits on prescription patterns

Physicians' perception as to whether or not their prescribing is influenced by PRs is very important since it can determine their attitudes towards PRs [37].

Wang et al. reported that 36% (n = 32) of ophthalmology trainees reported having changed prescribing behaviour based on the information provided by a PRs, 77% (n = 94) stated that they changed prescribing behaviour based on the availability of medicine samples [27].

Research shows, however, that the majority of physicians are convinced that PR visits do not influence their prescribing behaviour [24, 26, 27, 29, 31, 32, 34, 36]. De Ferrari et al. reported that about 88% of study respondents disclosed that they believe receiving gifts or going for company sponsored lunches does not affect their prescribing [9]. All 15 included studies illustrated one common point: that physicians almost always believe that such interactions can influence their colleagues' prescription patterns but not theirs; Roy et al. has for example, revealed that most physicians usually do not admit having accepted gifts from PRs and even if they do, they usually believe it does not affect their prescribing. Almost all of them, however, claim to know colleagues who accept gifts and whose prescribing behaviour is influenced by this [30, 38].

> *"I think drug reps are a good thing...Just because I have a pen with the name of a drug on it, doesn't mean I'm going to prescribe it"* [33].

The other reason stated by the physicians for their perceived immunity against biased information is the friendship between them and the PR over the years:

> *"I think if you see a rep who you know well ... it's the same rep who you've seen for several years, they don't try and pull the wool over your eyes. They know that if they tell you lies you'll be seeing them again in six months and you'll find them out"* [33].

On the contrary, some other physicians found this very same social bond to be the main reason their prescribing behaviour being affected; they felt they were sometimes influenced to prescribe a particular medicine due to their long term and continuous relationship with the representative [33].

Theme 5.0: Reasons to accept/reject PRs

Understanding the reasons behind physicians accepting PRs would be a breakthrough in understanding the overall nature of the interaction between PRs and prescribers [35].

5.1 Reasons for accepting PRs

5.1.1 Sponsorship, gifts One incentive behind meeting PRs is the sponsorship, gifts and products provided by them.

> *"We were building a new surgery and, you know, we needed some sponsorship"* [33].
> *"I don't mind a nice hotel for a weekend. You don't get many perks unfortunately as a GP, and I don't see a problem in that"* [33].
> *"I work in non-profit...you know [reps] do provide me with pens...[and] somehow my administrator doesn't want to spend too much money on office supplies"* [34].

5.1.2 Social aspect of the interaction Friendship and the social bonds made between physicians and PRs over the years has been proven to have a direct effect on the physicians' decisions on whether or not to accept a PR. Some physicians considered these meetings as a chance for social interaction and as a break from their busy work routine [21, 33].

The social aspect of the interaction is even strong enough that the physicians who have stopped seeing PRs still make exceptions for the ones who are their friends:

> *"Some reps I've known for donkey's years and they know all about my life and I know all about their life and you have a chat about things which are totally unrelated to why they came, but it does make life more interesting and you're probably more likely to actually retain what they came in to tell you if you've had a pleasant time talking to them about your kids or something"* [33].

Participants reported that they sometimes accepted the PRs not because they want to hear about new drugs but just to enjoy the social aspect of the visits.

> *"Sometimes we don't even talk about drugs, we just chat about the kids and it's good to have a relaxed and friendly lunch"* [34].

5.1.3 Courtesy and tradition Another reason for physicians to agree to meet PRs is the matter of courtesy, where physicians accept to meet a PR just so that they are not rude; some of the sample comments are as follows:

> *"I think they have a very difficult job. There will be an element of empathy for somebody who comes and says can I talk to you about something. Out of politeness, really"* [33].

"I know it's just the guy's job, and if I don't talk to him then he may lose it, so I talk to him" [33].
"The other side is to facilitate services for colleagues as they do this task [to support] their families. This refers to a social and economic situation for colleagues because he gets a payoff to spend on his family" [21].

Some physicians accepted representatives simply because it was tradition or, in other words, part of the job of a physician. Some reported 'inheriting' such visits from their previous colleagues, the practice then becoming part of their routine [23].

5.2 Reasons for avoiding/rejecting PRs

Not all physicians readily accept PRs, there are a few physicians who either have a certain criteria for choosing PRs or choose to avoid them completely [23]. The criteria used by some physicians are: personal style, company and the kind of drugs PRs offer.

"I have specific criteria for selection. I mean, whether I like this representative or not, whether I am comfortable with him or not and whether his style is true or not true. Is he logical or not logical? There are companies that [I] do not care about them. For example, a new company whose products are widely available such as popular products. I often do not meet them because they do not give us new ideas" [21].

One of the physicians who avoids PRs' comments:

"Really, from the time that I came here to work, I [have tried] to avoid meeting them because my use is limited, but I have to meet my colleagues. I try to avoid the interview because I know that I will not prescribe his product. I am a surgeon and my use is limited. Just I have painkiller. There is no other choice" [21].

Physicians cited many reasons for refusing to meet PRs, such as bad experience with PRs and commercial context (e.g., disagreements about some commercial deal), obligations to other companies, lack of conviction about the product, lack of credibility of PRs and workload or inappropriate timing of visits [21, 33].

"The other thing, I may refuse to meet [a] representative if the owner of the company behaves with our colleagues [in an] inhuman or dishonorable [way], so this forces us to stop prescribing its product and prescribe a similar alternative that exists in the market" [21].

Reasons for avoiding PRs, other than the ones mentioned above, were: commercially-biased information, pushy and argumentative approach, and a lack of accuracy in the information provided, and, finally, the PR's influence on prescribing behaviour.

"I have been very influenced in the past by my prescribing so I don't see them anymore now. I was getting no advantage from it at all, it was skewing my prescribing and I was losing a lot of time, so I stopped seeing them" [33].

Theme 6.0: Guidelines

6.1 Guidelines and their impact

Over the years, there have been a number of guidelines developed by different healthcare societies regarding the interaction between physicians and PRs such as; the American College of Obstetricians and Gynecologists (ACOG), the American Medical Association (AMA) and the Association of American Medical Colleges, Canadian Medical Association (CMA). Morgan et al. [25] and Anderson et al. [28] have each investigated the use and effect of guidelines in the US. Anderson et al. reports that 154 (62%) of participants in the US were familiar with guidelines on interacting with the pharmaceutical industry, of whom 81 (33%) had read guidelines developed by ACOG, 86 (35%) had read AMA guidelines, and 49 (21%) had read guidelines from other sources such as hospital guidelines, journal articles, and continuing medical education programmes [28].

Studies show that those who had read the guidelines would actually provide fewer free samples to patients or have less frequent meals with the PRs. They were also less likely to receive first hand news on medical products from PRs or include PRs in the decision as to whether to prescribe a new drug, compared to those who had not read the guidelines [25, 28].

According to Anderson et al., there was no significant difference between those who reported reading ethical guidelines and those who did not do so pertaining to using PRs for obtaining drug information [28]. It is postulated that having read guidelines did not affect the perceived value of PRs [28].

6.2 Physician's opinion on guidelines that restrict physician-PR interactions

The opinion of physicians on the policies that limit or prohibit the physician-PR interaction varied significantly. Some participants believed such restrictions to be unfair to prescribers and patients; some welcomed them with open arms. While others reported having doubts about policies, particularly those related to prohibition of free drug samples. These physicians however, disclosed that, over time they realized that their prescribing behaviour had actually been affected by the visits of PRs and availability of free drug samples, and they eventually started supporting policies that prohibit/restrict PR visits. In a study done in the US in 2003, 39.9% of participants stated that they disagreed with placing limitations on the interaction between physicians and PRs, while roughly the same percentage (33.3%) agreed with the policy. In Germany the data is slightly different, over half of the German physicians (n = 108; 52%) indicated that they would regret the cessation of the visits while the remaining 45% (n = 94) supported it [29, 34].

> *"I was really hesitant about getting rid of the sample closet years ago, but now I think it was really, definitely the right thing because I would reach for the best non-steroidal that was in there and at that point it was [brand name]. So I give a patient [brand name] thinking I did a good thing because he told me he didn't have any money, but often they would come back wanting [brand name] where I just could have given him Ibuprofen. ...Once we didn't have it anymore, I realized that..."* [34].

Discussion

As part of the health care system, pharmaceutical manufacturers have benefited countless people through their investment in research and product development. Their ultimate responsibility, however, is to their shareholders, who expect a reasonable profit from their investments [6]. The pharmaceutical industry, therefore, cannot be entirely blamed for trying to increase returns, within legal boundaries. Inappropriate marketing practices that may arise from this profit-led competition have been proven, however, to have the potential to influence physician prescribing.

Policymakers have therefore tried to restrict the interaction between physicians and PRs, which is where most of the marketing occurs, by developing guidelines and making relevant policies. The World Health Assembly, in an attempt to tackle the issue, adopted the WHO Ethical Criteria for Medicinal Drug Promotion in 1988, which requires PRs to have an appropriate educational background and be adequately trained with sufficient medical and technical knowledge and integrity to present information on products in an accurate, unbiased, and responsible manner. WHO also holds employers responsible, for not only the basic and continuing training of their representatives, but also for their statements and activities [39]. Many critics, however, have complained that these guidelines have been largely disregarded, including the voluntary Code of Pharmaceutical Practices developed by the industry's own International Federation of Pharmaceutical Manufacturers' Associations (IFPMA) [1]. While the development of guidelines and policies has proven helpful, therefore, it certainly is not enough..

As demonstrated by this meta-synthesis, the attitude of physicians towards PRs is a very crucial determinant of the potential of PRs to indirectly influence the health of patients in a positive or negative way. The studies included in this meta-synthesis were undertaken in nine different countries with significantly different economies, cultures, education/healthcare systems, and health policies, yet the positive attitude of physicians towards PRs was evident in all of them.

As stated earlier, there are a number of reasons behind this positive attitude with the one-to-one medium of interaction being one of them; the results of the research conducted by McGettigan et al. showed that the information sources most frequently rated important by physicians were not those most used in practice. The sources of practical importance were those involving the transfer of information through personal face-to-face contact, indicating the importance of the medium through which information is conveyed [40] which poses an advantage for direct pharmaceutical detailing.

Lack of time to read and keep abreast of the myriad of new medical information is another important facilitator for physicians to meet PRs. PRs are seen as convenient and timely sources of medicine related information. Physicians perceive the information provided by PRs as factual but in some cases biased. Our findings are in line with that of the systematic review conducted by Wazana et al. [11];physicians believe that they are immune from any potential marketing influence. This is mainly because most of physicians believe that they have the required expertise and knowledge to assess the presented information and distinguish the valid information from the exaggerated, biased information [21, 22, 24–27, 29, 32–34]. This is despite the clear evidence in the literature regarding the effect of PRs on prescribing behaviour [32].

Undeniably, detailing poses as a convenient face-to-face educational meeting [21, 23, 24, 26, 29, 33, 34],especially for newly launched medicines [33, 35]. Instead of seeking to ban these interactions, therefore, medical regulatory bodies could implement proactive measures to educate medical students about potential medical inducements [10]. Vinson et al. measured the effect of a one-hour lecture and discussion about the appropriateness of pharmaceutical gifts among second-year medical students. Findings from the survey have showed that these students had become statistically significantly more resistant to the gifts compared to the first-year students who served as a control group and had not experienced the lecture. This study strongly suggested that changes in students' attitudes towards marketing methods used by PRs may be fostered [41]. Similarly, positive long term effects were observed from educating trainees and physicians about understanding and responding to pharmaceutical promotion [42–44].

We believe that this meta-synthesis has given new insights into the PR-physician interaction. The findings of this meta-synthesis have implications for policy makers and educators. Future research should focus on practical education and policy interventions to better limit any potential conflict of interest that may arise from such interactions through education and informed policy development.

Limitations

This meta-synthesis focused on the recent literature and excluded studies published before 2000. This means that some relevant, important points might have been missed if they were published before 2000. Meanwhile, the themes were generated in such a way as to offer, in the authors' opinion, a useful insight into the different aspects of the PR-physician interaction. Drawing together data from multiple countries has some value, certainly. However, looked at from the opposite point of view, it is not entirely clear that the cultures of pharmaceutical companies and of physicians, and the regulatory/healthcare systems in countries as diverse as Peru, India, the Yemen, the UK and the US can be easily comparable. Direct to consumer advertising is, for example allowed in US but banned in other countries. Thus, there is a need for some further country specific studies.

Conclusions

The purpose of this meta-synthesis, was to highlight the detailing aspects of PR-physician interactions from the physician's point of view. This meta-synthesis shows that physicians generally see meetings with PRs as advantageous to everyone: the patients, because they receive free drug samples, the hospital/clinic, because they would receive stationery, books, and, most importantly, themselves, as these meetings help them to stay up-to-date and aware of newly launched medications. Future research should focus on educating medical students to correct their perception of immunity against marketing which may hold them back from critically appraising the information provided by PRs. This will ensure that patients do not bear the cost of competition between pharmaceutical companies.

Abbreviations

ACOG: American College of Obstetricians and Gynecologists; AMA: American Medical Association; CMA: Association of American Medical Colleges, Canadian Medical Association; GP: General Practitioner; IFPMA: International Federation of Pharmaceutical Manufacturers' Associations; MO: Medical officer; NA: Not applicable/available; PR: Pharmaceutical representative; SD: Standard deviation; UK: United Kingdom; US: United States; WHO: World Health Organization

Acknowledgements

We would like to acknowledge Johnathan from academic English editors for his services to check the language appropriateness of the paper.

Funding

None.

Authors' contributions

Conceived and designed the experiments: TMK and SS. Analyzed the data: SS, TMK and LCM. Wrote the paper: SS, TMK and LCM. Designed search strategies: TMK and SS. Critically reviewed the manuscript for important intellectual content: TMK and LCM. Read and approved the final version: SS, TMK and LCM. All authors read and approved the final manuscript.

Competing interests

The authors declare that they have no competing interests.

Author details

[1]Collaboration for Outcomes Research and Evaluation (CORE), Faculty of Pharmaceutical Sciences, The University of British Columbia, Vancouver, British Columbia, Canada. [2]Unit for Medication Outcomes Research and Education (UMORE), Pharmacy, School of Medicine, University of Tasmania, Hobart, Tasmania, Australia. [3]School of Pharmacy, Monash University, Sunway City, Selangor, Malaysia. [4]Department of Pharmacy, Abasyn University, Peshawar, Pakistan.

References

1. WHO. Trade, foreign policy, diplomacy and health. 2014. Available online: http://www.who.int/trade/glossary/story073/en/. Accessed 10 Aug 2014.
2. Othman N, Vitry AI, Roughead EE, Ismail SB, Omar K. Medicines information provided by pharmaceutical representatives: a comparative study in Australia and Malaysia. BMC Public Health. 2010;10:743.
3. Spurling GK, Mansfield PR, Montgomery BD, et al. Information from pharmaceutical companies and the quality, quantity, and cost of physicians' prescribing: a systematic review. PLoS Med. 2010;7:e1000352.
4. IMS Health. Global Pharmaceuticals Marketing Channel Reference. 2015. Available from: Global Pharmaceuticals Marketing Channel Reference. Accessed 24 Apr 2016.
5. Gagnon MA, Lexchin J. The cost of pushing pills: a new estimate of pharmaceutical promotion expenditures in the United States. PLoS Med. 2008;5:e1.
6. Brennan TA, Rothman DJ, Blank L, et al. Health industry practices that create conflicts of interest: a policy proposal for academic medical centers. JAMA. 2006;295:429–33.
7. Stark TJ, Brownell AK, Brager NP, Berg A, Balderston R, Lockyer JM. Exploring Perceptions of Early-Career Psychiatrists About Their Relationships With the Pharmaceutical Industry. Acad Psychiatry. 2015;40:249-54.
10. Blumenthal D. Doctors and drug companies. N Engl J Med. 2004;351:1885–90.
11. Wazana A. Physicians and the pharmaceutical industry: is a gift ever just a gift? JAMA. 2000;283:373–80.
12. Edwards DA. Gifts to physicians from the pharmaceutical industry. JAMA. 2000;283:2656. author reply 7–8.
13. Howard SM. Gifts to physicians from the pharmaceutical industry. JAMA. 2000;283:2655–6. author reply 7–8.
14. McKinney WP, Rich EC. Gifts to physicians from the pharmaceutical industry. JAMA. 2000;283:2656–7. author reply 7–8.
15. Tenery Jr RM. Gifts to physicians from the pharmaceutical industry. JAMA. 2000;283:2655–8.
16. Tenery Jr RM. Interactions between physicians and the health care technology industry. JAMA. 2000;283:391–3.

17. Vollmann J. Gifts to physicians from the pharmaceutical industry. JAMA. 2000;283:2656. author reply 7–8.
18. Liesegang TJ. Physicians and the pharmaceutical industry: is a gift ever just a gift? Wazana A. JAMA 2000;283:373–380. Am J Ophthalmol. 2000;130:261.
19. Green J, Thorogood N. Chapter 10 Reading, Appraising and Integrating Qualitative Research. In: Qualitative Methods for Health Research. London: Sage; 2013.
20. Walsh D, Downe S. Meta-synthesis method for qualitative research: a literature review. J Adv Nurs. 2005;50:204–11.
21. Al-Areefi MA, Hassali MA, Ibrahim MI. Physicians' perceptions of medical representative visits in Yemen: a qualitative study. BMC Health Serv Res. 2013;13:331.
22. Alssageer MA, Kowalski SR. A survey of pharmaceutical company representative interactions with doctors in Libya. Libyan J Med. 2012;7: 18556. http://dx.doi.org/10.3402/ljm.v7i0.18556.
23. Brett AS, Burr W, Moloo J. Are gifts from pharmaceutical companies ethically problematic? A survey of physicians. Arch Intern Med. 2003;163:2213–8.
24. Misra S, Ganzini L, Keepers G. Psychiatric resident and faculty views on and interactions with the pharmaceutical industry. Acad Psychiatry. 2010;34:102–8.
25. Morgan MA, Dana J, Loewenstein G, Zinberg S, Schulkin J. Interactions of doctors with the pharmaceutical industry. J Med Ethics. 2006;32:559–63.
26. Saito S, Mukohara K, Bito S. Japanese practicing physicians' relationships with pharmaceutical representatives: a national survey. PLoS One. 2010;5:e12193.
27. Wang Y, Adelman RA. A study of interactions between pharmaceutical representatives and ophthalmology trainees. Am J Ophthalmol. 2009;148: 619–22.e3.
28. Anderson BL, Silverman GK, Loewenstein GF, Zinberg S, Schulkin J. Factors associated with physicians' reliance on pharmaceutical sales representatives. Acad Med. 2009;84:994–1002.
29. Lieb K, Brandtönies S. A survey of German physicians in private practice about contacts with pharmaceutical sales representatives. Dtsch Arztebl Int. 2010;107:392–8.
30. Roy N, Madhiwalla N, Pai SA. Drug promotional practices in Mumbai: a qualitative study. Indian J Med Ethics. 2007;4:57–61.
31. Alssageer MA, Kowalski SR. What do Libyan doctors perceive as the benefits, ethical issues and influences of their interactions with pharmaceutical company representatives? Pan Afr Med J. 2013;14:132.
32. Sarikaya O, Civaner M, Vatansever K. Exposure of medical students to pharmaceutical marketing in primary care settings: frequent and influential. Adv Health Sci Educ. 2009;14:713–24.
33. Prosser H, Walley T. Understanding why GPs see pharmaceutical representatives: a qualitative interview study. Br J Gen Pract. 2003;53:305–11.
34. Fischer MA, Keough ME, Baril JL, et al. Prescribers and pharmaceutical representatives: why are we still meeting? J Gen Intern Med. 2009;24:795–801.
35. Mintzes B, Mangin D, Hayes L and Organization WH. Understanding and responding to pharmaceutical promotion: a practical guide. World Health Organization; 2009. Available from: http://haiweb.org/wp-content/uploads/2015/05/Pharma-Promotion-Guide-English.pdf. Accessed 2 May 2016.
36. World Health Organization/Health Action International. Understanding and responding to pharmaceutical promotion- a practical guideline. 2010. Available from: http://www1.paho.org/hq/dmdocuments/2011/drugpromotion-manual-CAP-3-090610.pdf. Accessed 10 June 2016.
37. Theodorou M, Tsiantou V, Pavlakis A, et al. Factors influencing prescribing behaviour of physicians in Greece and Cyprus: results from a questionnaire based survey. BMC Health Serv Res. 2009;9:150.
38. Cialdini RB. Influence: Science and practice. 2009.
39. World Health Organisation. Ethical criteria for medicinal drug promotion. Geneva: WHO; 1988. Available from: http://apps.who.int/medicinedocs/documents/whozip08e/whozip08e.pdf. Accessed 10 Jun 2015.
40. McGettigan P, Golden J, Fryer J, Chan R, Feely J. Prescribers prefer people: The sources of information used by doctors for prescribing suggest that the medium is more important than the message. Br J Clin Pharmacol. 2001;51:184–9.
41. Vinson DC, McCandless B, Hosokawa MC. Medical students' attitudes toward pharmaceutical marketing: possibilities for change. Fam Med. 1993;25:31–3.
42. King M, Essick C, Bearman P, Ross JS. Medical school gift restriction policies and physician prescribing of newly marketed psychotropic medications: difference-in-differences analysis. BMJ. 2013;346:f264.
43. Epstein AJ, Busch SH, Busch AB, Asch DA, Barry CL. Does exposure to conflict of interest policies in psychiatry residency affect antidepressant prescribing? Med Care. 2013;51:199–203.
44. McCormick BB, Tomlinson G, Brill-Edwards P, Detsky AS. Effect of restricting contact between pharmaceutical company representatives and internal medicine residents on posttraining attitudes and behavior. JAMA. 2001;286: 1994–9.

Assessing medication packaging and labelling appropriateness in Sri Lanka

N. Athuraliya[1], E. J. Walkom[2*], S. Dharmaratne[3] and J. Robertson[2]

Abstract

Background: There is substantial evidence of poor dispensing practices with inadequate packaging and labelling of medicines, and limited advice on their usage in low and middle-income countries (LMICs). We examined the labelling and packaging of medicines identified during a survey of 1322 households in six regions of Sri Lanka between 2010 and 2013 conducted using the World Health Organization (WHO) methodology for household surveys. We compared medicines obtained from public and private sources and asked interviewees if they understood how to take the medicines.

Methods: Packaging was considered adequate when the primary package was an envelope or closable container holding only one medicine. Adequate labels were legible and included medicine name, dose and expiration date. Interviewers assessed whether respondents knew how to take the medicines.

Results: Of 1322 households, 1253 households (94.8%) had at least one medicine; 84% were classified as western medicines and 16% traditional medicines. Of 5756 western medicines identified, 82.1% were adequately packaged, 43.3% adequately labelled and 41.4% both adequately packaged and labelled. Participants stated that they understood the label and knew how to take 96% of the medicines. Private medicine sources had more adequately packaged medicines than public sources (87.7% vs 73.5%; OR 2.58, 95% CI 2.23, 2.99) and more adequately labelled medicines (52.2% vs 27.4%; OR 2.90, 95% CI 2.57, 3.26).

Conclusions: Inadequate packaging and labelling of medicines remain a concern in Sri Lanka. Commitment to Good Pharmacy Practices, investments in staff education and training and adequate dispensing resources (containers and labels), particularly in the public sector, are needed to address sub-optimal dispensing practices. Ageing populations with more chronic diseases requiring polypharmacy and complex medicine regimens increase the need for appropriately packaged and labelled medicines.

Keywords: Medicines, Packaging, Labelling, Dispensing, Pharmacy practice, Low-middle income countries

Background

Medicines are central to health care and the most commonly used therapeutic intervention to manage acute and chronic conditions. The rational or responsible use of medicines depends on an appropriate clinical diagnosis and selection of the appropriate medicines in the correct dose and duration at the lowest cost to patients [1]. Good dispensing practices ensure that the medicine is delivered to the patient with clear instructions in a package that maintains the potency of the medicine up to the time of use [2]. Desirable and acceptable forms of packaging for different pharmaceutical dosage forms have been defined, however the high costs and poor availability of suitable containers can compromise dispensing practices in some settings [2].

Medicine containers should provide a surface for attaching or writing a label with identifying details and instructions for use. In addition, dispensers have a responsibility to ensure that patients understand how to take their medicines [2]. However, there is substantial evidence of poor dispensing practices, inadequate packaging, labelling, instruction and advice on usage and, storage of medicines in low and middle-income countries (LMICs) [3].

* Correspondence: Emily.Walkom@newcastle.edu.au
[2]Department of Clinical Pharmacology, School of Medicine and Public Health, The University of Newcastle, Newcastle, Australia
Full list of author information is available at the end of the article

Country situational analyses conducted in South East Asia in Bhutan, India, Indonesia, Myanmar, Nepal, and Timor-Leste have documented the frequent use of small plastic bags as packaging, sometimes writing the number of tablets per day and dosage frequency on a separate, unattached slip of paper, or no labelling of dispensed medicines at all [4]. Studies conducted in Egypt, Northern Nigeria, Pakistan and Ethiopia have reported between 0 and 13.7% of dispensed medicines with adequate labels [5–8]. Yet in these same studies 55 to 94% of patients were reported to have adequate knowledge of the correct dose of the medicine.

In many LMICs the private sector is an important source of medicines, and may be the first point of contact with the health care system and preferred channel for purchasing medicines [3]. However, questions have been raised about the quality of services provided. There is evidence of a lack of pharmacists or other trained personnel in these facilities, provision of advice that is not in accord with treatment guidelines, inappropriate supply of medicines and insufficient counselling [3, 9, 10].

The aim of this study was to examine the situation in Sri Lanka with regards to medicines labelling and packaging and to determine if there were differences in dispensing practices between public and private sources of medicines. In addition, we assessed interviewees' knowledge of how to take the medicines identified.

Methods

We conducted a study of access to medicines for acute and chronic illness in 2010/2011 (Kandy district) and 2012/13 (Colombo, Ampara, Monaragala, Polonnaruwa and Rathnapura districts), using the World Health Organization (WHO) methodology for household surveys [11]. Six administrative divisions (districts) were chosen from the 25 districts of Sri Lanka. An initial feasibility study was conducted in Kandy district. Colombo (capital) district was chosen as per the WHO guidelines. The remaining districts were divided into clusters based on the poverty level criteria, childhood anaemia, population density, and percentage of rural and urban populations within the district and selected to ensure inclusion of districts of different socio-economic status.

Thirty public health care facilities distributed across the six districts were randomly selected. The study population consisted of clusters of households at a given distance (<5, 5–10 and >10 km) from the reference health facilities. Thirty households in six clusters around each reference health care facility are recommended to be interviewed, i.e. a national sample of 900 households.

We used six pairs of interviewers who were Sociology, Biology or Pharmacy graduates and trained to collect the information. Training was guided by the WHO training tools (WHO Manual for household surveys; PowerPoint slide presentation). Supervision of interviewers and review of completed questionnaires were undertaken by two of the researchers (SD, NA).

As part of the data collection for household surveys, participants were asked by the interviewers to show all the medications present in their home at the time of the interview. Details were recorded for up to 20 medicines per household. The medicine was identified where possible and respondents were asked where they obtained the medicine: family/friend; public hospital; NGO/mission hospital; public health centre or dispensary; private health care provider; traditional healer; private pharmacy; drug seller and 'Other'. Medicines were classified as western or traditional. We report here on packaging and labelling of medicines obtained in the public and private sector, i.e. public hospital; public health centre or dispensary; private health care provider; private pharmacy. The labelling of traditional medicines is more complex and less subject to regulation and standardization, therefore a detailed analysis of the packaging and labelling of traditional medicines was beyond the scope of this study.

WHO household study definitions of adequate packaging and labelling were applied. The primary packaging for the medication was assessed and considered adequate if the package was an envelope or a closable container, and contained only one medicine. The interviewer recorded whether the label on the medicines was legible (included medicine name, dose and expiration date), and also whether the interviewee could understand the label and how to take the medicine.

Descriptive statistics (%) are used to summarise results. Differences between groups are presented as Odds Ratios (OR) with 95% confidence intervals (CI) and were calculated using StatsDirect Version 3 (2016).

Results

There were 1322 households from six regions of Sri Lanka included in the study. Most households had at least one medication to show the interviewer (94.8%, average 5 medicines per household, 4 western and 1 traditional). A total of 6856 medicines were identified; 84% (5756) were classified as western medicines and 16% (1085) traditional medicines (Table 1). Data used to conduct this analysis are available in Additional File 1.

Of the 5756 western medicines, the majority ($n = 4725$, 82.1%) were deemed adequately packaged, while less than half of the medicines assessed (43.3%) were adequately labelled. Only 2385/5756 (41.4%) medicines had both adequate packaging and labelling. Participants reported understanding the instructions for using almost all medicines (95.6%).

A greater proportion of western medicines sourced from private facilities were adequately packaged compared to

Table 1 Household characteristics and medicines by surveyed district

	Ampara	Colombo	Kandy	Monaragala	Polonnaruwa	Rathnapura	Total
Households surveyed (*N*)	216	213	210	216	255	212	1322
Persons per household (mean, range)	4.3 (1–9)	4.3 (1–8)	4.4 (1–9)	4.1 (1–9)	4.1 (1–8)	4.2 (1–9)	4.2 (1–9)
Western medicines (*N*)	765	1074	980	989	847	1101	5756
Western medicines per household (mean, range)	3.5 (0–14)	5.0 (0–15)	4.7 (0–15)	4.6 (0–15)	3.3 (0–15)	5.2 (0–14)	4.4 (0–15)
Traditional medicines per household (mean, range)	0.8 (0–5)	0.9 (0–5)	0.5 (0–5)	1.3 (0–7)	0.7 (0–9)	0.8 (0–4)	0.8 (0–9)

those obtained from public facilities (87.7% vs 73.5%; OR 2.58, 95% CI 2.23, 2.99; Table 2). Medicines issued from both private and public sectors were mostly contained in envelopes, plastic bags or glass bottles (see Figs. 1 and 2). In some of the public facilities, the packaging was unsatisfactory. Although not very frequent, an example of unsatisfactory packaging included the use of a sheet of paper to wrap tablets and capsules (Fig. 3).

Private health facilities were more likely to have supplied medicines with adequate labels than public facilities (52.2% vs 27.4%; OR 2.90, 95% CI 2.57, 3.26); often with the label written on the envelope containing the medicine. The use of slips of paper inside medicine containers was common in public hospitals. In some public facilities where papers were used to wrap medicines, the label was usually written directly on the folded paper.

Only 25.9% of medicines issued by public sector facilities were determined to be both adequately packaged and adequately labelled compared to 50% of medicines obtained from the private sector. This observation of better packaging and labelling in the private sector was consistent across the six regions (Table 2). A greater proportion of medicines issued by public sector facilities were correctly labelled in Colombo region (41.5%) compared to other regions (20.2–31.8%).

Discussion

The results of this study confirm previous observations of problems in dispensing practices in Sri Lanka and other LMICs, with notable differences in the quality of dispensing practices in the public and private sectors. In absolute terms the level of adequately labelled medicines was better than reported in studies conducted in Egypt, Northern Nigeria, Pakistan and Ethiopia [5–8], however labelling of medicines remains sub-optimal (<50%).

In general, medicines packaging was better than medicines labelling, however the criteria set for 'adequate' in both cases was quite low. An adequate label was one that was considered legible with the medicine name, dosage regimen and expiry date. This level of detail falls well short of current recommendations for labelling of outpatient medicines in high-income countries [12].

An adequate package was an envelope or closable container and containing only one medicine. We could not assess how long the medicines may have remained packaged this way; in busy health facilities staff may pre-package medicines into smaller units for individual patient use to facilitate the dispensing process. The implications of longer-term storage in envelopes and plastic bags on medicine potency are unclear. The use of folded sheets of paper to package some medicines from public facilities may indicate an acute shortage of

Table 2 Adequacy of packaging and labelling of western medicines issued by public and private facilities and by district

	Surveyed districts in Sri Lanka (*n*, %)						
	Ampara	Colombo	Kandy	Monaragala	Polonnaruwa	Rathnapura	Total
Medicines obtained from Public facilities							
Total medicines	453	284	336	439	478	425	2415
Adequate Label	106 (23.4)	118 (41.5)	68 (20.2)	100 (22.8)	152 (31.8)	117 (27.5)	661 (27.4)
Adequate Packaging	320 (70.6)	213 (75.0)	234 (69.6)	322 (73.3)	359 (75.4)	325 (76.5)	1773 (73.5)
Both Adequate	106 (23.4)	109 (38.4)	64 (19.0)	97 (22.1)	134 (28.0)	115 (27.1)	625 (25.9)
Medicines obtained from Private facilities							
Total medicines	232	687	549	473	287	590	2818
Adequate Label	128 (55.2)	440 (64.0)	288 (52.5)	229 (48.4)	138 (41.8)	247 (41.9)	1470 (52.5)
Adequate Packaging	217 (93.5)	655 (95.3)	492 (89.6)	412 (87.1)	251 (87.5)	444 (75.3)	2471 (87.7)
Both Adequate	127 (54.7)	438 (63.8)	266 (48.5)	219 (46.3)	127 (44.3)	234 (39.7)	1411 (50.1)

Public = public hospital, health centre or dispensary; Private = private health care provider or pharmacy

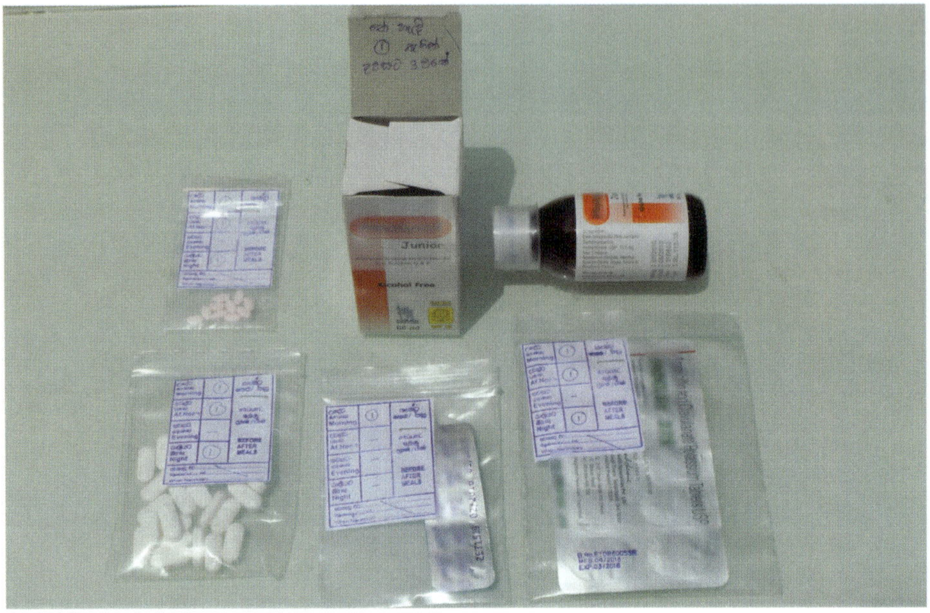

Fig. 1 Example of medicines sourced from private facilities

proper material for dispensing at least in some facilities. Such practices may not be limited to public facilities, with a previous WHO situational analysis in Sri Lanka reporting instances of private pharmacies dispensing medicines in envelopes, sometimes made of old newspaper; and in a few of the facilities there was no labelling of medicines [13].

The high proportion of respondents indicating they understood the label and how to take the medicines was in contrast to the findings on adequate packaging and labelling. However, this is a consistent finding of published studies—in spite of poor labelling and presumably little time for contact with dispensing personnel. It is difficult to compare our results with other studies due to differences in definitions. In some studies, patients stating they knew the dose was considered a positive response [7], while in others, patients had to be able to repeat at least the dose and frequency of medication administration [6]. We did not have the level of detail to compare awareness of dosing for prescription medicines

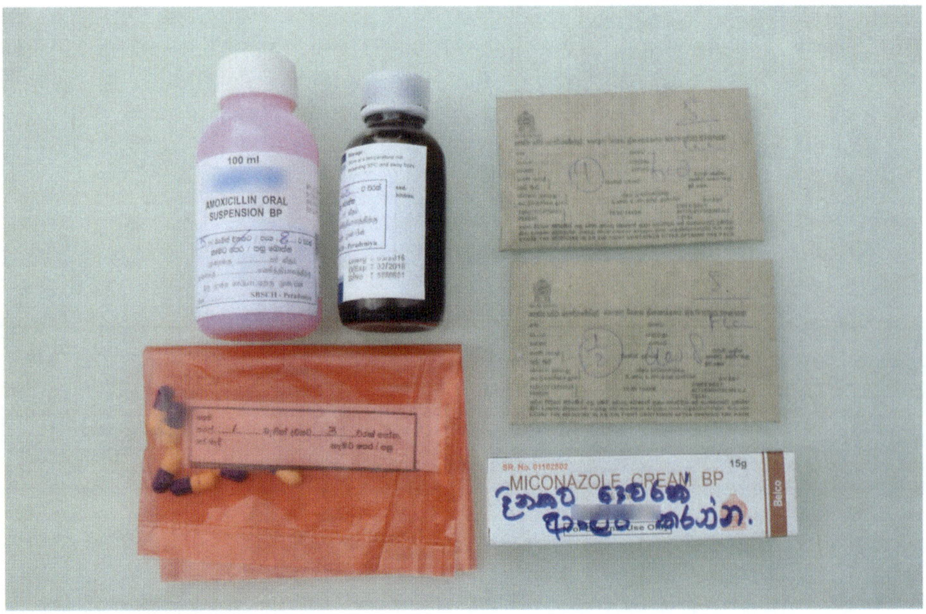

Fig. 2 Example of medicines sourced from public facilities

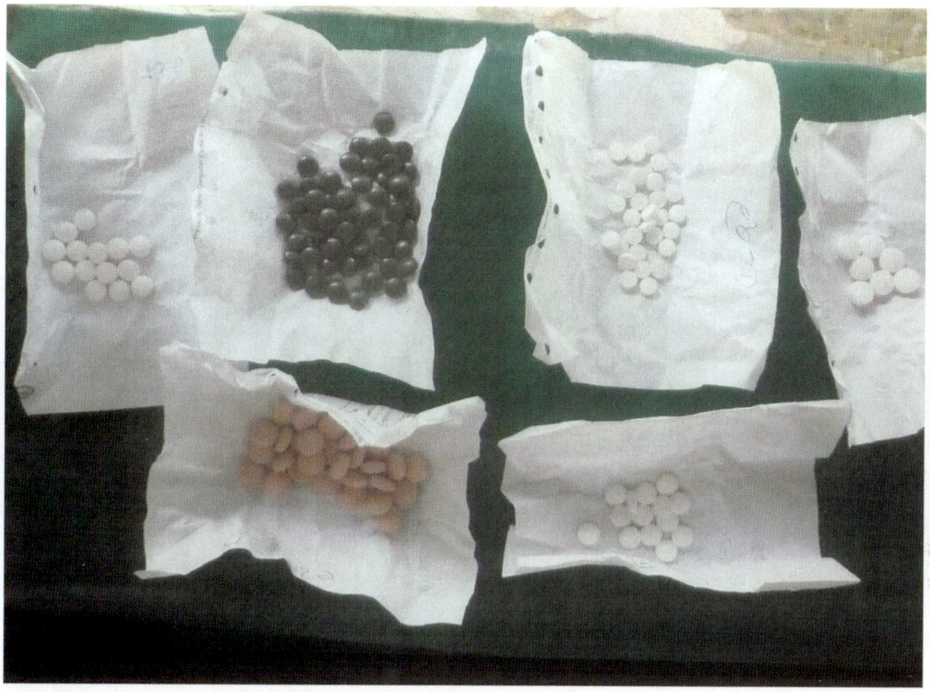

Fig. 3 Example of unsatisfactory packaging using paper to wrap medicines

versus other medicine types in the household or levels of knowledge of dosage regimens for new medicines compared to medicines taken previously. Babu et al. reported that only 57.3% of patients taking antihypertensive medicines had adequate knowledge of their dosage schedule [14]. Adherence to prescribed medicine regimens is important if patients are to achieve the desired clinical benefits of their treatment. We made no assessment of the appropriateness of the medicines present in the household.

There were a number of limitations inherent in the design of this primarily descriptive survey. The assessment of medicines packaging and labelling occurred in family homes, and it is possible that medicines may have been re-packaged for convenience by household members and not kept in original packaging. Assessment of the household members' understanding of how to take their medicines was limited to a simple yes/no response. There was no objective assessment of understanding of dosage instructions. Assessment of adequate labelling and packaging was made according to the WHO Manual for Household Surveys [11]. The standard for adequate labelling and packaging may not be considered adequate in other developed countries.

There has been increasing emphasis on effective drug regulatory procedures and good manufacturing practices (GMP) in medicines production and improved procedures for medicines storage and distribution to try to ensure that only quality-assured medicines are in circulation. However problems in dispensing practices remain [3, 15]. A notable feature of many of the studies is the short dispensing times and minimal interactions between dispensers and patients reported [13]. Syhakhang and colleagues found no differences in medicines adequately labelled in public and private pharmacy practices in one province of Lao PDR [16]. We cannot account for the differences observed in this study but there were suggestions of more acute shortages of appropriate dispensing materials in some of the public sector institutions.

There is evidence that training can improve dispensing practices [17]. However, education alone is unlikely to produce sustainable changes. Incentives, greater compliance with agreed professional pharmacy practice standards and technology solutions including electronic prescription systems that generate labels with standard patient information will all contribute to improved dispensing practices. Good Pharmacy Practice guidelines provide a quality management framework and a strategic plan for developing pharmacy services [18]. Preparing, obtaining, storing, securing, distributing, administering, dispensing and disposal of medical products are key functions. Much work and investment in staff and resources will be required in LMICs for pharmacists to fulfil these functions. However, as LMICS face ageing populations, the double burden of communicable and non-communicable chronic diseases, polypharmacy and more complex medicine regimens, the imperatives to provide quality pharmacy services grows.

Conclusions

There were significant differences in the quality of labelling and packaging of western medicines in the public and private sectors in this study. In general, medicines packaging was better than medicines labelling, however the criteria set for 'adequate' in both cases were quite low, and well below those in current recommendations for Good Pharmacy Practices. Organizational constraints are likely to have contributed to the problems observed with inadequate dispensing resources (containers and labels), particularly in the public sector. Low staffing levels will also limit the ability of trained staff to provide instructions to patients and carers on how to take the medicines.

The results of this study highlight the need for training and continuing education in Good Pharmacy Practices in Sri Lanka and other LMICs with similar problems with packaging and labelling of dispensed medicines. The goal is to ensure that medicines are delivered to the patient with a label providing clear instructions on administration and a package that maintains the potency of the medicine up to the time of use. Ageing populations with more chronic diseases requiring polypharmacy and complex medicine regimens increase the need for appropriately packaged and labelled medicines.

Abbreviations

CI: Confidence intervals; GMP: Good manufacturing practices; LMIC: Low and middle-income countries; OR: Odds ratio; WHO: World Health Organization

Acknowledgements

We would like to thank all the participants who gave their time freely for this research and the data collectors who conducted the interviews for this study.

Funding

Funding for this study was provided from research funds from the University of Newcastle.

Authors' contributions

All authors contributed to the design of the study and analysis and interpretation of the data. JR wrote the first draft of the manuscript. EJW, NA and SD provided critical comment on the manuscript. All authors approved the submission of the final manuscript.

Competing interests

The authors declare that they have no competing interests.

Author details

[1]Department of Medicine, The Maitland Hospital Clinical School, 550-560 High Street, Maitland 2320, NSW, Australia. [2]Department of Clinical Pharmacology, School of Medicine and Public Health, The University of Newcastle, Newcastle, Australia. [3]Medical Education Unit, Faculty of Medicine, University of Peradeniya, Peradeniya, Sri Lanka.

References

1. World Health Organization. Rational use of medicines. http://www.who.int/medicines/areas/rational_use/en/. Accessed 12 Apr 2016.
2. Management Sciences for Health (2012). Ensuring good dispensing practices. In Managing Drug Supply (MDS-3), Chapter 30. http://apps.who.int/medicinedocs/documents/s19607en/s19607en.pdf. Accessed 12 Feb 2016.
3. Miller R, Goodman C. Performance of retail pharmacies in low- and middle-income Asian settings: a systematic review. Health Policy Plan. 2016;31:940–53. doi:10.1093/heapol/czw007.
4. World Health Organization South East Asian Regional Office. Country situational analyses of medicines management in health care delivery. http://www.searo.who.int/entity/medicines/country_situational_analysis/en/. Accessed 17 April 2016.
5. Akl OA, El Mahalli AA, Elkahky AA, Salem AM. WHO/INRUD drug use indicators at primary healthcare centers in Alexandria, Egypt. J Taibah Univ med sci. 2014;9(1):54–64.
6. Geresu B, Kumar R, Beyene Y. Drug use pattern in Dessie Referral Hospital, north east Ethiopia. Afr j pharm pharmacol. 2014;8(45):1132–7.
7. Chedi BAZ, Abdu-Aguye I, Kwanashie HO. Drug use pattern in out-patient children: a comparison between primary and secondary health care facilities in northern Nigeria. Afr j pharm pharmacol. 2015;9(4):74–81.
8. Aslam A, Khatoon S, Mehdi M, Mumtaz S, Murtaza B. Evaluation of rational drug use at teaching hospitals in Punjab, Pakistan. J pharm pract community med. 2016;2(2):54–7.
9. Smith F. The quality of private pharmacy services in low and middle-income countries: a systematic review. Pharm world sci. 2009;31:351–61.
10. Hussain A, Ibrahim Mohamed IM. Perceptions of dispensers regarding dispensing practices in Pakistan: a qualitative study. Trop j pharm res. 2011;10:117–23.
11. World Health Organization. Manual for the household survey to measure access and use of medicines. http://www.who.int/medicines/areas/coordination/household_manual_february_2008.pdf. Accessed 17 April 2016.
12. Institute for Safe Medication Practices. Principles of designing a medication label for community and mail order pharmacy prescription packages. https://www.ismp.org/tools/guidelines/labelFormats/comments/default.asp. Accessed 17 April 2016.
13. World Health Organization South East Asian Regional Office. Medicines in Health Care Delivery: Sri Lanka—Situational Analysis. 16–27 March 2015. http://www.searo.who.int/entity/medicines/sri_lanka_mar_2016.pdf?ua=1. Accessed 28 April 2016.
14. Babu RH, Reddy MM, Vidyadhar S. Drug utilization study of antihypertensive agents in an urban primary health care center in south India. Int j innov pharmres. 2012;3(3):244–6.
15. Wolffers I. Drug information and sale practices in some pharmacies of Colombo, Sri Lanka. Soc sci med. 1987;25:319–21.
16. Syhakhang L, Stenson B, Wahlström R, Tomson G. The quality of public and private pharmacy practices. Eur j clin pharmacol. 2001;57:221–7.
17. Chaudhury RR, Parameswar R, Gupta U, Sharma S, Tekur U, Bapna JS. Quality medicines for the poor: experience of the Delhi programme on rational use of drugs. Health policy plan. 2005;20:124–36.
18. Joint FIP/WHO guidelines on good pharmacy practice: standards for quality of pharmacy services. WHO Technical Report Series, No. 961, 2011. Geneva: World Health Organization, 2011. http://www.fip.org/good_pharmacy_practice. Accessed 17 April 2016.

8

Structured pharmaceutical care improves the health-related quality of life of patients with asthma

Philip O. Anum[1*], Berko P. Anto[2] and Audrey G. Forson[3]

Abstract

Background: Asthma as a chronic health condition can be controlled when in addition to clinical care, adequate education and support is provided to enhance self-management. Like many other chronic health conditions improved self-management positively impacts the health-related quality of life (HRQoL). It can therefore be said that a well-structured pharmaceutical care delivery that addresses the issues related to patient education and support towards self-management stands a good chance of positively impacting asthma control.
This study evaluated the impact of a structured pharmaceutical care delivery on asthma control.

Methods: A prospective pre-/post- intervention study of a single cohort of 77 adult out-patients visiting specialist asthma clinics in Ghana were assessed for HRQoL and peak expiratory flow rates (PEFR) one month after pharmaceutical care intervention. Pharmaceutical care intervention covered education on the health condition, pharmacotherapy and self-management issues as well as correction of inhaler-use technique, where necessary and when to urgently seek medical care. The mean difference of the HRQoL and PEFR values were subjected to paired samples *t*-test analysis.

Results: Delivery of a structured pharmaceutical care led to a significant improvement in asthma specific quality of life and PEFR. The mean paired difference of the HRQoL for a cohort of patients with asthma post- pharmaceutical care intervention was 0.697(95% CI: 0.490 - 0.900) at $t = 6.85$ ($p < 0.05$). The mean paired difference for PEFR post intervention was 17.533 (95% CI: 2.876 - 32.190) at $t = 2.384$ ($p = 0.02$).

Conclusion: This study identified important challenges with both the pharmacologic and the non-pharmacologic management of adult asthma patients. Inadequate inhaler-use skills, widespread occurrence of preventable adverse events and irregular use of preventer medicines were prevalent among patients. At one month after pharmaceutical care intervention, patients with asthma in a cohort follow-up study showed significant improvements with regard to asthma-specific quality of life, peak flow rates and knowledge

Keywords: Asthma, Health-related Quality of Life, Pharmaceutical Care

Background

In the year 2012, non-communicable diseases (NCDs) were responsible for 38 million (68%) of the 56 million global deaths as reported by the World Health Organization (WHO) [1]. This report classified more than 40% of these deaths as premature under the age of 70 years. In Ghana NCDs were reported to have accounted for 42% of total deaths of which about 2% were associated to chronic respiratory diseases [1].

Asthma is a chronic respiratory disease with a rising prevalence within the African region [2]. The Asthma Burden report has indicated that some 50 million cases of asthma are believed to prevail in Africa, with South Africa alone having a prevalence rate of about 8.1% [2]. The findings of the International Study of Asthma and Allergies in Childhood (ISAAC) report (2007) indicated that the international difference in asthma symptom prevalence has generally reduced, particularly in the 13–

* Correspondence: philipanum@gmail.com
[1]National Drug Information Centre, Ministry of Health, Accra, Ghana
Full list of author information is available at the end of the article

14 year age group and with decreases in prevalence in Western Europe [3]. The results however, indicated increases in prevalence in regions where prevalence was previously low, such as in Africa and parts of Asia [3]. These indications of growing trends of asthma in Africa were corroborated by Adeloye and colleagues [4] who also estimated a rising asthma prevalence in Africa,to be in the region of about 74 million to 119.3 million over the past two decades (1990–2010). The incidence rate of asthma in Ghana has however been estimated at 1.5/1000 per year by the WHO [5].

Notwithstanding these levels of occurrence, most health care systems are still organised around the acute care model which does not meet the management needs of patients with NCDs. The WHO-Innovative Care for Chronic Conditions report (2002) has suggested that supported self-management with regular follow-ups in addition to effective treatments improves the outcomes for chronically ill patients [6].

The main stay for asthma management that conforms to this innovative care for NCDs is the continuous monitoring of the patient for asthma control and therapy adjustments that are intended to minimize the symptoms regardless of the severity of the condition [7, 8]. Studies performed by Juniper and colleagues [9] have shown close correlation between the values of the Health-Related Quality of Life (HRQoL) of asthma patients and the levels of their asthma control. On the basis of these advances, various studies on asthma have used the HRQoL to assess the impact of interventions.

These trials, and especially those related to determination of effect of patient education by pharmacists on the outcomes of the disease have shown mixed results [10–16]. Some of these studies have indicated improvements in patient symptom scores [15], quality of life measurements, [15, 17–19] asthma severity [15, 17] and PFR [15, 17, 19]. The extent of the interventions was broad and may have introduced some bias into these studies. Various levels of bias could have been introduced from the drug therapy interventions and PEFR assessments and interpretations from the skills of the pharmacists at the multiple sites for the interventions. Some studies used only asthma severity [15] as primary outcomes measure, while others investigated only some aspects of asthma control [17]. Some of the studies protracted beyond 3 months, [15, 17–19] but did not reasonably resolve the issues of sustainability in such a chronic disease that is influenced by numerous intrinsic and extrinsic factors. The GINA [7] recommendations with regards to continuous monitoring and adjustments of therapy towards asthma control should apply here for pharmacy interventions as well.

Furthermore most of these studies used case–control methods in community settings where the participants in the "case" group cannot be totally isolated from those in the "control" group of the study. In cases where education impacts outcome, then it must be ensured that there is no exchange between the "case" and "control" participants.

It is for these reasons that this researchers opted for a single cohort study and fewer sites to allow only two trained pharmacists to undertake the interventions. The interventions were also only focused on patient understanding of the disease condition, the medications and the appropriate use of the prescribed medications. The study employed the use of the HRQoL instrument as the primary outcome measure of asthma control. Secondary outcomes were the measurements of PEFR and inhalation technique scores. This cohort trial was organised to study the hypothesis that provision of organised pharmaceutical care that focussed on patient education on prescribed medications, would improve asthma control in adult patients.

Methods

Design

A prospective pre-/post- intervention study of a single cohort of adult out-patients visiting specialist asthma clinics in Ghana were assessed for HRQoL and peak expiratory flow rates (PEFR) at baseline and one month after pharmaceutical care intervention. Pharmaceutical care intervention covered education on the health condition, pharmacotherapy and self-management issues as well as correction of inhaler-use technique, where necessary and self-referral for early unscheduled review for worsening asthma condition. The mean differences in HRQoL and PEFR values were subjected to a paired samples *t*-test analysis.

Setting

Four out-patient clinical sites were used in the study. Two were teaching hospitals that managed referral cases from various health institutions and run specialist asthma clinics once a week. The two other hospitals were not teaching hospitals, but one runs specialist asthma clinics. All the clinical sites were located within the southern and middle belts of Ghana.

Sample-size estimation

Assuming a mean HRQoL difference size of 0.5 (the minimum important difference of clinical significance) [20] and a standard deviation of HRQOL score of 0.8 from previous studies in the literature, the calculated standardized effect size (the mean difference / standard deviation) was estimated to be approximately 0.6. To estimate the sample size to test the hypothesis, a power (β) of 0.9 and the level (two-sided) of statistical significance (α) of 0.05 were set. Using these settings, the estimated sample size required for the cohort, when using the paired samples *t*-test to compare means of continuous variables to determine the minimum important difference of 0.5 was 60 patients. A convenience sample of 92 patients was used recruited for the study.

Data collection instrument

Two sets of data collection instruments were used in this study. The Model Pharmaceutical Care Instrument was used to collect data on participant demographics, medication profile, inhaler-use technique, perceived adverse medication events, peak expiratory flow rates symptoms and environmental trigger factors. This was used to guide participant education. Review of this data identified care-needs of every participant in the study. Care needs addressed included: understanding of disease condition and the role of the various medications; inhaler-use technique; issues of medication adherence; availability of medications; management of trigger-factors; management of adverse events, and peak flow meter assessment of lung function.

The standard Asthma Quality of Life Questionnaire (AQLQ(S)) and the Peak Expiratory Flow Meter ("Airzone" flow meter by Clenment Clarke International) were used to assess participant HRQoL and lung function pre and post pharmaceutical care intervention..It was adopted to measure the functional problems (physical, emotional, social and occupational) that are most troublesome to adults (17–70 years) with asthma. The AQLQ(S) is an asthma-specific instrument that had been validated in clinical trials [21]. The AQLQ(S) contains 32 questions (items) comprising four domains: Activity Limitations, Asthma Symptoms, Emotional Function and Environmental Exposure. Each item was scored based on a 2-week recall of activities on a 7-point Likert scale with Point 1 indicating severe impairment and point 7 indicating no impairment. The overall score for HRQoL was the mean score of the 32 items.

A change in mean overall or domain score of 0.5 had been shown to represent the smallest change of importance to the patient (the "minimal important difference"), and a change in score of 1.0 represents a moderate change [20]. However, a maximum overall AQLQ(S) score of 7 represents no impairment in QOL due to asthma, and scores approaching 7 imply a minimal impact of asthma on QOL.

Ethical clearance

Having obtained an ethical clearance from the Ghana Health Service (GHS-ECH: 08/9/11) and participant consent, ninety two (92) adults with symptomatic asthma, without other active co-morbidities, who visited the out-patient clinic, were recruited into the study.

Data collection and intervention

Asthma patients attending regular clinical review in 4 selected hospitals located in the middle and southern belts of Ghana were recruited into the study. Eligibility for participation was limited to patients aged 17–70 years who have been medically diagnosed with asthma and had no active co-morbidities. Excluded in the study were patients whose medications were changed in their previous review visit prior to the recruitment. After giving their consent to participate in the study, a convenience sample of 92 patients was selected by

Table 1 Background characteristics of participants at baseline

	Participants %
Education ($n = 77$)	
Primary School	2.6
High School	48.1
Tertiary	49.4
Symptoms Occurrence ($n = 77$)	
Less than or 2 days in a week	71.4
More than 2 days per week but not daily	16.9
Daily occurrence	11.7
Night-time Awakenings ($n = 77$)	
Less than two times in a month	67.5
Three to four times in a month	15.6
More than once in a week, but not every night	16.9
Use of Reliever Medications for Control ($n = 77$)	
Less than or 2 days in a week	58.4
More than two days in a week but not daily	23.4
Daily use	18.2
Adherence to Prescribed Preventer Medications ($n = 69$)	
Regular usage	56.5
Irregular usage	43.5
Adverse Drug Events Reported ($n = 77$)	
Yes	42.9
No	57.1
Reported Adverse Events with Preventer Medications ($n = 69$)	
Regular Preventer Medicine Usage with Adverse Events	48.7
Regular Preventer Medicine Usage with No Adverse Events	51.3
Irregular Preventer Medicine Usage with Adverse Events	40.0
Irregular Preventer Medicine Usage with No Adverse Events	60.0

Table 2 Incidence of adverse events reported by participants

Adverse Events	Number of Participants	Adverse Events	Number of Participants
Coughs	8	Headache	2
Dry Mouth	6	Palpitations	1
Light Headedness	3	Sweating	1
Chest Burns	3	Phlegm	1
Sore Throat	3	Nasal Congestion	1
Itching	3	Blurred Vision	1
Sneeze	2	Pins & Needles	1
Nausea	2	Neck Pains	1

selecting 10 patients out of a mean attendance of 30 patients per week from 4 hospitals for a period of 12 weeks. These participants were administered with the baseline questionnaires and provided educational intervention. These participants were followed up one month after the interventions. Fifteen (15) participants were lost to follow up. They did not show up for the post-intervention assessments. Therefore data for a total number of 77 patients from the baseline intervention were used for analysis.

Two clinical pharmacists, who were trained for the study, undertook the patient assessment and provided educational intervention. The HRQoL instrument was self-administered by participants. All other participant data was collected with the "Model Pharmaceutical Care" forms. The best of 3 PEFR assessments were entered for each participant. The total score for inhaler-use technique was collated for each participant. Inhaler-use technique score was the sum of one (1) point per each correct step undertaken by participant and observed by the study pharmacist. The maximum total of 7-points score marks were based on the extension of the manufacturers' inhalation steps as found in product leaflets. Based on their inhaler-use technique scores, participants were coached to perform all the steps correctly. The "Model Pharmaceutical Care" forms were used to administer questionnaire on "perceived" environmental trigger factors on individual participant's asthma and adverse effects from their prescribed medications. The impact of asthma with regards to airway narrowing and the roles of "reliever" and "preventer" medicines on the airways were explained to each participant. Participant's knowledge, PEFR and HRQoL were consecutively reassessed in one month after the provision of the interventions.

Data analysis

Data from the study were subjected to both descriptive and inferential statistical analysis. Data were analyzed to generate various tables and charts to demonstrate similar themes, frequencies, trends and number counts under the following themes:

- Baseline Characteristics of Asthma Out-patient Clinic Participants
- Comparison of Asthmatic Patients' Characteristics Post Pharmaceutical Care Intervention

Data collected demonstrated normal distribution with same values for central tendency. Data were therefore analyzed to test the study hypothesis using a paired

Table 3 Participant asthma medication profile

Inhaled Medication(s)	Number of Participants (%)	Patients on Prednisolone with Inhaler Medication(s)
Salbutamol Only	5 (6.5)	-
Salbutamol + beclomethasone	1 (1.3)	-
Salbutamol + pulmicort	8 (10.4)	1
Salbutamol + budesonide/formoterol	37 (48.1)	2
Salbutamol + fluticasone/salmeterol	22 (28.6)	3
Budesonide/Formoterol only	2 (2.6)	-
Fluticasone/salmeterol only	1 (1.3)	-
Salbutamol + Fluticasone/salmeterol + ipratropium	1 (1.3)	1

Table 4 Participant inhaler medication usage

Years of Inhaler Usage	Participant's Inhaler Type (*n* = 77)	
	Reliever (%)	Preventer (%)
≥10 years	31 (42.3)	3 (3.9)
6 –9 years	8 (10.4)	7 (9.1)
1-5 years	27 (35.1)	42 (54.5)
≤1 year	5 (6.5)	18 (23.4)
Cannot recollect	6 (7.8)	7 (9.1)

samples *t*-test; the mean differences in the baseline and post pharmaceutical care intervention HRQoL were analyzed.

Results

General background characteristics at baseline

Study participants were predominantly female (61%) and had a mean age of 46 (±15) years. The mean peak expiratory flow rate was 284(±103) for the 77 participants. Most participants in the study had a minimum of high school education (97.5%) as in Table 1. The daily symptoms occurrence (11.7%) and the night-times awakenings (16.9%) frequencies were similar to reliever medication usage rates (18.2%), however there was a high irregular use (43.5%) of preventer medications (Table 1). Many participants (42.9%) reported one form or the other of various adverse events perceived to be associated to their asthma medicines.

Incidence of adverse events

Participants reported of widespread incidence of adverse drug events perceived to by associated with their asthma medications. Coughs and dry mouth were the most frequently reported incidence of events (Table 2).

Participants' inhaler medication profile

Almost all participants (96%) used Salbutamol inhalers. In addition, Budesonide/formoterol (51%) and Fluticasone/salmeterol (31%) inhalers were used in various combinations (Table 3).

Table 4 presents the number of years participants had used various inhaler types. While 42% of participants had used "Reliever" inhalers for 10 years or more, only 4% of participants had used "Preventer" inhaler for that long. However, 55% of participants had used a "Preventer" for a minimum of one year. Some 6 participants on "Reliever" inhalers and 7 other participants on "Preventer" inhalers could not recollect for how long they had used these medicines.

Participants' inhaler-use technique

Baseline inhaler-use technique score captured using an inhaler-use technique assessment questionnaire, shown in Table 5 indicate that only 12% and 17% of participants on dry powder inhalers (DPI) and metered dose inhalers (MDI) respectively scored the maximum score of 7 points. The mean inhaler-use technique scores were 4.66 (1.3) for the use of DPIs and 5.03(1.43) for the use MDIs.

Environmental trigger-factors affecting participants

Dust (78%), perfume/and strong scents (78%) and smoke (70%) were the most commonly mentioned environmental trigger-factors that worsened the asthma of participants (Table 6). Other trigger-factors like room air-conditioning, fresh cut grass, and alcohol and beer intake affected about 5% of participants.

Post-pharmaceutical care comparison of participant characteristics

The quantum of change in HRQoL is displayed in Table 7. About 56% of participants had a positive change in HRQoL, while 9% had a negative change after the pharmaceutical care intervention. However, about 35% of participants had changes that were not significant.

From Table 8, the paired mean difference values for the HRQoL and all the domains were above 0.5, the mean important difference. The overall paired mean difference for the HRQoL at 95% CI was 0.697 (0.490-0.900) at 95% CI, with a T- value of 6.845 (2-tailed $p < 0.001$). The paired mean difference at 95% CI was highest for the Symptoms domain 1.134 (0.910 – 1.360) and lowest for the Activity Limitation domain 0.548 (0.340 - 0.760).

The mean (PEFR) at baseline was 266.5 L/min (SD 85.9), which increased to 284.0 L/min (SD 103.3) after the intervention (Table 9). The paired mean difference between baseline and post-pharmaceutical care intervention PEFR was 17.5 L/min. (95% CI: 2.876-32.190, $p < 0.05$).

Table 5 Participant inhaler-use technique score

Inhaler Type	Inhaler-use Technique Score (7-point scale)								
	1	2	3	4	5	6	7	*Percentage with Adequate Technique*	*Mean Score (SD)*
DPI[a] (*n* = 66)	0	2	10	23	16	9	8	12.12	4.66(1.3)
MDI[b] (*n* = 63)	0	4	3	13	19	13	12	17.46	5.03(1.43)

[a]*PDI* dry powder inhaler, [b]*MDI* metered dose inhaler

Table 6 Number of participants affected by environmental trigger-factors

Trigger-factor type	Participants Affected (*n* = 77)	Frequency (%)
Dust	60	77.92
Perfume /Scent	60	77.92
Smoke	54	70.13
Food / Spices	21	27.27
Weather Changes	19	24.68
Stress / Tiredness/Emotions	14	18.18
Cold Drinks	11	14.29
Others (beer, fresh cutting grass, alcohol & air-conditioner)	4	5.19

Discussion

Overall participant Inhaler-use technique assessments revealed low scores. Over half of participants in this study had used Salbutamol metered-dose inhaler for more than 5 years, and yet very few had adequate inhaler-use technique to either the dry powder type of inhalers or the metered dose type of inhalers. It is possible that most of the participants had progressed up the therapeutic steps to the use of Salbutamol with Budesonide/formoterol or Fluticasone/salmeterol (step 3) as a result of poor asthma control due to inadequate use of inhalers. In conformity with third Expert Panel Review (EPR-3, 2007) and Global Initiative for Asthma (GINA, 2014) recommendations, usually after a 3-month period of well-controlled asthma there should have been a step down in therapy, [7, 21] but only 12% of patients were on ICS inhalers alone as controller medication. Poor inhaler-use technique and /or poor compliance could be the reason why patient's asthma was not stable enough to be stepped down. The GINA guidelines have suggested that before increasing pharmacologic therapy, one must first consider poor inhaler technique, poor adherence and co-morbidities as targets for intervention [7].

The degree of poor inhaler-use technique identified among study participants indicates that not enough consideration has been given to the role of inhaler-use technique in patient management. It further suggests that there is insufficient patient education and counselling at the clinic and at the pharmacy, and that any education and counselling provided to the study participants in the past clearly did not adequately impact on their skills, or its impact might have diminished with time.

The common major environmental trigger-factor affecting participants in this study were exposure to dust, smoke and perfume or strong scents, which suggests that another major need for intervention is education on the improved control of environmental triggers by patients within their environment.

Previous studies by Mangiapane,and colleagues [18], using a single cohort design, observed significant changes in both HRQoL, and PEFR, among others. This study also, using a single cohort design found significant changes in the HRQoL and the PEFR. Whilst more than half of the study participants' perceived improvements in HRQoL, 9% of them perceived worsened HRQoL and 35% did not perceived any changes in their HRQoL. Though no factual reasons could be assigned immediately, issues related to patient adherence to inhaler medications and the influence of environmental trigger-factors may have played a role. However, the deterioration and the non-significant change in HRQoL might also be explained by the "phenotype of asthma theory". The EPR-3 [8] suggests that very specific patterns of inflammation exist in some individuals that require different treatment approaches in addition to the usual steroid-based anti-inflammatory treatment.

The paired mean difference values for the overall general HRQoL and its various domains were both clinically and statistically significant, showing benefit of the pharmaceutical care intervention to the patients in all aspects of their quality of life. The Symptoms domain had the highest mean change difference of 1.134 (95% CI: 0.910 - 1.360) and the Activity Limitation had the lowest of 0.548 (95% CI: 0.340 – 0.760). This is an indication that the various domains were impacted to different extents within the composite overall HRQoL. Barbanel and colleagues [13] did not use the HRQoL as the outcomes measure when they studied the impact of pharmacists' intervention on asthma patients. They used asthma symptoms and observed significant improvements. This study also observed more significant improvements within the symptoms domain than the other various domains that constituted the composite HRQoL.

However, Mancuso and colleagues [22] found out that these favourable results from pharmacy interventions

Table 7 Quantum changes in quality of life post-pharmaceutical care

Change	Health Related Quality of Life (*n* = 77)						
Quantum	−3	−2	−1	0	1	2	3
Range	−3.49-(−2.50)	−2.49- (−1.50)	−1.49- (−0.50)	−0.49-0.49	0.50-1.49	1.50-2.49	2.50-3.49
Number of Participants (%)	0 (0.00)	1 (1.30)	6 (7.79)	27 (35.06)	29 (37.66)	12 (15.58)	2 (2.60)
Change rate (%) in HRQoL	7 (9.09)			27(35.06)	43(55.84)		
	Negative Change			No Change	Positive Change		

Table 8 Paired mean difference statistics of the health related quality of life of participants after intervention

Health-Related Quality of Life Domain		Mean (SD)	Paired Differences			T	Df	Sig. (2-tailed)
			Mean (SD)	*95% CI of the Difference*				
				Lower	Upper			
HRQoL	Pre-	4.15 (1.132)	0.697 (0.891)	0.490	0.900	6.845	76	0.000
	Post-	4.85 (1.271)						
Activity Limitation	Pre-	4.37 (1.143)	0.548 (0.921)	0.340	0.760	5.256	76	0.000
	Post-	4.92 (1.224)						
Symptoms	Pre-	3.998 (1.086)	1.134 (0.985)	0.911	1.358	10.104	76	0.000
	Post-	5.132 (1.304)						
Emotional Function	Pre-	3.907 (1.453)	0.714 (0.938)	0.501	0.927	6.684	76	0.000
	Post-	4.621 (1.583)						
Environmental Stimuli	Pre-	3.289 (1.562)	0.776 (1.099)	0.526	1.025	6.195	76	0.00
	Post-	4.065 (1.685)						

tended to wane with time if follow-ups were not pursued with participants, as may have been the case with our patients.

This study observed improvements in participants' values at the end of the intervention as with their HRQoL.when PEFR measurements were used as a secondary measure of asthma control. However, analytical exploration of the values indicated only a weak positive correlation between the changes in the overall HRQoL and PEFR from baseline as a result of the intervention. Previous studies by [15, 19] among others, also observed significant improvements in the PEFR within the intervention groups.

PEFR are known to have an a diminished correlation with the FEV1 in patients with asthma, [23] however the EPR- 2007 recommends PEFR monitoring, using the patient's best peak flow in an asthma action plan [21]. The weak correlation between the PEFR with the HRQoL therefore is a reflection of their controversial role in assessing airway obstruction rather than voluntary effort and muscular strength of the patient [23].

Outstanding are the economic implications of such intervention on the cost of asthma management. Further to any clinical significance of educational intervention, patients and health insurance schemes might make savings on asthma-related health care, cost of medications, hospitalization and emergency department visits as envisaged by [24–26]. Future studies may be needed to cost and reflect in monetary terms the savings from the impact of educational interventions in asthma.

Limitations to the study

This study has some limitations. First, the duration of the study did not allow for the participants to be followed-up further to assess duration of the impact of the intervention or to ascertain whether the therapies of the participants with significant improvements in HRQoL were subsequently adjusted in the post- intervention months. The design of this study did not factor duration of impact of the intervention since asthma is a dynamic condition that would require continuous re-evaluation and further education in conformity to the recommendations of GINA and the EPR. Secondly, the AQLQ used in the study to assess HRQoL were not translated into any of the local languages for patients who may not be able to read and write English and thereby limited the scope of patient participation. Furthermore the study covered the southern and middle belts of the country and that may to some extent also limit the overall generalizability of the findings.

Conclusion

This study identified important challenges with both the pharmacologic and the non-pharmacologic management of adult asthma patients. Inadequate inhaler-use skills, widespread occurrence of preventable adverse events and

Table 9 Paired mean difference statistics of peak expiratory flow rate after intervention

		Mean (SD) L/min.	Paired Differences			T	Df	Sig. (2-tailed)
			Mean (SD) L/min.	*95% CI of the Difference*				
				Lower	Upper			
Peak Flow Rate	Pre-	266.467 (85.857)	17.533 (63.705)	2.876	32.190	2.384	74	0.020
	Post-	284.000 (103.294)						

irregular use of preventer medicines were prevalent among patients. At one month after pharmaceutical care intervention, patients with asthma in a cohort follow-up study showed significant improvements with regard to asthma-specific quality of life, peak flow rates and knowledge.

Significance of pharmaceutical services in the hospital

A well-structured pharmaceutical care delivery in the hospital would contribute to patient knowledge and management and eventually improve the health-related quality of life of asthma patients. This study has shown that hospital Pharmacists would need to be properly trained to assess patients with asthma and to provide the needed education to address their individual challenges associated with the condition and the management.

Abbreviations

AQLQ(S): Standardized asthma quality of life questionnaire; DPI: Dry powder inhaler; EPR: Expert panel report; GHS: Ghana Health Service; GINA: Global initiative for asthma; HRQoL: Health related quality of life; MDI: Metered dose inhaler; NCD: Non-communicable disease; PEFR: Peak expiratory flow rate; WHO: World Health Organization; WHO-ICCC: World Health Organization-innovative care for chronic conditions; WHOQOL: World Health Organization Quality of Life

Acknowledgements

The authors wish to acknowledge the Faculty of Pharmacy, Kwame Nkrumah University of Science and Technology, the Komfo Anokye and Kole-bu Teaching hospitals, the Trust Hospital and the Cocoa Clinic for making their facilities, staff and patients available for the study. The authors wish to thank Prof. Juniper for granting us permission to use the Asthma Quality of Life Questionaire in this study.

Funding

This study was self-funded as part of a PhD project.

Authors' contributions

POA, BPA and AGF contributed to the conception and the study design. Acquisition of data was by POA, and the analysis by POA and BPA. POA and AGF drafted the manuscript, and all authors reviewed and approved the final manuscript for submission.

Competing interests

The authors declare that they have no competing interests.

Author details

[1]National Drug Information Centre, Ministry of Health, Accra, Ghana. [2]Department of Clinical and Social Pharmacy, Kwame Nkrumah University of Science and Technology, Accra, Ghana. [3]Department of Medicine, School of Medicine and Dentistry, University of Ghana, Accra, Ghana.

References

1. WHO. Global status report on non-communicable diseases. Geneva. 2014. (http://www.who.int/nmh/publications/ncd_report_full_en.pdf) (Accessed 08 Feb 2016).
2. GINA. (Global Initiative for Asthma). Global Burden of Asthma – Report. 2003. (http://www.globalasthmareport.org/burden/burden.php) (Accessed 08 Feb 2016).
3. ISAAC Group. Worldwide trends in the prevalence of asthma symptoms: Phase III of the International Study of Asthma and Allergies in Childhood (ISAAC). Thorax. 2007;62(9):758–66.
4. Adeloye D, Chan KY, Rudan I, Campbell H. An estimate of asthma prevalence in Africa: a systematic review. Croat Med J. 2013;54(6):519–31.
5. WHO. Public Health and the Environment. Geneva: World Health Organization; Country Profile of Environmental Burden of Disease: Ghana. 2009. (http://www.who.int/quantifying_ehimpacts/national/countryprofile/ghana.pdf) (Assessed 05 Jan 2015).
6. WHO-ICCC. Innovative care for chronic conditions: building blocks for action: World Health Organization- global report, 2002. (http://www.who.int/chp/knowledge/publications/icccreport/en/) (Accessed 10 Dec 2015).
7. GINA (Global Initiative for Asthma). Global Strategy for Asthma Management and Prevention 2014. (http://ginasthma.org/wp-content/uploads/2016/01/GINA_Report_2015_Aug11-1.pdf) (Accessed 12 Mar 2015).
8. EPR-3 (Expert Panel Report). Guidelines for the diagnosis and management of asthma (1997 report). Department of Health and Human Services; National Institutes of Health; National Heart, Lung, and Blood Institute; National Asthma Education and Prevention Program. Bethesda, MD: U.S. 2007. (https://www.nhlbi.nih.gov/health-pro/guidelines/current/asthma-guidelines/full-report) (Accessed 15 Nov 2015).
9. Juniper EF, Chauhan A, Neville E, Chatterjee A, Svensson K, Mörk AC, Ståhl E. Clinicians tend to overestimate improvements in asthma control: an unexpected observation. Prim Care Respir J. 2004;13:181–4.
10. Bynum A, Hopkins D, Thomas A, Copeland N, Irwin C. The effect of telepharmacy counseling on metered-dose inhaler technique among adolescents with asthma in rural Arkansas. Telemed J E Health. 2001;7(3):207–17.
11. Cordina M, McElnay JC, Hughes CM. Assessment of a community pharmacy-based program for patients with asthma. Pharmacotherapy. 2001;21(10):1196–203.
12. Stergachis A, Gardner JS, Anderson MT, Sullivan SD. Improving pediatric asthma outcomes in the community setting: does pharmaceutical care make a difference? J Am Pharm Assoc (Wash). 2002;42(5):743–52.
13. Barbanel D, Eldridge S, Griffiths C. Can a self-management programme delivered by a community pharmacist improve asthma control? A randomized trial. Thorax 2003. 2003;58(10):851–4.
14. McLean W, Gillis J, Waller R. The BC Community Pharmacy Asthma Study: a study of clinical, economic and holistic outcomes influenced by an asthma care protocol provided by specially trained community pharmacists in British Columbia. Can Respir J. 2003;10(4):195–202.
15. Saini B, Krass I, Armour C. Development, implementation, and evaluation of a community pharmacy-based asthma care model. Ann Pharmacother. 2004;38(11):1954–60.
16. Basheti IA, Reddel HK, Armour CL, Bosnic-Anticevich SZ. Counseling about turbuhaler technique: needs assessment and effective strategies for community pharmacists. Respir Care. 2005;50(5):617–23.
17. Armour C, Bosnic-Anticevich S, Brillant M, Burton D, Emmerton L, Krass I, Saini B, Smith L, Stewart K. Pharmacy Asthma Care Program (PACP) improves outcomes for patients in the community. Thorax. 2007;62:496–502.
18. Mangiapane S, Schulz M, Muhlig S, Ihle P, Schubert I, Waldmann HC. Community pharmacy-based pharmaceutical care for asthma patients. Ann Pharmacother. 2005;39(11):1817–22.
19. Schulz M, Verheyen F, Mühlig S, Müller JM, Mühlbauer K, Knop-Schneickert E, Petermann F, Bergmann KC. Pharmaceutical care services for asthma patients: a controlled intervention study. J Clin Pharmacol. 2001;41:668–76.
20. Juniper EF, Guyatt GH, Willan A, Griffith LE. Determining a minimal important change in a disease-specific quality of life instrument. J Clin Epidemiol. 1994;47:81–7.

21. EPR-3 (Expert Panel Report). Guidelines for the diagnosis and management of asthma –a report). Bethesda, Maryland: Department of Health and Human Services; National Institutes of Health; 2007.
22. Mancuso CA, Sayles W, Allegrante JP. Randomized trial of self-management education in asthmatic patients and effects of depressive symptoms. Ann Allergy Asthma Immunol. 2010;105:12–9.
23. Neuspiel DR. Peak flow rate measurement –Medscape (http://emedicine.medscape.com/article/1413347-overview) [Accessed 08 Feb 2015].
24. Teach SJ, Crain EF, Quint DM, Hylan ML, Joseph JG. Improved asthma outcomes in a high-morbidity pediatric population: results of an emergency department–based randomized clinical trial. Arch Paed Adolesc Med. 2006; 160(5):535-51.
25. Cicutto L, Murphy S, Coutts D, O'Rourke J, Lang G, Chapman C, Coates P. Breaking the access barrier: evaluating an asthma center's efforts to provide education to children with asthma in schools. Chest. 2005;128(4):1928–35.
26. Morgan WJ, Crain EF, Gruchalla RS, O'Connor GT, Kattan M, Evans R III, Stout J, Malindzak G, Smartt E, Plaut M, Walter M, Vaughn B, Mitchell H. Inner-City asthma atudy group: Resultsof a home-based environmental intervention among urban children with asthma. N Engl J Med; 2004;351(11):1068–80.

Capacity for ethical and regulatory review of herbal trials in developing countries: a case study of Moringa oleifera research in HIV-infected patients

Tsitsi G. Monera-Penduka[1*], Charles C. Maponga[1], Gene D. Morse[2] and Charles F. B. Nhachi[3]

Abstract

Background: Lack of regulatory capacity limits the conduct of ethical and rigorous trials of herbal medicines in developing countries. Sharing ethical and regulatory experiences of successful herbal trials may accelerate the field while assuring human subjects protection. The methods and timelines for the ethical and regulatory review processes for the first drug regulatory authority approved herbal trial in Zimbabwe are described in this report.

Methods: The national drug regulatory authority and ethics committee were engaged for pre-submission discussions. Six applications were submitted. Application procedures and communications with the various regulatory and ethics review boards were reviewed. Key issues raised and timelines for communications were summarized.

Results: There was no special framework for the approval of herbal trials. One local institutional review committee granted an exemption. Key issues raised for revision were around pre-clinical efficacy and safety data, standardization and quality assurance of the intervention as well as consenting procedures. Approval timelines ranged between eight and 72 weeks.

Conclusions: In the absence of a defined framework for review of herbal trials, approval processes can be delayed. Dialogue between researchers and regulators is important for successful and efficient protocol approval for herbal trials in developing countries.

Keywords: Herbal trial, Regulation, Developing countries

Background

Clinical trials are considered the gold standard in terms of evidence of efficacy and safety of herbal medicine, yet very few trials are conducted in developing countries. Insufficient capacity, including establishment of ethical and regulatory frameworks to support the conduct of herbal trials are often cited as a contributing factor [1, 2].

Current strategies to enhance capacity of researchers in developing countries to conduct ethical and rigorous herbal trials are focused on research training and resource mobilization and have not included sharing experiences involved in successful ethical and regulatory review processes [2, 3].

Clinical studies of herbal medicines should be designed to produce new, beneficial and generalizable knowledge that will improve health outcomes while assuring human subjects protection. However, difficulties in determining shared concepts of social value, scientific validity and favorable risk–benefit ratio, make this challenging. Nevertheless, herbal medicine research must endeavor to achieve a balance between scientific validity and ethics [4]. Public dissemination of ethical and regulatory processes, issues and challenges by researchers involved in herbal trials in developing countries will provide a platform to learn and build capacity for other researchers. In January 2013, the Zimbabwean national

* Correspondence: moneratg@yahoo.co.uk
[1]Drug and Toxicology Information Services (DaTIS), School of Pharmacy, University of Zimbabwe College of Health Sciences, Harare, Zimbabwe
Full list of author information is available at the end of the article

drug regulatory authority approved the first trial with a herbal intervention; the Moringa oleifera supplementation by patients on antiretroviral therapy (MOART) study. In this article we describe the ethical and regulatory processes that were involved; including the human subject protection issues raised and the time taken to acquire the requisite approvals. This experience should stimulate discussion and facilitate the set up of regulatory and ethical frameworks to support the conduct of herbal trials in other developing countries.

Methods

Description of the herbal trial

The MOART study was conducted by scientists from the University of Zimbabwe to determine if antiretroviral drugs are affected by concurrent intake of *Moringa oleifera* Lam, a frequently taken dietary supplement in Zimbabwe. This is important because herbal medicines may interact with conventional medicine resulting in increased or decreased drug exposure. The drugs nevirapine and efavirenz were studied. Both drugs are routinely used as part of combination therapy for treating HIV. The study was an intensive pharmacokinetic sampling study which compared pre- and post *Moringa oleifera* Lam. plasma concentration profiles of efavirenz and nevirapine in HIV-infected people on antiretroviral therapy. Moringa was administered as a standardized dry leaf powder in a one sequence cross-over, open label, phase I/IIa, observational study that was conducted over 35 days. Venous whole blood and urine were sampled after a 21-day washout period as well as on day 35 following 14 days of moringa supplementation. Compliance to medication and supplementation restrictions was assessed through reported adherence, pill counts and evaluation of a food/herb/medication diary. The trial is registered with clinicaltrials.gov NCT01410058.

Ethical and regulatory framework

In Zimbabwe, there are three regulatory bodies involved in clinical research, namely the Medicines Control Authority of Zimbabwe (MCAZ), the Medical Research Council of Zimbabwe (MRCZ) and the Research Council of Zimbabwe (RCZ). MCAZ is the national drug regulatory (NDRA) authority which approves and monitors all clinical trials in Zimbabwe in terms of Part III of the Medicines and Allied Substances Control Act [Chapter 15:03]. It has a well-established framework encompassing trial approval procedures and conduct guidelines, reporting standards and access to clinical trial and pharmacovigillence experts.

Before an application for the conduct of a conventional trial can be submitted to the NDRA, the protocol needs to go through ethical review by the ethics committees of the institutions responsible for the trial (IERC). Thereafter, parallel submissions to the the national ethics committee (NEC) and the NDRA may be made. The MRCZ is the NEC. It was established by the Government of Zimbabwe Notice No. 225 of 1974 and approves and provides ethical oversight for all health research.

When the protocol has a foreign co-investigator or planned bio-specimen shipment outside Zimbabwe, additional review and approval by the national research council (NRC) is required. The RCZ is the NRC. It is a statutory body established by the Research Act [Chapter 10:22] which promotes research in all fields and coordinates foreign/and or foreign funded research. All applications involving health research made to the NRC must go through the MRCZ.

The MCAZ, the MRCZ and the RCZ have publicly available guidelines based on the Declaration of Helsinki, the Council of International Organizations of the Medical Sciences (CIOMS) Guidelines as well as the International Conference on Harmonization for Good Clinical Practice guidelines.

Herbal protocol review procedures

At the onset, we engaged the MCAZ and the MRCZ in pre-submission discussions and established that there was no special framework for the approval of herbal trials. We were advised to work within the framework for conventional trials.

Following the conventional trial framework, four ethical and regulatory approvals were required for the MOART trial. First, ethical approval was sought from the principal investigator's institution. Upon approval by the IERCs, further applications were made to the national ethics committee, followed by the national drug regulatory authority. Due to unplanned bio-specimen shipment necessitated by limited capacity for one of the analyses, bio-specimen shipment approval also had to be sought from the NRC.

During the course of the applications the funding collaborators also indicated that their institutions required the protocol to be submitted to them for ethical review. Subsequently, two further ethical review applications were submitted to the institution of the foreign collaborating funder; as well as the institution of a local collaborating funder, bringing the total number of ethical and regulatory review submissions to six. However, the IERC for the local collaborator granted an exemption for ethics review. The exemption was based on the fact that another local IERC (IERC1) had already granted approval and the NEC was also reviewing the protocol.

The local regulatory and ethics committees reviewed a draft of the manuscript for accuracy.

Results and discussion

Feedback from the presubmission discussions

During the presubmission discussions the NDRA and NEC personnel directed the researchers to the complete set of forms and submissions required for the conventional trial application. Guidance was sought on how to best adapt our responses to fields on the forms that were originally intended for conventional trials. Discussions regarding fields related to the trial (herbal) intervention as well as existing preliminary data were particularly useful in marrying our planned approach to that of the regulators. This improved the efficiency with which the application package was submitted.

Further information requested to support initial applications

The researchers were requested to provide additional information on several aspects by the 5 bodies (Table 1). Some issues were raised as recommendations to improve understanding of the study documents while others were required as corrections. The three ethics committees recommended that more detailed descriptions of study procedures be given in both the protocol and the informed consent document. In addition, the IREC2 required a more detailed plan for adverse events monitoring and reporting. Both the requests were straightforward and constituted standard clarification and detail issues applicable in any clinical trial protocol. The initial protocol therefore was not complete and the oversight of the ethics committee was valuable. The missing details were all addressed satisfactorily in the first responses.

In addition, the NDRA, NRC and the IERC2 required justification and corrections around pre-clinical efficacy and safety data, standardization and quality assurance of the intervention as well as consenting procedures. These requests constitute the more challenging issues around scientific validity of research, risk-benefit assessments and informed consent that are commonly cited as core considerations for herbal trial protocols [4, 5]. Regarding preclinical data, the issue raised was that there were no published studies assessing the effect of moringa on efavirenz or nevirapine whose positive findings would typically inform the need for a human study. In response, reference was made to two World Health Organization (WHO) guidelines for research on traditional medicine, which recommend a rapid response research mechanism for herbs. The guidelines cite prior voluntary use of herbal medicines and documented experience of long-term use without evidence of safety problems as is the case with *Moringa oleifera,* as a basis of the risk assessment [6, 7]. Additional preclinical studies assessing the effect of Moringa on metabolic pathways shared by efavirenz and nevirapine with positive findings were also added to the protocol to augment the safety data.

In the initial application, we had proposed to use a single batch of Moringa from the most commonly cited local supplier to maintain generalizability of the findings. The NDRA however highlighted the need to use *Moringa oleifera* of verified and reproducible quality and required that measures be put in place and stated explicitly that would guarantee the integrity of the intervention. Previous herbal medicine reviews have cited product quality and standardization as a common challenge, particularly in light of the need to preserve external validity [4, 8]. At the time of the application, the NDRA did not regulate herbal medicine and did not cite any specific quality criteria to address the quality issue. Following the WHO Guidelines for assessing herbal medicines we assessed three different batches of moringa from the local market for microbial contamination and heavy metal content. Unfortunately, all three failed to meet the WHO criteria [9]. We then proposed an alternative approach which involved processing a batch of moringa leaf powder using good manufacturing practice (GMP) principles specifically for the trial, which would then be externally assessed for quality before proceeding with the trial. This was acceptable to the NDRA. The batch was subsequently processed by the School of Pharmacy and externally assessed for microbial and heavy metal contamination in the Departments of Biological Sciences and Chemistry laboratories respectively.

At the time of protocol approval all analysis was planned locally and as a result the consent form did not

Table 1 Further information requested to support initial applications

Domain	IERC 1	IERC 2	NDRA	NEC	NRC
Details of research procedures	X	X	X	X	
Details of informed/storage consent	X	X		X	
Reimbursement		x	x		
Details of research design		X	X		
Pre-clinical data to justify human studies			X		
Details of adverse event monitoring		X			
Details of product standardization and quality		X	X		
Adequacy of clinical trial site infrastructure			X		
Re-consenting of participants for specimen shipment					X

cover aspects of specimen shipment. When application was made to the NRC for bio specimen shipment approval, the NEC required additional consent from participants with the affected analysis before approval could be granted. This was done through targeted contact at routine HIV clinic visits and support group meetings.

Divergent requirements

The IERC2 required the use of their 'standard statement for reimbursement' for consent which stated that, *"In the unlikely event that you become ill or injured as a direct result of participating in this study, you understand that you may receive medical care, but it will not be free of charge even if the injury is a direct result of my participation"*. This request was not necessarily unique to herbal trials but comes up often in collaborative trials. It becomes important to discuss in this context because many herbal trials in developing countries will be collaborative with developed countries coming in as the funders [10].

While the statement was consistent with consent documents for other studies conducted in the United States of America [11], it was not compliant with the Helsinki declaration and CIOMS. It was also not in line with the NEC recommendation, which states *"In the event of injury resulting from your participation in this study, treatment shall be offered by the study"*. Globally, there is no consensus on the issue of compensation for research related injuries [12]. One school of thought says that because a participant has accepted that there may be risks and harms that can occur as a part of the study, they should not be compensated in case of an injury [13]. The other says that the consent process cannot be extrapolated to argue that the participant also consents to be harmed during the trial, as risk and harm are often unknown and unexpected and should be compensated [13, 14]. In response we highlighted the differences in health insurance frameworks in the local context that made the NEC require free medical treatment or participant insurance for all research participants. In addition, we highlighted that the requirements of the ethics committee of the study setting should take precedence over the foreign collaborator ones. The response was acceptable to the IERC2. In fact, current versions of their 'standard statement for reimbursement' now incorporate some exemptions for covering costs for research-related injurues. Our experience supports previous publications that have recommended democratic deliberations between researchers and regulators to resolve challenges in herbal medicine research [4].

Approval timelines

Figure 1 shows the distribution of the time taken to get approval between researchers and reviewers. The data incorporates weekends and public holidays.

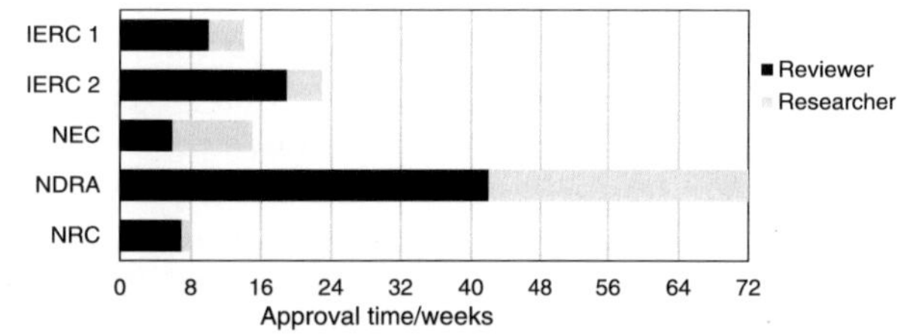

Fig. 1 Time taken to obtain approvals. The *black bars* represent the time taken by the reviewer, while the *grey bars* represent the researcher's response time

Delay in ethical and regulatory approval extends the duration of a trial, thereby increasing its cost and potentially risk losing relevance. This often causes tension between researchers and ethics committees [15]. The NEC review had the shortest review committee turnaround time. Ethics committee turnaround time is usually implicated in protocol approval delays [15]; contrary to the current experience in the NEC time was shorter that the respective researcher time. This could be attributed to it being the only committee that had published turnaround times for review of applications, indicating that they have put some thought and effort into improving their efficiency.

The deliberations with the NDRA however took over a year. The NDRA had the responsibility to thoroughly assess existing evidence and quality assurance. The apparent delay may have therefore have improved the protection of participants. Delays in meeting review timelines maybe justified complex protocols where there is need to study the application in-depth, or to get additional essential information from the applicant and to avoid unjustified risks. The distribution in the response time between the researchers and the regulators was 59:41% indicating that the issues raised demanded significant processing time from both reviewers and researchers. For instance, the issue of guaranteeing product quality required assessing several possible options before reverting to the NDRA. This mirrors the current global debate on the complex regulation issues associated with trials of herbal medicines [4, 8].

At the end of 2016, the Ministry of Health and Child Care in Zimbabwe set up a Complementary and Traditional Medicine Research Committee that would going forward, sit to review traditional medicine research including clinical trials. The move will go long way to promote successful and efficient protocol approval for future herbal trials in Zimbabwe.

Some time was also lost due to slow administrative procedures such as delays in delivery responses of interim communications or notification of researchers to collect the same. The results should be interpreted in light of the limitation that the data is from one study, being the only clinical trial of a herbal medicine approved by the NDRA.

Recommendations

There is a need to develop some guidance for the ethical and regulatory review of clinical trials with herbal interventions. The WHO guidelines on research on traditional medicine could be used as a reference to develop an adapted national regulation. This is particularly important for aspects of clinical trials that differ between "modern" and "traditional" medicines, such as pre-clinical data, standardization and quality assurance of the intervention.

Pre-submission discussions to clarify correct application procedures and identification of key areas can facilitate efficient and successful reviews.

Open and transparent engagement between researchers, ethics committees and regulators during the application process can facilitate resolution of ethical challenges in herbal trial protocols. This is applicable to deliberations between researchers and local as well as international regulators.

Publication of target turn around times for the different type of applications is a strategy that could be employed by other regulatory and ethics review bodies to monitor their efficiency and assist with researchers planning.

Conclusion

As far as can be ascertained, this report is the first to describe the ethical and regulatory approval processes of setting up a herbal clinical trial in a developing country. The experiences highlight the importance of dialogue between researchers and regulators for successful and efficient protocol approval for herbal trials in developing countries.

Abbreviations

IERC: Institutional ethics review committee; IERC1: Local institutional ethics review committee; IERC2: Foreign collaborating institutional ethics review committee; MCAZ: Medicines Control Authority of Zimbabwe; MOART: Moringa oleifera supplementation by patients on antiretroviral therapy; MRCZ: Medical Research Council of Zimbabwe; NDRA: National drug regulatory authority; NEC: National ethics committee; NRC: National research council; RCZ: Research Council of Zimbabwe; WHO: World Health Organization

Acknowledgements

The authors thank Alan Wolfe who provided insight that greatly assisted the research.

Funding

This publication was made possible by grant numbers 2U2RTW007367 and D43TW007991-01A2 from the Office of Global AIDS Coordinator and the U. S. Department of Health and Human Services, (National Institutes of Health (Fogarty International Centre). The two agencies funded the data collection. Its contents are solely the responsibility of the authors and do not necessarily represent the official views of the government.

Authors' contributions

TM was responsible for the conception of the study, its design, data collection, drafting of the manuscript and analysis of data. CN assisted in the design of the study, supervised the work, contributed to the analysis of data, revised the draft critically and gave final approval of the version to be published. GM contributed to the design of the study, the analysis of data, revised the draft critically and gave final approval of the version to be published. All authors read and approved the final manuscript.

Competing interests

The authors declare that they have no competing interests.

Author details

[1]Drug and Toxicology Information Services (DaTIS), School of Pharmacy, University of Zimbabwe College of Health Sciences, Harare, Zimbabwe. [2]Center for Integrated Global Biomedical Sciences, University at Buffalo, Buffalo, New York, USA. [3]Department of Clinical Pharmacology, University of Zimbabwe College of Health Sciences, Harare, Zimbabwe.

References

1. Siegfried NL, Hughes G. Herbal medicine, randomised controlled trials and global core competencies. S Afr Med J. 2012;102(12):912–3.
2. Willcox M, Siegfried N, Johnson Q. Capacity for clinical research on herbal medicines in Africa. J Altern Complement Med. 2012;18(6):622–8.
3. Davies J, Mullan Z. Research capacity in Africa—will the sun rise again? Lancet Glob Health. 2016;4(5):e287.
4. Tilburt JC, Kaptchuk TJ. Herbal medicine research and global health: an ethical analysis. Bull World Health Organ. 2008;86(8):594–9.
5. Koonrungsesomboon N and Karbwang J. Ethical considerations in clinical research on herbal medicine for prevention of cardiovascular disease in the ageing. Phytomed. 2015;doi: 10.1016/j.phymed.2015.10.017.
6. World Health Organisation. Guidelines for Clinical Study of Traditional Medicines in the WHO Africa region, WHO Regional Office for Africa: India. 2004. http://apps.who.int/medicinedocs/en/d/Js21350en/. Accessed 27 April 2016.
7. Stohs SJ, Hartman MJ. Review of the safety and efficacy of Moringa oleifera. Phytother Res. 2015;29(6):796–804.
8. Smith CA, Priest R, Carmady B, Bourchier S, Bensoussan A. The ethics of traditional Chinese and Western herbal medicine research: views of researchers and human ethics committees in Australia. Evid Based Complement Alternat Med. 2011;doi:10.1155/2011/256915.
9. Mudzengi J, Monera TG, Nhachi CFB. Microbial and heavy metal content of selected herbal medicines commonly used by HIV patients in Zimbabwe. J Appl Sci South Afr. 2013;19(i):28–42.
10. Ravinetto R, De Nys K, Boelaert M, Diro E, Meintjes G, Adoke Y, etal. Sponsorship in non-commercial clinical trials: definitions, challenges and the role of Good Clinical Practices guidelines. BMC Int Health Hum Rights. 2015;15 (34).doi: 10.1186/s12914-015-0073-8.
11. Hochhauser M. Paying for research related injuries in the US. BMJ. 2006; 332(7541):610.
12. Pandya M, Desai C. Compensation in clinical research: the debate continues. Perspect Clin Res. 2013;4(1):70–4.
13. Munshi R and Thatte U. Compensation for research related injury. Perspect Clin Res. 2013. doi: 10.4103/2229-3485.106392.
14. Grant RW, Sugarman J. Ethics in human subjects research: Do incentives matter? J Med Philos. 2004;29:717–38.
15. Adams P, Kaewkungwal J, Limphattharacharoen C, Prakobtham S, Pengsaa K, Khusmith S. Is your ethics committee efficient? Using "IRB Metrics" as a self-assessment tool for continuous improvement at the Faculty of Tropical Medicine, Mahidol University, Thailand. PLoS One. 2014;9(11):e113356.

10

Individual capacity-building approaches in a global pharmaceutical systems strengthening program

Niranjan Konduri[1*], Megan Rauscher[2], Shiou-Chu Judy Wang[1] and Tanya Malpica-Llanos[1]

Abstract

Background: Medicines use related challenges such as inadequate adherence, high levels of antimicrobial resistance and preventable adverse drug reactions have underscored the need to incorporate pharmaceutical services to help achieve desired treatment outcomes, and protect patients from inappropriate use of medicines. This situation is further constrained by insufficient numbers of pharmaceutical personnel and inappropriate skill mix. Studies have addressed individual capacity building approaches of logistics, supply chain or disease specific interventions but few have documented those involving such pharmacy assistants/professionals, or health workers/ professionals charged with improving access and provision of pharmaceutical services. We examined how different training modalities have been employed and adapted to meet country-specific context and needs by a global pharmaceutical systems strengthening program in collaboration with a country's Ministry of Health and local stakeholders.

Methods: Structured, content analysis of training approaches from twelve selected countries and a survey among conveniently selected trainees in Bangladesh and Ethiopia.

Results: Case-based learning, practice and feedback, and repetitive interventions such as post-training action plan, supportive supervision and mentoring approaches are effective, evidence-based training techniques. In Ethiopia and Bangladesh, over 94% of respondents indicated that they have improved or developed skills or competencies as a result of the program's training activities. Supportive supervision structures and mentorship have been institutionalized with appropriate management structures. National authorities have been sensitized to secure funding from domestic resources or from the global fund grants for post-training follow-up initiatives. The Pharmaceutical Leadership Development Program is an effective, case-based training modality that motivates staff to develop quality-improvement interventions and solve specific challenges. Peer-to-peer learning mechanisms than traditional didactic methods was a preferred intervention among high level government officials both within country and between countries.

Conclusion: Interventions must involve local institutions in the design and delivery of content for both pre-service and in-service training as well as web-based methods where feasible. Such efforts would meet the changing demand in the pharmaceutical system, and promote the ownership of the human capacity development interventions. The cost-effective partnership with universities demonstrate that competency based pre-service training will prepare the future pharmaceutical workforce with a critical foundation of knowledge and skills required to meet the growing demand for patient-centered pharmaceutical services in resource-constrained countries.

Keywords: Human resources, Pre-service training, In-service training, Pharmaceutical systems, Pharmaceutical services, Capacity building

* Correspondence: nkonduri@msh.org
[1]Systems for Improved Access to Pharmaceuticals and Services (SIAPS) Program, Management Sciences for Health, Arlington, VA, USA
Full list of author information is available at the end of the article

Background

The Sustainable Development Goal 3.8 of the 2030 Agenda for Sustainable Development specifies that in order to achieve universal health coverage, national development strategies must include "access to safe, effective, quality and affordable medicines and vaccines for all" [1]. The Lancet commission on essential medicines for universal health coverage acknowledged that professionals such as pharmacists and prescribers as well as dispensers need specialized training and information to assure the appropriate use of medicines in the interest of patients and caregivers [2]. Beyond access, medicines use related challenges such as inadequate adherence [3], high levels of antimicrobial resistance [4] and the impact of preventable adverse drug reactions [5] have underscored the need to incorporate patient-oriented pharmaceutical services that help to achieve desired treatment outcomes and protect patients from harm [6, 7]. This situation is further constrained by insufficient numbers of pharmaceutical personnel and incomplete or inappropriate skill mix to respond to the needs of local populations [8, 9].

The Systems for Improved Access to Pharmaceuticals and Services program (the 'program') funded by the U.S. Agency for International Development (USAID) works in partnership with local governments and partners to build resilient pharmaceutical systems that deliver safe, timely, and quality pharmaceuticals and healthcare services, through a pharmaceutical systems strengthening approach [10, 11]. The program's overall capacity building approach was adapted from Potter and Brough's "Pyramid of Effective Needs" and includes nine interrelated components [12, 13]. The components are categorized into individual (performance capacity and personal capacity) and institutional (workload, facility, supervisory, support service, structural, systems, and role capacity). Potter and Brough assert that developing a common definition of capacity building is challenging because of different sociocultural settings. Instead, establishing a hierarchy of capacity-building needs is more useful for designing and implementing activities to address varied capacity gaps.

Pharmaceutical systems in resource-constrained countries are challenged by limited number of institutions for pharmaceutical training and lack of up-to-date training curricula. Using locally relevant and context specific training approaches, the program aims to build and augment individual capacity building interventions to ensure that the pharmaceutical health workforce has the right skill mix and distribution to meet population needs and the appropriate tools to do so. Published studies have addressed individual capacity building approaches of logistics, supply chain [14] or disease specific interventions [15]. However, to our knowledge, from a global program implementer perspective, few have documented the programmatic approach of building individual capacity involving pharmacy professionals, pharmacy assistants or health workers charged with improving access and provision of pharmaceutical services. The objective of this paper is to summarize the various approaches that have been implemented by the program in collaboration with a country's Ministry of Health and local stakeholders, and examine the influence of the training on individual capacity, as defined by Potter and Brough. Using selected, specific country examples, we examined how different training modalities have been employed and adapted to meet country-specific context and needs.

Methods

Twelve program implementing countries were selected for review based on internal funding availability during the study period June to December 2015: Angola, Bangladesh, Burundi, Cameroon, Democratic Republic of the Congo [DR Congo], Ethiopia, Mali, Namibia, Philippines, South Africa, Swaziland, and Ukraine. We retrieved documentation from the first 3 years of program implementation that was available between 2012 and 2015. We performed a structured, content analysis of training activities from the program's topic specific technical reports, quarterly and annual reports. Internal reports from a one-off training event or multi-event training series were reviewed, which typically provide the training objectives and training methods employed. Country-specific technical reports that contained information on an intervention with a training component were reviewed. After desk review of project documents, each country or portfolio was contacted for the purpose of clarifying content or seeking elaboration on any training methodologies if not documented in sufficient detail. Through our country program, we conducted a survey among conveniently selected trainees in Bangladesh and Ethiopia due to the large number of pharmaceutical personnel trained (Additional file 1 provides details on the methodology). In-country program staff also conducted key informant interviews with 11 authorities in Bangladesh and 19 authorities in Ethiopia who were part of the training initiatives. Institutional permission was obtained from the Ministry of Health personnel based on our country program's ongoing monitoring and evaluation mechanism.

Results

The program's individual capacity building approaches can broadly be grouped into three categories: pre-service, in-service and proven approaches for individual capacity building. Pre-service training is defined as activities that take place before a person starts a job that requires specific training [16], i.e., before a person "enters service" whereas in-service training is considered training of persons who are already employed, e.g., health care providers working in the public or private sector [17]. Drawing upon lessons learned from our predecessor Strengthening Pharmaceutical Systems program (2007–2011) [18], this paper presents the following proven approaches to individual capacity building as applied to either pre-service or in-service training approaches: supportive supervision [19, 20], team based and peer-to-peer learning mechanisms [21, 22], e-learning and blended learning [23]. The program has utilized blended learning models (a combination of face-to-face and virtually facilitated sessions) to scale up the delivery of training activities in a cost-effective, sustainable manner, especially in collaboration with local institutions.

Pre-service training approaches

A key impediment to the scale-up of pharmaceutical services to address the HIV burden in Namibia was the shortage of skilled pharmaceutical personnel, including pharmacists and pharmacy assistants [24]. To increase the number of qualified pharmaceutical professionals, the program supported two major pre-service activities: the development of a local Bachelor of Pharmacy (B Pharm) degree [25], and revamping accompanying training curricula and supporting the training efforts of the National Health Training Centre (Fig. 1) [26]. By 2014, the number of enrolled B Pharm students increased to 107, and the first 14 graduated received their B Pharm degree in 2015. Details on the process of establishing Namibia's first school of pharmacy is available in the program website [27, 28]. A wide range of support to improve the quality of pre-service training for B Pharm students and pharmacist assistants was provided, including curriculum revision, recruitment of pharmacy lecturers, information technology assistance, accreditation and quality management system support [29, 30].

In DR Congo, the program's partner, the Accreditation Council for Pharmaceutical Education (ACPE) [31], reviewed the pharmacy school curriculum at the University of Kinshasa and developed a road map for updating and implementing a revised curriculum that meets international standards [32]. DR Congo's vision is to prepare competent pharmacists who can better address public health priorities, particularly in the areas of supply chain management, appropriate use of medicines, pharmaceutical services, pharmacovigilance and antimicrobial resistance. National stakeholders recognized this intervention as a high-impact activity with the results spinning off on the other three faculties of pharmacy in the country and the National Pharmacy Council, thereby influencing pharmacy education and practice in the whole country, including the private sector. Thereafter, the program supported the University of Kinshasa to develop a 5-year strategic plan to improve the coordination, monitoring, and evaluation of faculty operations and to develop a competency framework [33], which defines required cognitive, procedural, and behavioral competencies that graduated pharmacists should have upon completion of their degree (Fig. 2) [34].

This competency framework was a major step in overhauling current training curricula and recognized by the USAID's Mission Director in DR Congo (quote): "*To improve the pharmaceutical sector, we must address the root of the problem, which is pharmacist training*" [35]. Table 1 summarizes key results in Namibia and DR Congo.

In-service training approaches

Globally, as of December 2015, 35 in-service training curricula had been developed or revised in 11 countries with the program's support. Nearly 39,000 individuals (31% female, 62% male) in over 24 countries (Table 2) had been trained in various aspects of pharmaceutical management, including: financing, leadership, regulatory systems, quality assurance, pharmaceutical care, medicine safety, antimicrobial resistance, and supply chain management.

The program seeks to ensure that its capacity-building efforts address immediate country needs to empower and enable country governments and local institutions to develop, implement, and own the technical assistance and capacity-building efforts. Globally, as of December 2015, the program facilitated 394 local institutions or organizations to provide training or technical assistance in pharmaceutical management.

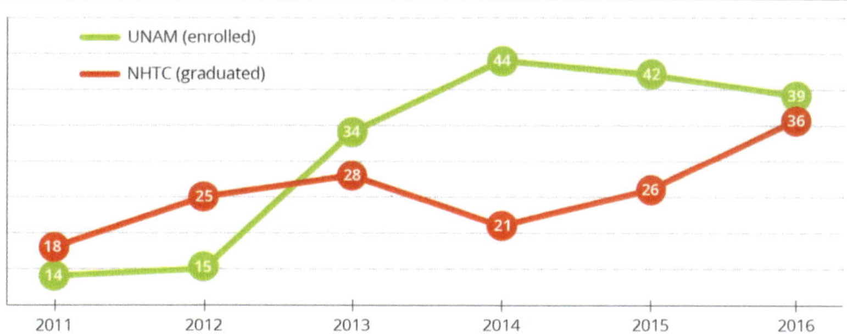

Fig. 1 Number of pharmacist assistants graduating from the National Health Training Center, by year of graduation

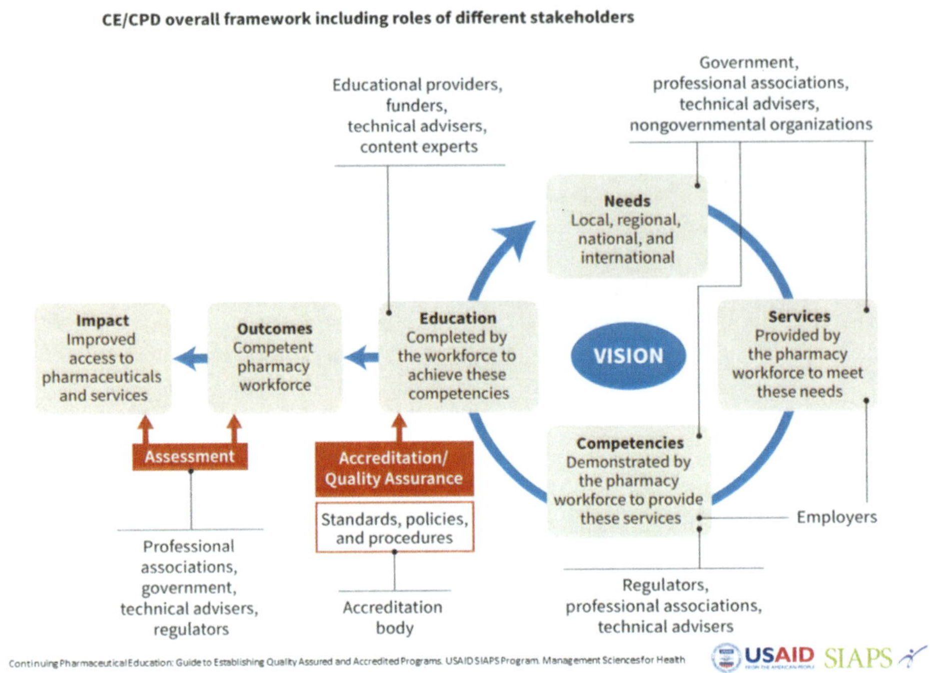

Fig. 2 Continuing Education and Continuing Professional Development Framework, including Roles of Different Stakeholders

Cascade training approaches

To strengthen sustainability efforts, the program often employs a cascade training approach to rapidly develop new knowledge or skills in specific pharmaceutical management topics and capacitate national staff in local

Table 1 Relevant Results (Namibia and DR Congo)

	As of December 2015	Key Results
Namibia	41% increase in the number of certified pharmacy personnel 97% of public health facilities are staffed with certified pharmacy personnel	• B Pharm and PA competency framework developed • Accreditation for B Pharm program and PA courses received • B Pharm program launched in 2011 • The majority (75%) of the pharmacist assistants reported overall satisfaction with their PA training at the NHTC • Over 90% of the employers and supervisors were satisfied with the pharmacist assistants' performance at work
DR Congo	1103 persons trained in pharmaceutical management 2 health or allied health professional associations or councils receiving TA in pharmaceutical management education	• Pre-service competency framework developed with 5-year strategic plan

Table 2 Number of Personnel Trained in Pharmaceutical Management, as of December 2015

Country/portfolio	Number trained
Angola	251
Bangladesh	15,594
Burundi	2890
Cameroon	741
Dominican Republic	2232
DR Congo	1103
Ethiopia	5110
Guinea	796
Latin America and Caribbean Amazon Malaria Initiative	554
Lesotho	438
Mali	1593
Mozambique	579
Namibia	501
Neglected tropical diseases core portfolio	35
Philippines	358
South Africa	1087
South Sudan	864
Swaziland	1092
Tuberculosis core portfolio	2695
Turkmenistan	22
Ukraine	280
West Africa Regional	120
Total	38,935

institutions. In an effort to address the high burden of multidrug-resistant tuberculosis, the program and National Tuberculosis Program (NTP) staff piloted training on the e-TB Manager (web-based tool for managing all the information needed by national TB control programs) in three oblasts (states) of Ukraine, which resulted in a decision to scale up the use of e-TB Manager nationwide [36]. Given the country's large size and the resource intensive nature of scale up, a training of trainers (TOT) approach was selected to more efficiently cascade the training across the country. The program engaged a local Ukrainian group specializing in adult learning techniques and TOT methodologies and paired it with NTP staff, with the objective of developing the competencies of oblast-level officials who would run the e-TB Manager educational programs and also assure ownership of the intervention. While interactive methods of training are generally quite new to Ukraine's public-sector health professionals, competency-based methodologies were employed. The TOT session was conducted over a 5-day period, with the first half focusing on adult learning methodologies and the second half on the core technical content of e-TB Manager. A series of six TOT sessions were organized and carried out, involving more than 100 key officials and the NTP program staff. Results of the trainings are summarized in Table 3 [37].

In Mali, essential medicines and health commodities are frequently unavailable at various levels of the health system due to inefficient and poorly coordinated forecasting and quantification processes. To address these challenges, the program intervened to improve the individual capacity of senior leaders and administrators of key pharmaceutical institutions to redesign and roll out an improved Logistics Management Information System (LMIS). Training activities focused on strengthening the technical capacity of managers at all levels in the LMIS-related activities. During training activities, individuals and teams developed plans to support activity implementation. As a key follow-up activity, a joint government and program team visited several health districts to collect information on the status of individual implementation plans. Using coaching and supervision techniques, individual plans were evaluated by the team and shortcomings addressed. In many of the facilities, trained staff satisfactorily implemented at least one activity in their action plan, including: 1) good storage practices; 2) correct filing; and 3) management and submission of LMIS reports. Table 4 includes selected indicators related to training activities in Mali from 2013 to 2014.

Table 3 Relevant Results (Ukraine)

By December 2015	Milestones
225,000 MDR-TB cases were in the e-TB Manager system More than 100 oblast officials reached over 1200 users in 26 oblasts Consistency between paper-based and electronically generated reports was about 99%	• TOT curriculum developed • E-TB Manager training scaled up nationally • Full transfer of the operation, administration, and development support of the e-TB manager was transferred from the program to the Government of Ukraine in 2015

Proven approaches for individual capacity building

The program has applied participatory, team-oriented learning approaches that incorporate continuous feedback processes and group problem-solving by using local human resources and skillsets. These include task shifting structures, implementing continuous quality improvement measures, engaging the private sector, exploring online learning platforms, and placing an emphasis on effective knowledge sharing and exchange.

Supportive supervision

The program assists governments and in-country counterparts to design and implement a supportive supervision plan and helps to conduct supportive supervision visits [38]. For example, in Lesotho, the program mentored 24 health care workers in the management of laboratory commodities, and conducted 135 supportive supervision visits to health facilities for LMIS and nutrition assessment counseling in three implementing districts, contributing to improved reporting rates, from 4 to 95% between two quarters [39]. In Swaziland 12 annual supportive supervision visits and mentorship in

Table 4 Relevant Results (Mali)

By December 2015	Milestones
1593 persons trained in pharmaceutical management	• Developed new LMIS that includes the community level • Developed training materials, tools, and job aids for the new LMIS • Increased percentage of stock records that correspond with physical counts for a set of indicator medicines in Ministry of Health storage and at health facilities, from 16% in 2013 to 42% in 2014 • Decreased percentage of warehouses with stock-outs of a pre-selected group of medicines for 3 days or more in the last 3 months, from 89% in 2013 to 66% in 2014 • Increased percentage of health facilities that completed and submitted an LMIS report for the most recent reporting period, from 7% in 2013 to 33% in 2014

131 health facilities contributed to increased LMIS reporting rate from 55% in 2012 to 95% in 2015. As a result of improved information quality, national authorities were able to make timely decisions and saved the government close to 6.25 million dollars in unnecessary procurement of medicines and commodities [40].

Peer-to-peer learning mechanisms

Peer-to-peer learning mechanisms have been applied in specific circumstances. In Ukraine, the program facilitated a practical, interactive training approach rather than employing a traditional didactic method to train individuals in framework contracting in the pharmaceutical sector [41]. In Dnipropetrovsk oblast, authorities launched eight bids in framework contracting; six were successful. Thereafter the program brought the Dnipropetrovsk authorities to Poltava oblast, so that Poltava oblast authorities could hear lessons learned and ask relevant questions from Dnipropetrovsk authorities directly, rather than conducting a formal training program on framework contracting. By facilitating knowledge exchange among high-level government authorities, Poltava oblast authorities learned practical tips and successfully relaunched the tender process in framework contracting after a failed first attempt. The program facilitated a similar approach for high-level government officials in Bangladesh to learn from their peers in India for managing complex World Bank funded selection and procurement of medicines and commodities; and facilitated a partnership with the Korean International Cooperation Agency to enable peer learning with the Korean Ministry of Food and Drug Safety in medicines regulatory systems strengthening.

Electronic information sharing

The program's approach to capacity building recognizes the growing importance of electronic and new media for widespread access to learning and knowledge exchange [42]. New courses on good governance in the management of medicines and a two-part course on antimicrobial resistance are available on the global health eLearning center [43]. The World Health Organization's dedicated information portal on Essential Medicines and Health Products has more than 5000 pharmaceutical management related documents [44]. In collaboration with the South Africa program, the University of Western Cape developed an online rational medicines use module [45]. An online course for the program's electronic quantification and early warning system (Quan TB) provides access to learning resources with user guides available in six languages [46].

Team-based learning approaches

To address critical leadership, management and governance skill gaps in South Africa [47], the program applied the Pharmaceutical Leadership Development Program (PLDP). The PLDP brings together health care professionals, including clinicians, pharmacists, facility managers, and operational managers, to strengthen their leadership, management, and governance skills, while engaging them in analyzing a persistent challenge they face at the health facility they serve. Adapted from Management Sciences for Health's Leadership Development Program [48–50], the PLDP is designed to strengthen leadership, governance, and management capacity for health managers in public health service. The PLDP adaption includes additional content on legislation, ethics, governance, financial management, and human resources. It combines pharmaceutical management knowledge and sound leadership practices to better equip pharmacy managers to respond to challenges in their workplaces (Table 5).

An external, independent evaluation of the program stated "the people and institutions [in South Africa] who received this capacity building [including the PLDP] and tools [are] independently capable of managing and making improvements to their programs with minimal technical assistance [...] from the program" [51]. With long-term sustainability in mind, the PLDP/LDP approach has been institutionalized at district and facility levels [52]. Several trained teams have continued to scale up their initial interventions. The management of team mentoring activities has been transitioned from the program to sub-district level teams.

Survey findings from trainees in Bangladesh and Ethiopia

Over 94% of respondents indicated that they have improved or developed skills or competencies as a result of the program's training activities (Fig. 3).

In Bangladesh, an example of systems performance improvements include improved efficiency of supply chain systems in more than 29,000 service delivery points, improved use of data for decision making in 488 sub-districts, and greater customer satisfaction [53, 54]. One respondent stated the following in relation to LMIS [55] training efforts:

> "[A] *higher authority is now aware, due to the online report, of increased transparency and quality of work; able to identify issues and make timely decisions; improving data quality in LMIS reports though improved inventory management (takes less time, get online* [and] *on to server easily); timely recovery of information from archive to satisfy information seekers,* i.e., *audit; etc.*"

Key informant interviews with supervisors cited staff performance improvements on reporting data and report preparation, including reduced time required to complete a reporting task and improved accuracy in data entry and

Table 5 Selected Results from the Pharmaceutical Leadership Development Program (South Africa) [85]

Priority Areas	Province	Facility	Results
Waiting time	Western Cape	Kraaifontein Community Health Centre	Reduced average patient wait time at the pharmacy from 41 to 19 min over a 6 month period
Ensuring medicine accessibility	KwaZulu-Natal	Umzinto Primary Healthcare Clinic	Reduced the defaulter rate of patients collecting pre-dispensed chronic medicine from 28 to 23%
	Eastern Cape	Midlands Hospital and nearby clinics	Developed referral system which facilitated delivery of chronic diseases medicines from Midlands Hospital to feeder clinics
Improving medicine supply management	Eastern Cape	Cecilia Makiwane Hospital	Implemented a batch management system that cut the percentage of money wasted due to expired stock from 3.8% (as a percentage of expenditure) in April 2012 to 0.7% in June 2012, which is in keeping with international norms
	KwaZulu-Natal	Multiple clinics	Reduced the quantity of expired stock from 3.4% to less than 0.5% of stock holding
Ensuring compliance with standards	KwaZulu-Natal	Stanger, Montebello hospitals and Sundumbili CHC	Improved compliance with standard treatment guidelines for prescribing non-steroidal anti-inflammatory agents from 57 to 94%, 60 to 68%, and 37 to 67%, respectively
	North West	10 primary health care facilities	Increased compliance with national core standards from 33 to 77% by developing SOPs, distributing reference manuals, and building capacity in good pharmacy practice and medicine supply management
Ensuring rational use of medicines	North West	Joe Morolong Memorial Hospital	Average number of patients initiated on isoniazid preventive therapy increased from 3 to 8 per month
	North West	Four facilities in Bojanala District	Increased reporting of adverse drug events from 26 to 45%
	KwaZulu-Natal	Imbalenhle Community Health Centre	Reduced inappropriate prescriptions by 53%

analysis. Another government official from Bangladesh's Directorate General of Drug Administration (DGDA) overseeing medicines registration and pharmacovigilance activities remarked on the benefits of training approaches linked to improved quality of work or performance of the system:

"Established a system for pharmacovigilance; publish regular medicine safety reports and newsletters; monthly field visits; uploading ADR-related data [adverse drug reactions] through Vigiflow system. Adverse Drug Reaction Monitoring cell of DGDA was

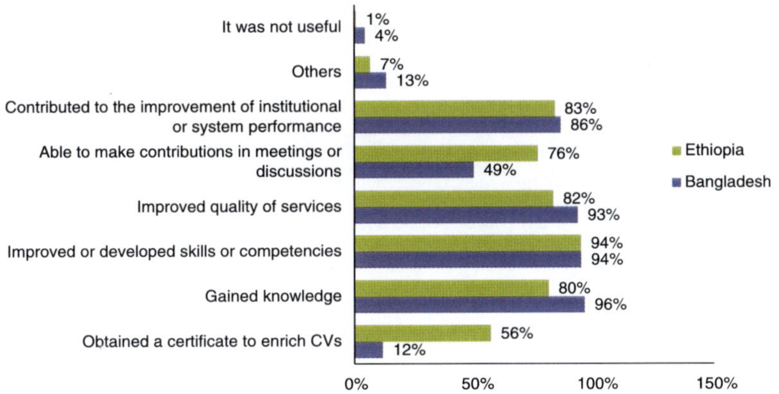

Fig. 3 Feedback on training: results from Ethiopia ($N = 153$) and Bangladesh ($N = 69$)

awarded the 120th full membership of the WHO International Drug Monitoring Centre."

Figure 4 indicates trainee reported post-training factors that contributed to the achievement of results. A small number of individuals indicated the reasons for training not being helpful (Table 6). Among respondents in both countries, the factors that promoted ongoing use of skills in daily on-the-job activities and those that incorporated group sharing and learning were mentioned the most frequently. Supportive supervision structures that enabled the implementation of post-training action plans were also frequently mentioned. One respondent in Ethiopia commented on the importance of having ongoing, interactive training to continue to move programmatic activities forward:

"*One can mention APTS* [Auditable Pharmaceutical Transaction and Services] [56] *where, with the creative approaches of* [the program], *10 hospitals could be able to start APTS shortly after APTS training, unlike the classic trainings we know where staffs see training as means of a retreat.* [The program's] *mentoring* [...] *serves as a recipe for moving best practices forward ...*"

Overall, the majority of the respondents cited systems-related support mechanisms and strong interpersonal support as important components related to the success of training efforts. Figure 5 provides a summary of the top eight preferred learning methods (see Additional file 2 for the entire list). The detailed reports for both Bangladesh and Ethiopia provides further information on the training approaches used and insights from key informant interviews [57].

Discussion

We provide a unique global implementer perspective regarding the variety of training approaches in the pharmaceutical system applied by country programs that fosters country ownership and sustainability consistent with other approaches [58]. Case-based learning, practice and feedback, and repetitive interventions such as post-training action plan, supportive supervision and mentoring approaches are effective, evidence-based training techniques applied by the program [59]. Individual capacity building efforts that include repetitive delivery and real-life case based trainings delivered positive results. South Africa's experience with the PLDP demonstrates that ongoing work-place based training that encourages people to solve real life work-related challenges is an effective, case-based training modality. Twenty years of lessons on capacity building from the World Bank Institute's Flagship Program also found that *"rather than a one-way dumping of information through repeated PowerPoint sessions,"* case-based learning and team approaches are crucial for learning and health systems improvement [60]. The PLDP in South Africa and implementation of post-training action plans in other countries applied similar principles to the monitoring-training-planning approach that emphasizes responsibility for

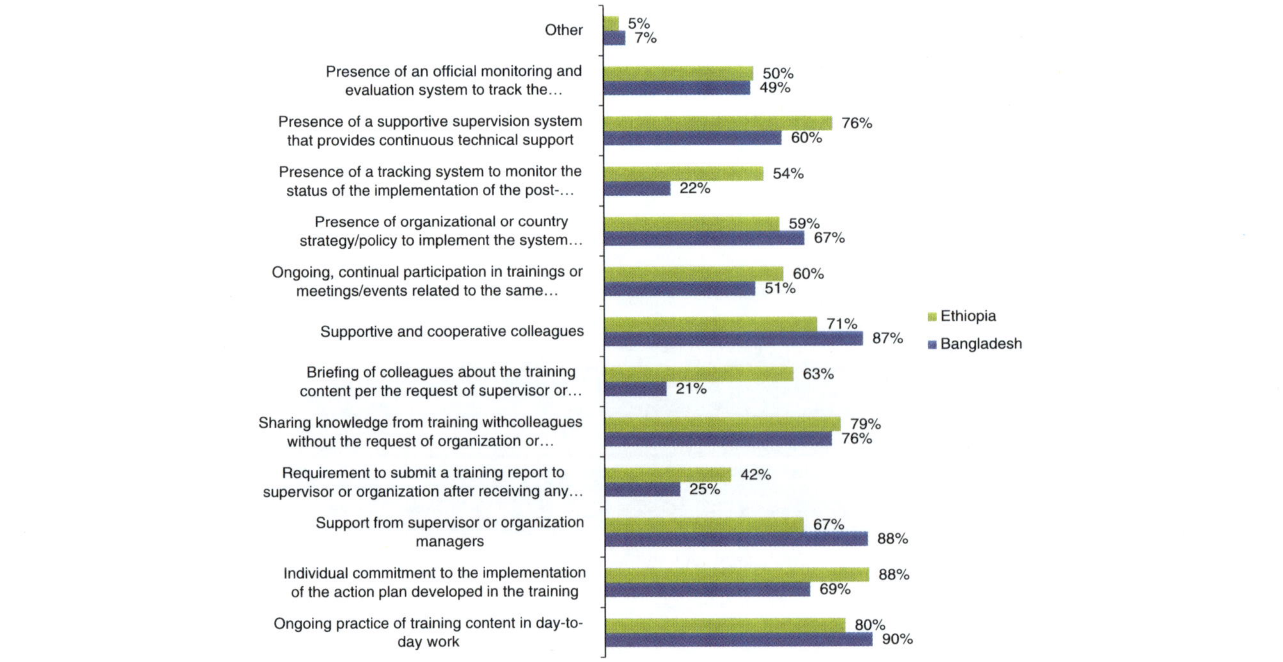

Fig. 4 Post-training factors that contributed to the results of the training in Bangladesh ($N = 69$) and Ethiopia ($N = 153$)

Table 6 Reasons why training was cited as not helpful

Reason provided by trainees surveyed	Bangladesh (*N* = 69)	Ethiopia (*N* = 153)
Training or capacity-building approach was not interesting	3	5
Training content was too challenging to understand and/or put into practice	2	9
Training content or technical area of the training did not correspond with the participants' work	3	3
Appropriate environment was not in place to enable participants to use the knowledge gained during the training	2	5

implementing the pharmaceutical management practices learned in the hands of local staff [61]. Individual capacity training design tailored to the work environment and local context permit staff to receive ongoing and consistent feedback through multiple interventions with ongoing support from supervisors and peers [62].

Ensuring that strong systems are set up to bolster training activities is critical for those who are implementing individual capacity building efforts. Respondents from Bangladesh and Ethiopia perceived that both interpersonal support networks such as supportive supervision, and systems-level support mechanisms, such as aligned national and/or subnational strategies, improve the results of training as similar to the experience in Angola [63]. Yet, supportive supervision and mentoring which cost an annual average of US $ 1.2 million in just one district of South Africa for instance, must be adequately funded and institutionalized to mitigate the risk of not being planned and implemented [64]. Based on the experience from Mali, Namibia, South Africa and from other countries, the program ensured that supportive supervision structures and mentorship have been institutionalized with appropriate management structures. National authorities have been sensitized to secure funding from domestic resources or from the global fund grants for post-training follow-up initiatives.

Tailoring training activities to fit the local context is imperative for successful individual capacity building. Among the 12 selected countries reviewed, training was provided in several local languages: Amharic, Bangla, French, Portuguese and Ukrainian by local staff with the subject matter expertise frequently in collaboration with national and regional authorities. Over the years, the program took substantial efforts to have local staff deliver training and technical assistance interventions. The latter was acknowledged as "ethically sound" and culturally sensitive by leading educators at the Consortium of Universities for Global Health [65]. For specific topics that required international technical expertise such as pharmaceutical services, pharmacovigilance, regulatory systems strengthening, medicines registration, health technology assessment or digital health initiatives, interpretation would be provided in concert with rapid accessibility of translated training materials and job aids.

High turnover of staff challenges efforts to increase individual capacity of the workforce because training efforts alone are not sufficient to address larger issues relating to

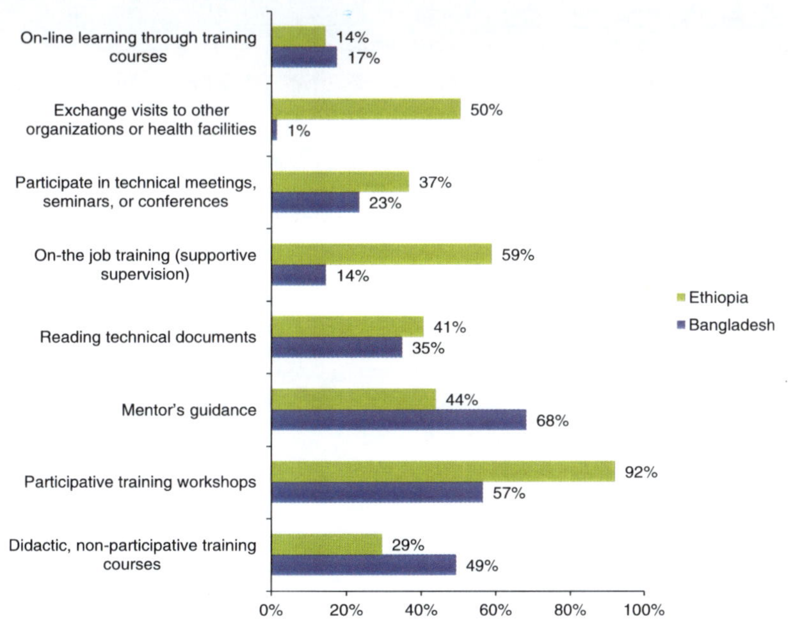

Fig. 5 Top eight preferred learning methods, as chosen by survey participants in Bangladesh (*N* = 69) and Ethiopia (*N* = 153)

long-term recruitment and retention challenges. The Latin America model on facilitated distance learning for pharmaceutical services managers for continuous professional development may be replicated in the context of right enabling conditions and contribute to retention of health workers [66]. Interventions must involve local institutions in the design and delivery of content for both pre-service and in-service training as well as web-based methods where feasible [67]. The Ethiopia program collaborated with several university teaching hospitals as a strategy to ensure sustained local capacity of pharmacists and health workers for the APTS intervention and supportive supervision activities [68, 69].

Our program experience has implications for those considering the future of pharmaceutical workforce development and training, given the High-Level Commission on Health Employment and Economic Growth's 10-point recommendations on investing in the health workforce to ensure progress towards the Sustainable Development Goals and to achieve Universal Health Coverage [70]. Effective pre-service training potentially reduces the need for future large-scale and expensive in-service trainings [71]. The program's experience demonstrate that competency based pre-service training will prepare students with a critical foundation of knowledge and skills required in the pharmaceutical system [72–74]. Sometimes, new topics such as pharmacovigilance [75], electronic medicines registration processes [76, 77], clinical pharmacy services [78, 79], patient-centered pharmaceutical care [80, 81], improving antibiotic prophylaxis [82] or medicines benefits package for universal health coverage [83] require comprehensive in-service and on-the-job training. The program's external evaluation found that national pharmaceutical system stakeholders are "*increasingly concerned about the development of sustainable human capacity to support the growing demand for more and more sophisticated pharmaceutical services*" and acknowledged the program's multi-pronged efforts [51]. The program's efforts complement the Nanjing statement on needs based approach through 13 global pharmaceutical workforce development goals for improving global health [84].

Limitations

Our selected review of the program's 12 implementing countries may be subject to selection bias because the program operated in more than 24 countries. Differences in training approaches and resulting data variation across countries and time contributes to limitations of this review. As a result, we are unable to compare data across countries. Moreover, because training events were developed for country-specific needs, training-related indicators were not applicable across all countries. Therefore, there was no way to compare training activities across countries and to generate trends at a global level. We do not elaborate the rationale in a country program's choice of a certain individual capacity building approach nor describe what did not work because there were multiple country-specific contextual factors that were not within the scope of this selected multi-country review. Because our focus was a selected review on modalities of training approaches in multiple countries based on the first 3 years of program implementation, we do not provide results on patient or health related outcomes associated with specific training interventions. The Bangladesh and Ethiopia trainee surveys included small sample sizes due to time and funding constraints. Yet our paper offers a unique implementer perspective supported with references to various country project documents.

Conclusion

Based on Potter and Brough's model, the program utilized a hierarchy of individual capacity building approaches that address the needs for tools (contextualized training curricula, job aids), skills (competency- and needs- based training design), and staff and facilities (training and post-training support). These three tiers build the foundation of improving the pharmaceutical system capacity. Program implementers must systematically collaborate with local institutions to provide coordinated training efforts that fill current skill shortage gaps, meet local needs in the pharmaceutical system, and promote the ownership of human capacity development interventions. Robust monitoring and evaluation efforts that are adequately funded must accompany individual capacity building programs to ensure that effective training methods are scaled up while those that are weak or ineffective are discontinued. Finally, training alone is not sufficient to address major human resource shortages and skill gaps. It must be paired with other system-level efforts to improve recruitment and retention of professionals.

Abbreviations

ACPE: Accreditation Council for Pharmaceutical Education; APTS: Auditable Pharmaceutical Transaction and Services; B Pharm: Bachelor of Pharmacy; DGDA: Directorate General of Drug Administration [Bangladesh]; DR Congo: Democratic Republic of the Congo; LMIS: Logistics Management Information System; NTP: National Tuberculosis Program; PLDP: Pharmaceutical Leadership Development Program; TOT: Training of trainers; USAID: United States Agency for International Development; WHO: World Health Organization

Acknowledgements

We thank Kimberly Grimmick, formerly with Management Sciences for Health for contributing to the study design and review. We appreciate the Bangladesh and Ethiopia country program team for their contribution in conducting the trainee survey. The contents of this manuscript would not have been possible without the dedicated and tireless efforts by the SIAPS country programs around the world who work in strong partnership with the Ministry of Health, private sector and local and international stakeholders to strengthen human capacity in pharmaceutical systems and services.

Authors' contributions

Country document content analysis design: SCW. Performed country desk review and analysis: SCW, TMLI, NK. Oversaw Bangladesh and Ethiopia survey data collection, interpretation and writing: SCW. Wrote the first draft of the manuscript: MR. Revised and finalized the manuscript: NK. Contributed to manuscript review: MR, SCW, TMLI. All authors read and approved the final version.

Authors' information

Megan Rauscher was affiliated with Pharmaceuticals and Health Technologies Group, Management Sciences for Health at the time of manuscript development.

Competing interests

The authors declare that they have no competing interests.

Author details

[1]Systems for Improved Access to Pharmaceuticals and Services (SIAPS) Program, Management Sciences for Health, Arlington, VA, USA. [2]Pharmaceuticals and Health Technologies Group, Management Sciences for Health, Arlington, VA, USA.

References

1. United Nations. Sustainable Development Goal 3: [Internet]. Sustainable Development Knowledge Platform. Available from: https://sustainabledevelopment.un.org/sdg3. cited 24 Jan 2017.
2. Wirtz VJ, Hogerzeil HV, Gray AL, Bigdeli M, de Joncheere CP, et al. Essential medicines for universal health coverage. Lancet. 2016. doi: 10.1016/S0140-6736(16)31599-9.
3. Shubber Z, Mills EJ, Nachega JB, Vreeman R, Freitas M, Bock P, et al. Patient-Reported Barriers to Adherence to Antiretroviral Therapy: A Systematic Review and Meta-Analysis. PLoS Med. 2016;13(11):e1002183.
4. United Nations. High level meeting on antimicrobial resistance. Endorsed Political Declaration on AMR [Internet]. 2016. Available from http://www.un.org/pga/71/wp-content/uploads/sites/40/2016/09/DGACM_GAEAD_ESCAB-AMR-Draft-Political-Declaration-1616108E.pdf. cited 13 Jan 2017.
5. Hakkarainen KM, Hedna K, Petzold M, Hägg S. Percentage of patients with preventable adverse drug reactions and preventability of adverse drug reactions—a meta-analysis. PLoS One. 2012;7(3):e33236.
6. Pande S, Hiller JE, Nkansah N, Bero L. The effect of pharmacist-provided non-dispensing services on patient outcomes, health service utilisation and costs in low- and middle-income countries. Cochrane Database Syst Rev. 2013;28(2):CD010398.
7. Systems for Improved Access to Pharmaceuticals and Services (SIAPS). Enhancing Health Outcomes for Chronic Diseases in Resource-Limited Settings by Improving the Use of Medicines: The Role of Pharmaceutical Care, Submitted to the U.S. Agency for International Development by the SIAPS Program. Arlington: Management Sciences for Health; 2014. Available from: http://apps.who.int/medicinedocs/en/d/Js21523en/.
8. World Health Organization. Tackling the crisis of workforce shortages in the pharmaceutical sector. Geneva: World Health Organization; 2011. Available from: http://apps.who.int/medicinedocs/en/m/abstract/Js17997en/.
9. Bates I, John C, Bruno A, Fu P, Aliabadi S. An analysis of the global pharmacy workforce capacity. Hum Resour Health. 2016;14:61.
10. Hafner T, Walkowiak H, Lee D, Aboagye-Nyame F. Defining pharmaceutical systems strengthening: Concepts to enable measurement. Health Policy Plan. 2016. Advance Access. doi: 10.1093/heapol/czw153.
11. Systems for Improved Access to Pharmaceuticals and Services (SIAPS) Program. | SIAPS Program [Internet]. Available from: http://siapsprogram.org. cited 24 Jan 2017.
12. Potter C, Brough R. Systemic capacity building: a hierarchy of needs. Health Policy Plan. 2004;19(5):336–45.
13. Systems for Improved Access to Pharmaceutical Services (SIAPS). Annual Report: Project Year 4, October 2014–September 2015, Submitted to the US Agency for International Development by the SIAPS Program. Arlington: Management Sciences for Health; 2015. Available from: http://apps.who.int/medicinedocs/en/m/abstract/Js22239en/.
14. Chandani Y, Andersson S, Heaton A, Noel M, Shieshia M, Mwirotsi A, et al. Making products available among community health workers: Evidence for improving community health supply chains from Ethiopia, Malawi, and Rwanda. J Glob Health. 2014;4(2):20405.
15. Oqua D, Agu KA, Isah MA, Onoh OU, Iyaji PG, Wutoh AK, et al. Improving pharmacy practice through public health programs: experience from Global HIV/AIDS initiative Nigeria project. SpringerPlus. 2013;2:525.
16. WHO EMRO. Pre-service education. Child health and development [Internet]. Available from: http://www.emro.who.int/child-health/IMCI-preservice-training/what-is-it. cited 24 Jan 2017.
17. Systems for Improved Access to Pharmaceuticals and Services (SIAPS). Revising Preservice Curriculum to Incorporate Rational Medicine Use Topics: A Guide, Submitted to the US Agency for International Development by the SIAPS Program. Arlington: Management Sciences for Health; 2013. Available from: http://apps.who.int/medicinedocs/en/d/Js21526en/.
18. Strengthening Pharmaceutical Systems. Strengthening Pharmaceutical Services Program Final Report: 2007–2012, Submitted to the US Agency for International Development by the Strengthening Pharmaceutical Systems (SPS) Program. Arlington: Management Sciences for Health; 2013. Available from: http://pdf.usaid.gov/pdf_docs/pdacy204.pdf.
19. Minh PD, Huong DT, Byrkit R, Murray M. Strengthening pharmacy practice in Vietnam: findings of a training intervention study. Trop Med Int Health. 2013;18(4):426–34. doi:10.1111/tmi.1206.
20. Bradley S, Kamwendo F, Masanja H, de Pinho H, Waxman R, Boostrom C, McAuliffe E. District health managers' perceptions of supervision in Malawi and Tanzania. Hum Resour Health. 2013;11:43. doi:10.1186/1478-4491-11-43.
21. Namagembe A, Ssekabira U, Weaver MR, Blum N, Burnett S, Dorsey G, Sebuyira LM, Ojaku A, Schneider G, Willis K, Yeka A. Improved clinical and laboratory skills after team-based, malaria case management training of health care professionals in Uganda. Malar J. 2012;11:44. doi:10.1186/1475-2875-11-44.
22. Swanson RC, Cattaneo A, Bradley E, Chunharas S, Atun R, Abbas KM, Katsaliaki K, Mustafee N, Mason Meier B, Best A. Rethinking health systems strengthening: key systems thinking tools and strategies for transformational change. Health Policy Plan. 2012;27 Suppl 4:iv54–61.
23. Frehywot S, Vovides Y, Talib Z, Mikhail N, Ross H, Wohltjen H, Bedada S, Korhumel K, Koumare AK, Scott J. E-learning in medical education in resource constrained low- and middle-income countries. Hum Resour Health. 2013;11:4. doi:10.1186/1478-4491-11-4.
24. Brock T, Wuliji T, Sagwa E, Mabirizi D. Technical Report: Exploring the Establishment of a Pharmacy Course at the University of Namibia, March 12–27, 2009, Submitted to the U.S. Agency for International Development by the Strengthening Pharmaceutical Systems (SPS) Program. Arlington: Management Sciences for Health; 2009. Available from: http://pdf.usaid.gov/pdf_docs/Pnadu430.pdf.
25. University of Namibia. Overview of the School of Pharmacy [Internet]. Available from: http://www.unam.edu.na/school-of-pharmacy. cited 24 Jan 2017.
26. Mazibuko G, Phulu B, Sagwa E, Kibuule D, Kagoya H, Mavu D. Support to local training institutions to address human resources shortages and capacity affecting ART service delivery in Namibia, Submitted to the US Agency for International Development by the Systems for Improved Access

to Pharmaceuticals and Services (SIAPS) Program. Arlington: Management Sciences for Health; 2014.

27. Rennie T, Kibuule D, Haoses-Gorases L, Nyarang'o P, Mabirizi D, Sagwa E, et al. Namibia's First School of Pharmacy: From Creation to Graduation, Systems for Improved Access to Pharmaceuticals and Services (SIAPS) Program. Arlington: Management Sciences for Health; 2015. Available from: http://siapsprogram.org/2015/04/27/namibias-first-school-of-pharmacy-from-creation-to-graduation/.
28. Systems for Improved Access to Pharmaceuticals and Services (SIAPS) Program. Technical Brief: Strengthening Namibia's Pharmacy Sector and Workforce. Arlington: Management Sciences for Health; 2016. Available from: http://siapsprogram.org/publication/technical-brief-strengthening-namibias-pharmacy-sector-and-workforce/.
29. Kibuule D, Lates J, Niaz Q, Mazibuko G, Phulu B, Kagoya HR, et al. Concept and Guidelines for Medicine Use Assessment during Students' Rural Placements. Submitted to the US Agency for International Development by the MoHSS-NHTC with support from the SIAPS program. Management Sciences for Health: Arlington; 2015. Available from: http://apps.who.int/medicinedocs/en/m/abstract/Js22148en/.
30. Kutenda O, Leboea J, Kambyambya K, Mavu D, Kagoya H, Mazibuko G, et al. Post-qualification Monitoring and Evaluation of Pharmacist Assistants Trained at the National Health Training Centre in Namibia, Submitted to the US Agency for International Development by the MoHSS-NHTC with support from the Systems for Improved Access to Pharmaceuticals and Services program. Arlington: Management Sciences for Health; 2015. Available from: http://siapsprogram.org/publication/post-qualification-monitoring-and-evaluation-of-pharmacist-assistants-trained-at-the-national-health-training-centre-in-namibia/.
31. Accreditation Council for Pharmaceutical Education (ACPE). About ACPE [Internet]. Available from https://www.acpe-accredit.org/about/. cited 24 Jan 2017.
32. Vlasses P, Grégoire J. Recommendations for Advancing Pharmacy Education in the Democratic Republic of the Congo, Submitted to the US Agency for International Development by the Systems for Improved Access to Pharmaceuticals and Services (SIAPS) Program. Management Sciences for Health: Arlington; 2014. Available from http://apps.who.int/medicinedocs/en/d/Js21918en/.
33. Anderson C, Bates I, Brock T, Brown AN, Bruno A, Futter B, et al. Needs-Based Education in the Context of Globalization. Am J Pharm Educ. 2012;76(4):56.
34. Rouse M, Vlasses P, Wadelin J, Zarembski D, Joshi MP, Mabirizi D, Saleeb S. Continuing Pharmaceutical Education: Guide to Establishing Quality Assured and Accredited Programs, Submitted to the US Agency for International Development by the Systems for Improved Access to Pharmaceuticals and Services (SIAPS) Program. Arlington: Management Sciences for Health; 2016. Available from http://apps.who.int/medicinedocs/en/m/abstract/Js22394en/.
35. USAID Works to Improve Quality of Pharmacist Training [Internet]. U.S. Embassy in the Democratic Republic of the Congo. 2015. Available from: https://cd.usembassy.gov/usaid-works-improve-quality-pharmacist-training/. cited 24 Jan 2017.
36. Systems for Improved Access to Pharmaceuticals and Services (SIAPS). e-TB Manager Promotes Treatment Quality and Evidence-Based Forecasting of TB Medicines. Arlington: Management Sciences for Health; 2015. Available from: http://siapsprogram.org/publication/e-tb-manager-promotes-treatment-quality-and-evidence-based-forecasting-of-tb-medicines-in-ukraine/.
37. Systems for Improved Access to Pharmaceuticals and Services (SIAPS). Institutionalizing e-TB Manager as a national TB registry in Ukraine [Internet]. Arlington: Management Sciences for Health; 2015. Available from: http://siapsprogram.org/2015/11/04/institutionalizing-e-tb-manager-as-a-national-tb-registry-in-ukraine/.
38. Systems for Improved Access to Pharmaceuticals and Services (SIAPS). Strengthening Pharmaceutical Services through Structured Supportive Supervision in Namibia. Arlington: Management Sciences for Health; 2015. Available from: http://siapsprogram.org/publication/strengthening-pharmaceutical-services-through-structured-supportive-supervision-in-namibia/.
39. Systems for Improved Access to Pharmaceutical Services (SIAPS). Annual Report: Project Year 3, October 2013–September 2014. Submitted to the US Agency for International Development by the SIAPS Program. Arlington: Management Sciences for Health. Available from: http://apps.who.int/medicinedocs/en/d/Js21707en/.
40. Systems for Improved Access to Pharmaceuticals and Services (SIAPS). Design, Implementation, and Use of Pharmaceutical Logistics Management Information Systems (LMIS): SIAPS Technical Brief. Arlington: Management Sciences for Health; 2016. Available from: http://siapsprogram.org/publication/lmis-technical-brief-the-usaid-siaps-best-practices-in-the-design-implementation-and-use-of-pharmaceutical-logistics-management-information-systems/.
41. Kniazkov S, Savchuk T. Framework Contracting in Ukraine: A Story of Success. Submitted to the US Agency for International Development by the Systems for Improved Access to Pharmaceuticals and Services (SIAPS) Program [Internet]. Management Sciences for Health; 2015. Available from: http://apps.who.int/medicinedocs/en/m/abstract/Js22280en/. cited 24 Jan 2017.
42. Sullivan TM, Limaye RJ, Mitchell V, D'Adamo M, Baquet Z. Leveraging the Power of Knowledge Management to Transform Global Health and Development. Glob Health Sci Pract. 2015;3(2):150–62.
43. USAID. Global Health e-Learning Center. Courses [Internet]. Available from: https://www.globalhealthlearning.org/courses. cited 24 Jan 2017.
44. Essential Medicines and Health Products Information Portal [Internet]. Available from: http://apps.who.int/medicinedocs/en/. cited 17 Jan 2017.
45. University of the Western Cape. Online Rational Medicines Use Module. Schools of Public Health and Pharmacy in collaboration with SIAPS program and other partners. South Africa. Available at https://www.uwc.ac.za/Faculties/CHS/soph/News/Pages/NEW-Online-Rational-Medicines-Use-Module.aspx.
46. Management Sciences for Health. LeaderNet. QuanTB online course. Systems for Improved Access to Pharmaceuticals and Services (SIAPS) Program [Internet]. Available from: http://leadernet.org/groups/courses/quantb/. cited 24 Jan 2017.
47. Bradley H, Lehmann U, Butler N. Emerging roles and competencies of district and sub-district pharmacists: a case study from Cape Town. Hum Resour Health. 2015;13:88.
48. Tools and Approaches: Developing Effective Leaders for Stronger Health Systems [Internet]. Medford, MA: Management Sciences for Health [Internet]. Available from: https://www.msh.org/sites/msh.org/files/msh_leadership_brochure.pdf. cited 24 Jan 2017.
49. Mansour M, Mansour JB, Swesy AHE. Scaling up proven public health interventions through a locally owned and sustained leadership development programme in rural Upper Egypt. Hum Resour Health. 2010;8:1.
50. Seims LR, Alegre JC, Murei L, Bragar J, Thatte N, Kibunga P, Cheburet S. Strengthening management and leadership practices to increase health-service delivery in Kenya: an evidence-based approach. Hum Resour Health. 2012;10:25.
51. Carrino C, Miralles M, Whitworth R. Interim evaluation of Systems for Improved Access to Pharmaceuticals and Services (SIAPS) Project. Submitted by GH PRO project to USAID; 2016 May. Report No.: 3001–083. Available from: http://pdf.usaid.gov/pdf_docs/pa00m7qr.pdf.
52. Putter S, Mkele G, Mkandawire T, Nene N, Payne K, Tindula C. Technical Report: South Africa Pharmaceutical Leadership Development Program (PLDP), Submitted to the US Agency for International Development by the Systems for Improved Access to Pharmaceuticals and Services (SIAPS) Program. Arlington: Management Sciences for Health; 2015. Available from: http://siapsprogram.org/publication/technical-report-south-africa-pharmaceutical-leadership-development-program/.
53. Systems for Improved Access to Pharmaceuticals and Services. Dashboard module reduces contraceptive stock-outs at SDPs in Bangladesh. SIAPS Technical Highlight. Arlington: Management Sciences for Health; 2016. Available from: http://siapsprogram.org/publication/technical-highlight-dashboard-module-reduces-contraceptive-stock-outs-at-sdps-in-bangladesh/.
54. Systems for Improved Access to Pharmaceuticals and Services. Video: Reducing Stock-outs and Saving Lives in Bangladesh, [Internet]. Arlington: Management Sciences for Health; 2016. Available from: http://siapsprogram.org/2016/11/30/video-reducing-stock-outs-and-saving-lives-in-bangladesh/.
55. Systems for Improved Access to Pharmaceuticals and Services (SIAPS). Logistics Management Units Improve Availability of Medicines in Bangladesh. Arlington: Management Sciences for Health; 2015. Available from: http://siapsprogram.org/publication/logistics-management-units-improve-availability-of-medicines-in-bangladesh/.
56. Sheckler A. How One Pharmacist Can Make a Difference: Transforming Ethiopia's Pharmaceutical Sector. Frontline Health Workers Coalition; 2014 Available from: https://www.frontlinehealthworkers.org/how-one-pharmacist-can-make-a-difference-transforming-ethiopias-pharmaceutical-sector/.
57. Systems for Improved Access to Pharmaceuticals and Services. Selected Review of Training Approaches in the SIAPS Program: Bangladesh and Ethiopia Country Reports. Arlington: Management Sciences for Health; 2016. Available from: http://siapsprogram.org/publication/selected-review-of-training-approaches-in-the-siaps-program-bangladesh-and-ethiopia-country-reports/.

58. Cancedda C, Farmer PE, Kerry V, Nuthulaganti T, Scott KW, Goosby E, et al. Maximizing the Impact of Training Initiatives for Health Professionals in Low-Income Countries: Frameworks, Challenges, and Best Practices. PLoS Med. 2015;12(6):e1001840.
59. Bluestone J, Johnson P, Fullerton J, Carr C, Alderman J, BonTempo J. Effective in-service training design and delivery: evidence from an integrative literature review. Hum Resour Health. 2013;11:51.
60. Reich MR, Yazbeck AS, Berman P, Bitran R, Bossert T, et al. Lessons from 20 Years of Capacity Building for Health Systems Thinking. Health Syst Reform. 2016;2(3):213–21.
61. Rational Pharmaceutical Management Plus Program. A Guide for Implementing the Monitoring-Training-Planning (MTP) Approach to Build Skills for Pharmaceutical Management, Submitted to the U.S. Agency for International Development by the Rational Pharmaceutical Management Plus Program. Arlington: Management Sciences for Health; 2009. Available from: https://www.k4health.org/toolkits/leadershipmgmt/guide-implementing-monitoring-training-planning-mtp-approach-build-skills.
62. Wang S, Hoohlo N, Tshabalala K, Ntoi K, Sepetla T. Capacity Needs Assessment for Pharmaceutical Services for the ART Program in Lesotho, Submitted to the US Agency for International Development by the Systems for Improved Access to Pharmaceuticals and Services (SIAPS) Program. Arlington: Management Sciences for Health; 2013. Available from: http://apps.who.int/medicinedocs/en/d/Js21831en/.
63. Joao L. Improving Supply Chain Management for Malaria: Lessons from Angola. Management Sciences for Health; 2015. Available from: https://www.msh.org/news-events/stories/improving-supply-chainmanagement-for-malaria-lessons-from-angola.
64. Johnson S. Cost implications and benefits of using Roving Mentor Teams to strengthen HIV and TB clinical management in public sector primary care clinics. Presentation at the PEPFAR partner dissemination meeting: Reaching 90-90-90 in South Africa Part III: Best Practices and Innovations in Linkage, Treatment and Viral Suppression. 2016. US Embassy South Africa. Available from: https://za.usembassy.gov/our-relationship/pepfar/partner-dissemination-meetings/reaching-90-90-90-south-africa-part-iii-presentations/.
65. Eichbaum Q, Evert J, Hall T. Will there be enough jobs for trained global health professionals? Lancet Glob Health. 2016;4(10):e692–3.
66. Emmerick IC, Chaves LA, Marin N, Luiza VL. Strengthening the capacity of managers in pharmaceutical services based on Primary Health Care (PHC) at different levels of the health system. Hum Resour Health. 2014;12:34.
67. Matowe L, Waako P, Adome RO, Kibwage I, Minzi O, Bienvenu E. A strategy to improve skills in pharmaceutical supply management in East Africa: the regional technical resource collaboration for pharmaceutical management. Hum Resour Health. 2008;6:30.
68. University of Gonder Teaching Hospital. University of Gondar Hospital Launches Auditable Pharmaceutical Transaction and Service (APTS). Available from: http://www.uog.edu.et/university-gondar-hospital-launches-auditable-pharmaceutical-transaction-service-apts/.
69. Tadeg H, Ejigu E, Geremew E, Adinew A. Auditable Pharmaceutical Transactions and Services (APTS): Findings of the Baseline Assessment at Federal, Addis Ababa, and Teaching Hospitals, Submitted to the US Agency for International Development by the Systems for Improved Access to Pharmaceuticals and Services (SIAPS) Program. Arlington: Management Sciences for Health; 2013. Available from: http://apps.who.int/medicinedocs/en/d/Js21704en/.
70. World Health Organization. UN Commission: New investments in global health workforce will create jobs and drive economic growth. 2016. Available from: http://www.who.int/mediacentre/news/releases/2016/global-health-workforce/en/.
71. Youmans S, Ngassapa O, Chambuso M. Clinical pharmacy to meet the health needs of Tanzanians: education reform through partnership across continents (2008–2011). J Public Health Policy. 2012;33 Suppl 1:S110–25.
72. General Directorate of Pharmaceutical Affairs and, General Directorate of Human Resources, General Directorate of Pharmaceutical Affairs and. Competency Framework for Pharmaceutical Services [Internet]. Islamic Republic of Afghanistan Ministry of Public Health; 2012. Available from: http://apps.who.int/medicinedocs/en/d/Js21747en/.
73. Joshi M, Ludman M, Kibuule D, Rennie T, Lates J, Knott M, et al. Strengthening Pre-service Pharmacy Training on Rational Medicine Use and Antimicrobial Resistance, Submitted to the US Agency for International Development by the Systems for Improved Access to Pharmaceuticals and Services Program. Arlington: Management Sciences for Health; 2014. Available from: http://apps.who.int/medicinedocs/en/m/abstract/Js21528en/.
74. Systems for Improved Access to Pharmaceuticals and Services (SIAPS). SIAPS' Capacity Building Efforts to Improve the Dominican Republic's Health Management System. Arlington: Management Sciences for Health; 2016. Available from: http://siapsprogram.org/publication/siaps-capacity-building-efforts-to-improve-the-dominican-republics-health-management-system/.
75. Systems for Improved Access to Pharmaceuticals and Services (SIAPS) Program. Strengthening Bangladesh's National Pharmacovigilance System: Lessons Learned and Opportunities. Arlington: Management Sciences for Health; 2016. Available from: http://siapsprogram.org/publication/strengthening-bangladeshs-national-pharmacovigilance-system-lessons-learned-and-opportunities/.
76. Kim EM. Strengthening the Medicine Regulatory System by Implementing an Electronic Medicine Registration Data Management System (Pharmadex) in Mozambique, Submitted to the US Agency for International Development by the Systems for Improved Access to Pharmaceuticals and Services (SIAPS) Program. Arlington: Management Sciences for Health; 2016. Available from: http://apps.who.int/medicinedocs/en/d/Js22438en/.
77. Aimiuwu J. Improving the Process of Medicines Registration in Bangladesh: Adoption of the Common Technical Document Format and Implementation of Pharmadex to Automate the Registration of Medicines, Submitted to the US Agency for International Development by the Systems for Improved Access to Pharmaceuticals and Services (SIAPS) Program. Arlington: Management Sciences for Health; 2016. Available from: http://apps.who.int/medicinedocs/en/d/Js23064en/.
78. Geremew E, Worku F, Hailu T, Ejigu E, Mekonnen N. Building Local Capacity for Clinical Pharmacy Service in Ethiopia through a Holistic In-Service Training Approach, Submitted to the US Agency for International Development by the Systems for Improved Access to Pharmaceuticals and Services (SIAPS) Program. Arlington: Management Sciences for Health; 2014. Available from: http://apps.who.int/medicinedocs/en/d/Js21810en/.
79. Agu KA, Oqua D, Agada P, Ohiaeri SI, Adesina A, Abdulkareem MH, et al. Assessment of satisfaction with pharmaceutical services in patients receiving antiretroviral therapy in outpatient HIV treatment setting. Int J Clin Pharm. 2014;36(3):636–47.
80. Systems for Improved Access to Pharmaceuticals and Services (SIAPS). Systems Improving Health Outcomes through Delivery of Patient-Centered Pharmaceutical Care by Pharmacists in Low- and Middle-Income Countries. Technical Brief. Arlington: Management Sciences for Health; 2016. Available from: http://siapsprogram.org/publication/technical-brief-improving-health-outcomes-through-delivery-of-patient-centered-pharmaceutical-care-by-pharmacists-in-low-and-middle-income-countries/.
81. Agu KA, Oqua D, Adeyanju Z, Isah MA, Adesina A, Ohiaeri SI, et al. The incidence and types of medication errors in patients receiving antiretroviral therapy in resource-constrained settings. PLoS One. 2014;9(1):e87338.
82. Gammouh S, Joshi M. Improving Antibiotic Prophylaxis in Cesarean Section in Jordanian Hospitals: SIAPS Technical Report, Submitted to the US Agency for International Development by the Systems for Improved Access to Pharmaceuticals and Services (SIAPS) Program. Arlington: Management Sciences for Health; 2013. Available from: http://apps.who.int/medicinedocs/en/d/Js21698en/.
83. Wagner AK, Quick JD, Ross-Degnan D. Quality use of medicines within universal health coverage: challenges and opportunities. BMC Health Serv Res. 2014;14:357.
84. International Pharmaceutical Federation. Pharmaceutical Workforce Development Goals. Global Conference on Pharmacy and Pharmaceutical Sciences Education. Nanjing; 2016. Available from: http://www.fip.org/nanjing2016/.
85. Systems for Improved Access to Pharmaceuticals and Services (SIAPS). Strengthening the Leadership and Management of Pharmaceutical Services in South Africa: SIAPS Technical Brief. Arlington: Management Sciences for Health; 2016. Available from: http://siapsprogram.org/publication/technical-brief-strengthening-the-leadership-and-management-of-pharmaceutical-services-in-south-africa/.

Drug utilization patterns among elderly hospitalized patients on poly-pharmacy in Punjab, Pakistan

Muhammad Rehan Sarwar[1], Muhammad Atif[1*], Shane Scahill[2], Anum Saqib[1], Muhammad Qamar-uz-Zaman[1] and Zaheer Babar[3]

Abstract

Background: Reports from drug utilization reviews are important tools employed in the assessment of healthcare practices. The objective of this study was to evaluate drug utilization patterns among elderly hospitalized patients on poly-pharmacy regimens in Pakistan.

Methods: A descriptive, non-experimental, cross-sectional study was carried out from December 2015 to March 2016 in six tertiary-care hospitals in the Punjab province of Pakistan. The population under study were patients aged ≥60 years, taking ≥5 medicines per day (i.e., patients on poly-pharmacy) and who were hospitalized in the selected tertiary-care hospitals. In this study, data was collected from 600 hospitalized elderly patients (100 patients per hospital). All medicines prescribed on each in-patient chart were noted on a pre-designed pro-forma sheet and were classified under the Anatomical Therapeutic Chemical (ATC) classification system. Multiple linear regression analysis was used to determine the independent factors associated with poly-pharmacy in this cohort. Statistical Package for Social Sciences (SPSS) was used to analyze the data. *P*-value < .05 indicated statistical significance.

Results: In 600 hospitalized in-patient (male 52.7% and female 47.3%) medication charts, 3179 medicines were prescribed. The most commonly prescribed drug classes were: A: alimentary tract and metabolism 80% (A02: drugs for acid related disorders 64.5%, A03: drugs for functional gastrointestinal disorders 21.5%), N: nervous system 66.3% (N02: analgesics 67.2%, N03: antiepileptic's 11.2%), J: anti-infectives for systemic use 62.2% (J01: antibacterial for systemic use 82.5%, J04: antimycobacterials 15.3%) and C: cardiovascular system 48.3% (C07: beta blocking agents 19.8%, C10: lipid modifying agents 16.5%), respectively. The most commonly prescribed active substances were: A02BC01 (omeprazole 51.3%), N02BE01 (paracetamol 50.8%) and J01DD04 (ceftriaxone 40.2%), respectively. In multiple linear regression analysis, male gender (95% CI −.205, −.006, *p* = .039, B = −.091), being divorced (95% CI −.604, −.136, *p* = .002, B = −.130) and presence of comorbidity (95% CI .068, .267, *p* = .001, B = .144) were the independent factors associated with increased drug use among elderly hospitalized patients on poly-pharmacy.

Conclusions: The rational use of medicines is of utmost importance, most particularly in the elderly population. More consideration should be given to rationalizing pharmacotherapy in elderly hospitalized patients who are on poly-pharmacy regimens in Pakistan.

Keywords: Drug use, Drug utilization pattern, Elderly, Hospitalized, Poly-pharmacy

* Correspondence: pharmacist_atif@yahoo.com; muhammad.atif@iub.edu.pk
[1]Department of Pharmacy, The Islamia University of Bahawalpur, Bahawalpur, Pakistan
Full list of author information is available at the end of the article

Background

Drug therapy serves as the commonest medical intervention reducing health related risks across numerous diseases [1]. A number of studies have been conducted globally to explore the socio-demographic [2, 3], medical related [3, 4] and health system factors [5] as substantial influencers of drug utilization. Despite this, a limited literature is available on drug utilization within a multivariate framework which considers all of the aforementioned variables [1, 6, 7]; particularly in Pakistan.

The elderly are more prone to chronic illnesses due to aging and physiological changes; with the majority of older people (up to about 80%) suffering from chronic illnesses [8]. Consequently, this group are more likely to have increased drug utilization over the general population [9]. Medical, social and financial changes, both at the individual and societal level, are the consequence of geographical differences and/or changes in medicine use over time, and there is a need to identify, explain and remedy these pharmaco-epidemiological differences.

There is scarce data available on drug utilization among elderly in Pakistan and the investigation of poly-pharmacy (taking ≥5 medicines per day) remains under studied. Elderly people in Pakistan comprise a large proportion drug use and this has led to an increase in total health expenditure. Pakistan's demographic trends demonstrate that between 1990 and 2010, the population aged ≥60 years increased by 75.1% [10]. A World Health Organization (WHO) report (1998) also reports that 5.6% of Pakistan's population was over 60 years of age, with a probability of doubling to 11% by the year 2025 [11]. With the lack of literature on drug utilization in older adults in the developing world and the rising global demographic of older adults, this points toward the need for drug utilization studies in this area. Drug utilization research is a valuable tool to guide health policy-makers in making their decisions. Similarly, this facilitates value-added communication amongst healthcare personnel, healthcare authorities and scientists [12]. Drug utilization research assesses the utilization and impact of medicines in the community and plays a key role in prioritizing the medical needs of a given country through guiding selection of medicines for national formularies. Reports from drug utilization reviews are important tools employed in the assessment of healthcare practices. The findings of drug utilization surveys also help to improve the rational use of medicines [13].

As such, the objective of this study was to investigate drug utilization patterns among elderly hospitalized patients on poly-pharmacy regimens in Punjab province, Pakistan. Furthermore, we evaluated the combined effect of various factors (for example, demographic, socioeconomic, and health-related factors) on patients on poly-pharmacy in a representative sample of hospitalized elderly patients.

Methods

Study design

A descriptive, non-experimental, cross-sectional study was carried out in six tertiary-care hospitals in the Punjab province of Pakistan, to evaluate drug utilization patterns among elderly hospitalized patients who were on poly-pharmacy regimens.

For this study, data was collected and evaluated according to the objectives of the study. Elderly patients who had been hospitalized for at least 3 days and who were on ≥5 medicines per day were included in this study. Nutritional supplements, other than vitamins and electrolytes were not considered to be drugs and were not recorded.

Study settings

Six tertiary care hospitals (1: Bahawal Victoria Hospital (BVH), 2: Nishtar hospital, 3: Allied hospital, 4: Mayo hospital, 5: District Headquarter (DHQ) Sargodha, 6: Benazir Bhutto hospital) from different areas of the Punjab province were selected as research sites.

The choice of tertiary-care hospitals was made through systematic random sampling. There are 23 tertiary-care hospitals in the Punjab province [14]. Out of these, six were randomly selected using the random number generator function in Microsoft Excel, thus negating the potential for selection bias. In Pakistan, the tertiary care hospitals are very similar in terms of staff and operations and consequently physicians follow the same prescribing practices. Similarly, the patient population is likely to be the same in tertiary care hospitals. Thus randomly selecting patients from these six hospitals is not expected to create issues with significant bias.

Study population and sample size

The population under study were patients of age ≥ 60 years, who were hospitalized in six selected tertiary-care hospitals. According to the latest Pakistani Census, the population of the surveyed province consists of 91,379,615 individuals [15]. The minimum required sample size was 385, as calculated using the Raosoft sample size calculator [16], with 95% confidence interval (CI) and 5% margin of error [Eq. 1].

$$n = Nx/((N-1)E2 + x) \quad (1)$$

Where N is the population size, x is the CI and E is the margin of error.

The study was conducted on the patients who were admitted in selected hospitals due to complications associated with their chronic illness rather than on the patients who were admitted due to an acute episode unrelated to their chronic condition.

Data collection

Over a 3 month period (15 December 2015 to 14 March 2016), a total of 3129 elderly patients were approached in-order to obtain consent from 600 to participate. Data was collected at different intervals from these tertiary-care hospitals irrespective of the date of admission of patients.

A data collection form was designed [Additional file 1], which consisted of four main parts: demographic, socio-economic, health-related characteristics and drug utilization patterns. The reliability and internal consistency of the data collection form was assessed by conducting a pilot study. Piloting was undertaken using data from 60 patients. After piloting, the data collection form was restructured by adding chronic conditions and an area for a list of prescribed medicines, which was not part of the original form. The Cronbach's alpha value was 0.84 demonstrating excellent reliability.

Measurements

Demographic characteristics

The following categorical variables were recorded; gender (male/female), age (60–74, 75–89, ≥90 years), and civil status (single, married, divorced, widowed).

Socioeconomic characteristics

Education level (primary, secondary and tertiary), annual income (low, middle, upper class), residence (rural, urban), employment status (employed, unemployed) were the four variables measuring the socio-economic status of participants. Those participants who were retired (taking a pension) or running a business were classified as employed. The data was obtained through face to face questioning of all 600 patients.

Health-related characteristics

In-patient charts/medical records were used to collect this data. However, if more information on socio-demographic or health-related characteristics were needed, then patients or caregivers were interviewed. Health-related characteristics included the following; self-reported health (good, moderate, poor), health risks (smoking, alcohol consumption, obesity, none), health service utilization [normal clinic visits (≤3/year), high clinic visits (≤4/year)], and chronic diseases (heart diseases, respiratory, gastrointestinal, diabetes mellitus, joint diseases, hypertension, central nervous system (CNS) disorders, others) and comorbidities (present, absent). Obesity was assessed by the body mass index (BMI), and respondents were regarded as either normal (BMI < 25 kg/m^2), overweight (25 ≤ BMI < 30 kg/m^2) or obese (BMI ≥ 30 kg/m^2) [1].

Drug utilization evaluation

All medicines in each prescription were noted on the pro-forma sheet. For the evaluation of drug utilization patterns, all the medicines from the 600 in-patient charts were classified under the Anatomical Therapeutic Chemical (ATC) classification system [17]. Furthermore, the most commonly prescribed active substances were categorized according to trends in use; low (prescribed to <10% of the selected patients), medium (prescribed to ≥10% of the selected patients but <40%) and high (prescribed to >40% of the selected patients).

Statistical analysis

Statistical Package for Social Sciences (IBM, SPSS Statistics for Windows, version 21.0. Armonk, NY: IBM Corp.) was used for data analysis. Simple linear regression analysis was adopted to determine the association between variables. Multiple linear regression analysis was then carried out for statistically significant variables from the univariate analysis to identify factors associated with increased drug use among elderly hospitalized patients who were on polypharmacy regimens [18]. The 95% CI, beta, standard error, and *p*-value were described for each factor. Pseudo R square values were included to describe the percentages of variance explained by the model. *P*-value < .05 was deemed to be statistically signifiant [18].

Results

A total of 3129 elderly hospitalized patients in six tertiary-care hospitals were approached and 600 consented patients (response rate: 19.2%) were included according to the inclusion & exclusion criteria. The response rate was low due to the frailty of the patients and their associated medical conditions meant they often opted not to participate in the study.

Just over half (52.7%, n = 316) of the participants were male and 70.3% (n = 422) were 60–74 years of age. Over three-quarters (77%, n = 462) were married and most (86.8%, n = 521) had primary education level and where of low annual income (79.5%, n = 477). Three-quarters (74.5%, n = 447) were unemployed (or on pensions) and a little over one half (55.8%, n = 335) were domiciled rurally. Self-reported health was moderate in 61.3% (n = 368) and a similar percentage (62%, n = 372) had attended ≤3 clinic visits in the previous year. Just over one-third (37.8%, n = 227) were smokers and comorbidity was present in over one half (54%, n = 324) of the patients (Table 1).

Table 1 Characteristics of hospitalized elderly population

Variables		Male (n = 316)	Female (n = 284)	Total (n = 600)
		n (%)	n (%)	n (%)
Age (years)	60–74	239 (75.6)	183 (64.4)	422 (70.3)
	75–89	57 (18)	76 (26.8)	133 (22.2)
	≥90	20 (6.3)	25 (8.8)	45 (7.5)
Civil Status	Single	15 (4.7)	6 (2.1)	21 (3.5)
	Married	284 (89.9)	178 (62.7)	462 (77)
	Widowed	13 (4.1)	78 (27.5)	91 (15.2)
	Divorced	4 (1.3)	22 (7.7)	26 (4.3)
Education level	Primary (≤10 years)	259 (82)	262 (92.3)	521 (86.8)
	Secondary (11–13 years)	54·(17.1)	21 (7.4)	75 (12.5)
	Tertiary (≥14 years)	3 (0.9)	1 (0.4)	4 (0.7)
Annual income	Low class (PKR0–299,999)	237 (75)	240 (84.5)	477 (79.5)
	Middle class (PKR300,000–999,999)	63 (19.9)	41 (14.4)	104 (17.3)
	Upper class (PKR ≥ 1,000,000)	16 (5.1)	3 (1.1)	19 (3.2)
Employment status	Employed	114 (36.1)	39 (13.7)	153 (25.5)
	Unemployed	202 (63.9)	245 (86.3)	447 (74.5)
Residence	Rural (an area outside of cities and towns)	177 (56)	158 (55.6)	335 (55.8)
	Urban (a city area considered as the inner city)	139 (44)	126 (44.4)	265 (44.2)
Self-reported health	Good	14 (4.4)	20 (7)	34 (5.7)
	Moderate	208 (65.8)	160 (56.3)	368 (61.3)
	Poor	94 (29.7)	104 (36.6)	198 (33)
Health Service Utilization	Clinic visits ≤3/year	207 (65.5)	165 (58.1)	372 (62)
	Clinic visits ≥4/year	109 (34.5)	119 (41.9)	228 (38)
Health Risks	Smoking	189 (59.8)	38 (13.4)	227 (37.8)
	Alcohol Consumption	5 (1.6)	0 (0)	5 (0.8)
	Obesity	48 (15.2)	166 (58.5)	214 (35.7)
	None	74 (23.4)	80 (28.2)	154 (25.7)
Co-morbidity	Present	163 (51.6)	161 (56.7)	324 (54)
	Absent	153 (48.4)	123 (43.3)	276 (46)
Number of drugs	5	251 (79.4)	204 (71.8)	455 (75.8)
	6	53 (16.8)	62 (21.8)	115 (19.2)
	7	11 (3.5)	15 (5.3)	26 (4.3)
	8	1 (0.3)	3 (1.1)	4 (0.7)

The most common chronic conditions among participants were; gastrointestinal (37.8%), hypertension (32%) and joint diseases (25.7%) (Table 2).

The most commonly prescribed drug classes were: A: alimentary tract and metabolism (80%), N: nervous system (66.3, J: anti-infectives for systemic use (62.2and C: cardiovascular system (48.3%), respectively. The detailed description about the drug utilization pattern is given in Tables 3 and 4.

The most commonly prescribed active substances were; A02BC01: omeprazole (n = 308, 51.3%), N02BE01: paracetamol (n = 305, 50.8%) and J01DD04: ceftriaxone (n = 241, 40.2%) (Table 5). A detailed description about the usage of all prescribed medicines can be found in Appendix.

After adjusting the factors associated with increased drug use among elderly hospitalized patients who were on polypharmacy regimens in the univariate analysis, the factors which remained significant in the multiple linear regression were; male gender (95% CI −.205, −.006, p = .039, B = −.091), being divorced (95% CI −.604, −.136, p = .002, B = −.130) and the presence of comorbidity (95% CI .068, .267, p = .001, B = .144) (Table 6).

Table 2 Chronic conditions associated with elderly hospitalized patients on polypharmacy

Male (n = 316)		Female (n = 284)		Total (n = 600)	
Chronic conditions	n (%)	Chronic conditions	n (%)	Chronic conditions	n (%)
Heart diseases[a]	62 (19.6)	Heart diseases[a]	43 (15.1)	Heart diseases[a]	105 (17.5)
Respiratory[b]	74 (23.4)	Respiratory[b]	69 (24.3)	Respiratory[b]	143 (23.8)
Gastrointestinal[c]	123 (38.9)	Gastrointestinal[c]	104 (36.6)	Gastrointestinal[c]	227 (37.8)
Diabetes Mellitus	41 (13)	Diabetes Mellitus	71 (25)	Diabetes Mellitus	112 (18.7)
Joint diseases[d]	75 (23.7)	Joint diseases[d]	79 (27.8)	Joint diseases[d]	154 (25.7)
Hypertension	89 (28.2)	Hypertension	103 (36.3)	Hypertension	192 (32)
CNS disorders[e]	63 (19.9)	CNS disorders[e]	46 (16.2)	CNS disorders[e]	109 (18.2)
Others	46 (14.6)	Others	49 (17.3)	Others	95 (15.8)

[a](Heart failure, Coronary ischemic disease, Atrial fibrillation, Stenosis)
[b](Chronic bronchitis, Asthma, Chronic obstructive pulmonary disease)
[c](Peptic ulcer, Irritable bowel syndrome)
[d](Osteoarthritis, Rheumatoid arthritis)
[e](Alzheimer's disease, Epilepsy, Depression, Anxiety)

Discussions

This large pharmaco-epidemiological study set out to determine drug utilization patterns of elderly patients on poly-pharmacy regimens within six hospitals in Punjab province, Pakistan. Furthermore, the study evaluated the combined effect of factors including; demographic, socioeconomic, and health-related issues on poly-pharmacy in this population. This Discussion compares a summary of the findings with the literature and notes the contribution, outlines the implications for policy, practice and future research and considers the limitations of the study.

Drug utilization patterns

Alimentary tract and metabolism category drugs were the most commonly prescribed class. Pakistan has been afflicted by alimentary tract disorders (ATDs) with an estimated prevalence of 45% [19]. It has been seen that ATDs affect a large number of people (approximately 60 to 70 million people in the US each year) and contribute substantially to morbidity and mortality [20]. According to one estimate, these disorders pose a significant fiscal and societal burden in the US [21]. In 2004 in the US, there were approximately 72 million ambulatory care visits, 4.6 million hospitalizations, 236,000 deaths and an estimated economic burden of $142 billion due to ATDs [22]. A study conducted in Finland reported that Alimentary tract and metabolism category drugs were prescribed to 77% of elderly patients who were on poly-pharmacy regimens [23]. Similarly, another study conducted in Italy reported that ATDs were prescribed to 42% of this population [24]. Thus the common prevalence of ATDs globally has led to increased utilization of alimentary tract and metabolism category drugs.

In the alimentary tract category, the most frequently prescribed sub-classes were; A02: drugs for acid related disorders (64.5%), A03: drugs for functional gastrointestinal disorders (21.5%), A01: stomatological preparations (20%) and A10: drugs used in diabetes (19.5%), respectively (Table 4). Drugs for acid related disorders are most commonly prescribed because they are generally safe and effective medicines used to treat gastric ulcers, heartburn, and gastro-oesophageal reflux disease (GORD). In this category, proton pump inhibitors (PPIs) are the highest-selling drugs worldwide. In addition to the treatment of gastritis, proton pump inhibitors are also very commonly prescribed as a gastro-protectant for patients prescribed antiplatelet and non-steriodal anti-inflammatory drugs (NSAIDs). In some countries they are available over-the-counter (OTC). Nexium (esomeprazole) in the US, earns nearly 6 billion USD and Risek (omeprazole) in Pakistan, earns close to 2 billion PKR, according to IMS Health data from 2012 [25]. It must be kept in mind that the chronic use of PPIs is associated with problems such as osteoporosis, hip fracture, escalated risk of infections, hypergastrinemia, decreased absorption of vitamins and minerals, kidney damage, dementia to name a few [26–28]. Healthcare professionals must adhere to prescribing guidelines and curb the excessive use of PPIs in-order to minimize associated adverse effects and reduce costs.

Nervous system drugs were the second most commonly prescribed class attributed to the high prevalence of neurologic and psychiatric disorders in this study. According to a World Health Organization Report, depression is the leading cause of health-related disability, globally [29]. Furthermore, a study on mood disorders in 30 European countries estimated that approximately 165 million elderly people (38% of the total population of these countries) suffer from significant mental illness [30]. In Pakistan, neurologic and psychiatric disorders are indeed prevalent [31]. A systematic review reported that the mean overall prevalence of anxiety and depressive

Table 3 Prescription drug utilization in study participants

Prescription Drug Utilization (%)																				
Pharmacologic groups	60–74 years				75–89 years				≥90 years				Total					
	Male (*n* = 239)	%	Female (*n* = 183)	%	Male (*n* = 57)	%	Female (*n* = 76)	%	Male (*n* = 20)	%	Female (*n* = 25)	%	Male (*n* = 316)	%	Female (*n* = 284)	%	Overall (*n* = 600)	%
A = Alimentary tract and metabolism	182	76.2	151	82.5	44	77.2	58	76.3	20	100	25	100	246	77.8	234	82.4	480	80
B = Blood and blood-forming organs	25	10.5	19	10.4	3	5.3	6	7.9	1	5	2	8	29	9.2	27	9.5	56	9.3
C = Cardiovascular system	102	42.7	81	44.3	36	63.2	44	57.9	12	60	15	60	150	47.5	140	49.3	290	48.3
D = Dermatologic	10	4.2	7	3.8	8	14	7	9.2	2	10	2	8	20	6.3	16	5.6	36	6
G = Genitourinary system	3	1.3	0	0	0	0	0	0	0	0	0	0	3	0.9	0	0	3	0.5
H = Systemic hormonal agents	10	4.2	18	9.8	2	3.5	2	2.6	2	10	2	8	14	4.4	22	7.7	36	6
J = Anti-infectives for systemic use	147	61.5	133	72.7	25	43.9	40	52.6	13	65	15	60	185	58.5	188	66.2	373	62.2
L = Antineoplastic and immune-modulating agents	7	2.9	2	1.1	1	1.8	3	3.9	0	0	0	0	8	2.5	5	1.8	13	2.2
M = Musculoskeletal system	70	29.3	56	30.6	18	31.6	26	34.2	2	10	12	48	90	28.5	94	33.1	184	30.7
N = Nervous system	160	66.9	134	73.2	34	59.6	48	63.2	12	60	10	40	206	65.2	192	67.6	398	66.3
P = Antiparasitic products	8	3.3	1	0.5	0	0	2	2.6	1	5	0	0	9	2.8	3	1.1	12	2
R = Respiratory system	65	27.2	54	29.5	20	35.1	29	38.2	5	25	9	36	90	28.5	92	32.4	182	30.3
V = Various	0	0	3	1.6	0	0	1	1.3	0	0	0	0	0	0	4	1.4	4	0.7

Table 4 Drug utilization pattern in study participants (ATC level 1–4)

Drug Utilization pattern (%[a])												
Level 1	*n*	%	Level 2	n	%	Level 3	*n*	%	Level 4	*n*	%
A	480	80	A01: Stomatological preparations	120	20	A01A: Stomatological preparations	120	20	A01AB: Anti-infectives and antiseptics for local oral treatment	120	20
			A02: Drugs for acid related disorders	387	64.5	A02B: Drugs for peptic ulcer and GERD	382	63.7	A02BA: H2-receptor antagonists	60	10
									A02BC: Proton pump inhibitors	309	51.5
			A03: Drugs for functional gastrointestinal disorders	129	21.5	A03F: Propulsives	116	19.3	A03FA: Propulsives	116	19.3
			A10: Drugs used in diabetes	117	19.5	A10B: Blood glucose lowering drugs	72	12	A10BB: Sulfonylureas	53	8.8
B	56	9.3	B01: Antithrombotic agents	26	4.3	B01A: Antithrombotic agents	26	4.3	B01AC: Platelet aggregation inhibitors	23	3.8
			B05: Blood substitutes	27	4.5	B05B:I.v. solutions	27	4.5	B05BC: Osmotic diuresis	27	4.5
C	290	48.3	C03: Diuretics	75	12.5	C03C: High-ceiling diuretics	68	11.3	C03CA: Sulfonamides, plain	68	11.3
			C07: Beta blocking agents	119	19.8	C07A: Beta blocking agents	119	19.8	C07AB: Beta blocking agents, selective	62	10.3
			C08: Calcium channel blockers	99	16.5	C08C: Selective calcium channel blockers	91	15.2	C08CA: Dihydropyridine derivatives	91	15.2
			C10: Lipid modifying agents	99	16.5	C10A: Lipid modifying agents, plain	97	16.2	C10AA: HMG CoA reductase inhibitors	97	16.2
D	36	6	D07: Corticosteroids	41	6.8	D07A: Corticosteroids, plain	41	6.8	D07AA: Corticosteroids, weak (group I)	30	5
G	3	0.5	G04: Urologicals	4	0.7	G04C: Drugs used in BPH	2	0.3	G04CA: Alpha-adrenoreceptor antagonists	2	0.3
H	36	6	H01: Pituitary and hypothalamic hormones	31	5.2	H01C: Hypothalamic hormones	31	5.2	H01CB: Somatostatin and analogues	31	5.2
J	373	62.2	J01: Antibacterials for systemic use	495	82.5	J01D: Other beta-lactam antibacterials	266	44.3	J01DD: 3rd-generation cephalosporins	255	42.5
						J01 M: Quinolone antibacterials	68	11.3	J01MA: Fluoroquinolones	68	11.3
			J04: Antimycobacterials	92	15.3	J04A: Drugs for tuberculosis	92	15.3	J04AK: Other drugs	48	8
L	13	2.2	L01: Antineoplastic agents	17	2.8	L01B: Antimetabolites	04	0.7	L01BA: Folic acid analogues	03	0.5
M	184	30.7	M01: Anti-inflammatory and antirheumatic products	188	31.3	M01A: Anti-inflammatory and antirheumatic products, non-steroids	188	31.3	M01AB: Acetic acid derivatives	159	26.5
N	398	66.3	N02: Analgesics	403	67.2	N02B: Other analgesics and antipyretics	359	59.8	N02BE: Anilides	305	50.8
			N03: Antiepileptics	67	11.2	N03A: Antiepileptics	67	11.2	N03AX: Other antiepileptics	32	5.3
P	12	2	P01: Antiprotozoals	13	2.2	P01B: Antimalarials	12	2	P01BF: Artemisinin and derivatives	9	1.5
R	182	30.3	R01: Nasal preparations	84	14	R01A: Decongestants and other	84	14	R01AD: Corticosteroids	61	10.2
			R03: Drugs for obstructive airway diseases	113	18.8	R03A: Adrenergics, inhalants	86	14.3	R03AC: Selective beta-2 agonists	43	7.2
			R06: Antihistamines for systemic use	67	11.2	R06A: Antihistamines for systemic use	67	11.2	R06AA: Aminoalkyl ethers	46	7.7
V	4	0.7	V03: Other therapeutic products	6	1	V03A: Other therapeutic products	6	1	V03AB: Antidotes	6	1

Note: A patient may be prescribed one or more than one drug from level 2, level 3 and level 4 categories
[a]Percentages given with respect to the total sample size of the patients. GERD Gastroesophageal reflux disease, BPH Benign prostate hyperplasia

Table 5 Top active substances prescribed to study participants (ATC level 5)

Name	ATC Code	Frequency (*n* = 3179)	Percentage[a]	Trend in use
Amlodipine	C08CA01	78	13	Medium
Aspirin	N02BA01	54	9	Low
Atenolol	C07AB03	62	10.3	Medium
Captopril	C09AA01	53	8.8	Low
Ceftriaxone	J01DD04	241	40.2	High
Dexamethasone	R01AD03	61	10.2	Medium
Diclofenac sodium	M01AB05	111	18.5	Medium
Furosemide	C03CA01	68	11.3	Medium
Lactulose	A06AD11	49	8.2	Low
Metformin	A10BA02	53	8.8	Low
Metoclopramide	A03FA01	86	14.3	Medium
Metronidazole	A01AB17	119	19.8	Medium
Omeprazole	A02BC01	308	51.3	High
Paracetamol	N02BE01	305	50.8	High
Simvastatin	C10AA01	63	10.5	Medium

[a]Percentages given with respect to the total sample size of patients

disorders in the Pakistani population is 34% (range 29–66% for women and 10–33% for men) [32]. Three studies conducted in the Finnish elderly population reported that nervous system drugs were prescribed to between 63% and 89% in this group of patients [23, 33, 34]. Another study in nearby Sweden reported that this class was prescribed to 37% of the elderly population [35]. Thus neurological disorders afflicts both high income and low income countries with comparatively high treatment rates in high income countries [36].

In the nervous system category, frequently prescribed sub-classes in this study were; N02: Analgesics (67.2%), N03: Anti-epileptics (11.2%), respectively (Table 4). Analgesics, main therapy for low back pain, were the most frequently prescribed agents because low back pain is commonplace in the elderly, due to ageing of intervertebral discs [37, 38] with a prevalence of 60–70% in industrialized nations [39]. In 2010 Global Burden of Disease Study estimated that low back pain was one of the top 10 injuries and diseases throughout the world [40]. An American study reported that an estimated 149 million work days were lost due to low back pain, with an economic burden of USD 100 to 200 billion [41, 42].

The third most frequently prescribed drugs in this study were from the anti-infectives for systemic use class. These medicines are prescribed for a variety of infections caused by bacteria, virus, fungi, viroids, prions, nematodes, arthropods and so forth. A range of medicines are used to treat infections including;

Table 6 Factors affecting number of prescribed drugs: multiple linear regression analysis

Variables	Unstandardized Coefficients	Standardized Coefficients	*p*-value	95.0% Confidence Interval for B	
	Std. Error	B		Lower Bound	Upper Bound
Male	.051	−.091	*.039*	−.205	−.006
Widowed	.073	−.008	.865	−.157	.132
Divorced	.119	−.130	*.002*	−.604	−.136
Low income class	.135	.051	.592	−.193	.339
Middle income class	.144	−.034	.716	−.335	.230
Moderate self-reported health	.105	−.075	.397	−.296	.118
Poor self-reported health	.127	−.034	.744	−.292	.208
≥4 clinic visits	.076	.075	.238	−.060	.240
Comorbidity	.051	.144	*.001*	.068	.267

P-value < .05 was considered statistically significant. Note: Only statistically significant variables in the univariate analysis were entered in the multiple linear regression analysis and are shown in the Table
Model summary: $R^2 = 0.052$, $p < 0.0005$

antivirals, antibiotics, antifungals, antihelminthics, and antiprotozoals. Infectious diseases accounted for 9.2 million deaths worldwide in 2013 (approximately 17% of all deaths) [43]. As in many other developing countries, infectious diseases are common in Pakistan and therefore anti-infectives are commonly prescribed and have a large market size [44]. A study conducted in Italy reported that anti-infectives for systemic use category drugs were prescribed to 41% of the elderly population [24]. Another study conducted in Sweden reported that anti-infectives were prescribed to just over one quarter (27.6%) of the elderly population [35]. It is likely that inter-country variability of infectious diseases is responsible for the varying patterns of global antibiotic use. In the Anti-infectives (for systemic use) category, the most frequently prescribed sub-classes were; J01: anti-bacterials for systemic use (82.5%) and J04: anti-mycobacterials (15.3%) (Table 4). Anti-bacterials/antibiotics are the most widely consumed pharmaceutical group, worldwide [45]. According to one estimate, the utilization of antibiotics has increased by 36% over the 10 years from 2000 to 2010. Russia, China, South Africa, India and Brazil are accountable for 76% of this of the prescribing and the growth [46]. In India, a rise from 29 to 57% was seen in Klebsiella pneumonia between 2008 and 2014. The concerning aspect here is that Klebseilla is becoming increasingly resistant to very potent antibiotics such as carbapenems [45]. The other concern is that this figure is considerably lower in the US and Europe i.e. less than 10% [45]. Generally, for most countries the usage of antibiotics varies with the season [46] and this appears to be no different in Pakistan.

The fourth most frequently prescribed medicines in this study were for cardiovascular diseases. These findings are in line with the fact that cardiovascular disorders (CVDs) are the most prevalent and leading causes of death worldwide [47], resulting in 17.3 million deaths in 2013 [43]. In 2010, the total costs of CVD globally was estimated to be in the vicinity of 315.4 billion USD [48]. Amongst the elderly population, 71% of people aged between 60 and 80 years, and 85% of people over 80 years are estimated to have CVD [49]. Similarly, in Pakistan, amongst the elderly population, 76% of people aged between 60 and 70 years, and 83% of people over 90 years are estimated to have CVD [50]. According to a Danish study of persons aged ≥70 years, cardiovascular drugs (35%) were the most frequently prescribed class [25]. A Danish study revealed that the most commonly prescribed medicines amongst 75 year olds were cardiovascular (25%) drugs [12] where it was almost double this in Sweden with 47% of elderly being prescribed cardiovascular drugs [41]. In the cardiovascular category, the most frequently prescribed sub-classes were; C07: beta blocking agents (19.8%), C08: calcium channel blockers (16.5%), C10: lipid-modifying agents (16.5%) and C03: diuretics (12.5%) respectively (Table 4). Beta-blocking agents are most widely prescribed because they are used to manage cardiac arrhythmias and myocardial infarction, as well as hypertension [51]. Diuretics were the most commonly prescribed class because they represent the first-line treatment for hypertension and the prevalence of hypertension is high throughout the world; it affected between 30 and 45% of the population of Europe in 2013 [52].

In summary, the most commonly prescribed active substances were; omeprazole, paracetamol and ceftriaxone. This follows the developed world with regards omeprazole and paracetamol but the excessive use of potent IV antibiotics such as ceftriaxone warrants serious review.

Factors associated with "poly-pharmacy"

Results from the multiple linear regression analysis revealed that male gender (negatively associated); being divorced (negatively associated) and comorbidity (positively associated) were the main factors associated with increased drug use among elderly hospitalized patients in Pakistan, who were on poly-pharmacy regimens.

The greater ratio of female to male gender amongst these elderly hospitalized patients on poly-pharmacy regimens could be attributed to physiological aspects, which differentially adjust the etiology patterns for females and males. These altered etiology patterns may represent illness behaviors such as being more sensitive to their health and consequently taking more medicines. It is also possible that there are more women in hospital because men simply die at an earlier age, often without even getting to hospital [53]. Such differences explain the use of specific types of medicines by women only. Simultaneously, the societal roles adopted by women in Pakistan, principally as housewives or paid employees also influence these gender differences [43]. Numerous studies have proposed that multiple roles for women, including home-maker, parent, and paid employees are likely to be hectic and harmful to their health [54–56]. Civil status, such as 'being divorced' played an important role in the illness behavior in this study. Amongst this subgroup of the elderly, psychological conditions such as depression and anxiety contributed towards poly-pharmacy [56]. Comorbidities are a significant factor associated with poly-pharmacy and increased mortality in older people. The elderly are significantly more prone to comorbidities due to aging and physiological changes; the majority of the older people (up to about 80%) suffer from chronic illnesses [8]. Consequently, they are more likely to have greater drug utilization to manage their chronic illnesses [9].

Implications for policy and practice

There are implications from the findings of this study for pharmaceutical policy and practice in Pakistan.

In terms of policy and practice, there has been very little evaluation of "poly-pharmacy" in the context of Pakistan and so this study contributes significantly to that understanding. This study raises the question of whether prescribing needs to change in some way? Omeprazole was the most commonly prescribed pharmaceutical, followed by paracetamol and this appears to follow the trends in developing countries. What is most concerning, is the very high use of powerful IV antibiotics such as ceftriaxone. A national policy and guidelines need to be put in place to ensure the rational prescribing of potent antibiotics such as this. Further, in Pakistan infrastructure for proper medicine dispensing and patient education is not available within the health system and the availability of pharmacists at public hospital and private pharmacies is negligible. Elderly people who are on polypharmacy regimens are at risk of medicines overuse and adverse effects associated with polypharmacy. There is a global trend to "de-prescribe" in the setting of hospitalized older adults and the government should take the appropriate measures to ensure skilled pharmacists are available to enact this.

Implications for future research

Future research could look at evaluating the impact of pharmacists around implementing and monitoring drug use indicators and clinical guidelines. Further, studies like the current one could be extended to assess potential drug interactions, trends in prevalence and determinants of potentially inappropriate medication use based on the Beer's Criteria among the elderly population. This study recruited hospitalized elderly patients and it cannot be assumed that the sample is representative in any form of the ambulatory primary care population. Studies need to be conducted in the general community to better understand pharmaco-epidemiological patterns across the wider population. It will be interesting to explore in more detail the impact of being divorced on medicines use in Pakistan as the data (un-expectantly) suggests this is a significant determinant.

Study limitations

There are a few study limitations. First, the population under study was elderly patients being hospitalized in the selected tertiary-care hospitals. Second, only those elderly patients were approached who are taking more than five prescribed medicines per day. Third, DDDs for the prescribed medicines to the hospitalized elderly patients were not calculated. Finally, the study did not investigate the ADRs associated with poly-pharmacy. However, this study provides the baseline information to the researchers regarding the drug utilization pattern among a cohort of hospitalized elderly patients in the Punjab province of Pakistan.

Conclusion and recommendations

The increased use of prescription medicines is commonplace amongst the elderly population worldwide, and this study suggests it is no different in Pakistan. Similarly, the average number of medicines being used by elderly women is on the rise. This study concludes that a series of factors are responsible for "poly-pharmacy" in older adults in Pakistan including; being male, being divorced and the presence of multiple comorbidities. The most common chronic conditions associated with these hospitalized elderly patients were; gastrointestinal, hypertension and joint diseases, respectively. In this study, the most commonly prescribed drug classes reflect that seen in developed nations including; Alimentary tract and metabolism, Nervous system, Antibacterial for systemic use and Cardiovascular system, respectively.

There is no doubt that the usage of medicines is essential; however, poly-pharmacy is likely to also compound in a cyclical manner the associated problems with the use of multiple medicines. It is highly recommended that greater consideration be given to elderly hospitalized patients who are on poly-pharmacy regimens, in Pakistan. To reduce the potential for ADRs associated with poly-pharmacy and to get the maximum benefit of therapy, there is a requirement to use medicines effectively and to evaluate progress at regular intervals based on diagnosis and expected treatment outcomes. The rational use of medicines is of utmost importance, most particularly in the elderly population and the responsibility lies with health-care professionals to regularly evaluate medicine use.

Unfortunately, geriatrics is not recognized as a specialized area of research in Pakistan and hospital pharmacists are not as commonplace; as they are in developed nations. Under the current scenario, the role of the pharmacist in the management of elderly patients must be enhanced in Pakistan and the impact of this intervention could be tested by employing experimental study designs. The contribution of this paper is that it provides baseline information about the prescribing patterns in the older hospitalized patients in Pakistan and provides a platform for evaluation of policy and practice interventions by Pakistani hospital pharmacists in the future.

Appendix

Table 7 Description about the usage of all prescribed medicines

Sr. No	Name	ATC Code	Frequency ($N = 3179$)	Percentage[a]	Trend
1	Aciclovir	J05AB01	11	1.8	Low
2	Acarbose	A10BF01	1	0.2	Low
3	Aclarubicin	L04AB04	1	0.5	Low
4	Adalimumab	L01DB04	3	0.2	Low
5	Alimemazine	R06AD01	2	0.3	Low
6	Allopurinol	M04AA01	17	2.8	Low
7	Amantadine	N04BB01	1	0.2	Low
8	Amiodarone	C01BD01	2	0.3	Low
9	Aminophylline	R03DA05	16	2.7	Low
10	Amitriptyline	N06AA09	2	0.3	Low
11	Amoxicillin	J01CA04	27	4.5	Low
12	Amlodipine	C08CA01	78	13.0	Medium
13	Anastrazole	L02BG03	2	0.3	Low
14	Artemether	P01BF01	08	1.3	Low
15	Aspirin	N02BA01	54	9.0	Low
16	Atenolol	C07AB03	62	10.3	Medium
17	Atropine	A03BA01	4	0.7	Low
18	Atorvastatin	C10AA05	15	2.5	Low
19	Attapulgite	A07BC04	1	0.2	Low
20	Azithromycin	J01FA10	13	2.2	Low
21	Beclomethasone	D07AC15	11	1.8	Low
22	Bisoprolol	C07AB07	1	0.2	Low
23	Bismuth subcitrate	A07BX05	1	0.2	Low
24	Benzyl penicillin	J01 CE01	7	1.2	Low
25	Bleomycin	L01 DC01	1	0.2	Low
26	Bromazepam	N05BA08	8	1.3	Low
27	Bromocriptine	G02CB01	3	0.5	Low
28	Calcium gluconate	A12AA03	1	0.2	Low
29	Captopril	C09AA01	53	8.8	Low
30	Carbamazepine	N03AF01	6	1.0	Low
31	Carvedilol	C07AG02	2	0.3	Low
32	Cefotaxime	J01DD01	14	2.3	Low
33	Ceftriaxone	J01DD04	241	40.2	High
34	Celecoxib	M01AH01	5	0.8	Low
35	Cephradine	J01DB09	4	0.7	Low
36	Cetirizine	R06AE07	2	0.3	Low
37	Cimetidine	A02BA01	3	0.5	Low
38	Chlorhexidine	A01AB03	1	0.2	Low
39	Chloramphenicol	J01BA01	6	1.0	Low
40	Chlorpheniramine	R06AB04	11	1.8	Low
41	Chlorpromazine	N05AA01	6	1.0	Low
42	Colecalciferol	A11CC05	6	1.0	Low

Table 7 Description about the usage of all prescribed medicines *(Continued)*

43	Ciprofloxacin	J01MA02	34	5.7	Low
44	Clarithromycin	J01FA09	25	4.2	Low
45	Clindamycin	J01FF01	7	1.2	Low
46	Clopidogrel	B01AC04	23	3.8	Low
47	Clonazepam	N03AE01	2	0.3	Low
48	Clonidine	C02AC01	2	0.3	Low
49	Codeine	R05DA04	2	0.3	Low
50	Colchicine	M04 AC01	21	3.5	Low
51	Cromolyn sodium	A07EB01	3	0.5	Low
52	Cyclosporine	N04 AD01	2	0.3	Low
53	Dacarbazine	L01AX04	2	0.3	Low
54	Darifenacin	G04BD10	1	0.2	Low
55	Drotaverine	A03AD02	5	0.8	Low
56	Dexamethasone	R01AD03	61	10.2	Medium
57	Diclofenac sodium	M01AB05	111	18.5	Medium
58	Dicyclomine	A03AA07	1	0.2	Low
59	Digoxin	C01AA05	3	0.5	Low
60	Diphenhydramine	R06AA02	46	7.7	Low
61	Diphenoxylate	A07DA01	3	0.5	Low
62	Diloxanide	P01AC01	1	0.2	Low
63	Diltiazem	C08DB01	1	0.2	Low
64	Divalproex sodium	N03AG01	25	4.2	Low
65	Dobutamine	C01CA07	2	0.3	Low
66	Domperidone	A03FA03	30	5.0	Low
67	Dopamine	C01CA04	2	0.3	Low
68	Doxycycline	J01AA02	2	0.3	Low
69	Epinephrine	B02BC09	4	0.7	Low
70	Ephedrine	R01AA03	1	0.2	Low
71	Erythromycin	J01FA01	1	0.2	Low
72	Escitalopram	N06AB04	18	2.8	Low
73	Ethambutol	J04AK02	25	4.2	Low
74	Ezitimibe	C10AX09	2	0.3	Low
75	Famotidine	A02BA03	20	3.3	Low
76	Fexofenadine	R06AX26	6	1.0	Low
77	Fluoxetine	N06AB03	2	0.3	Low
78	Formoterol	R03AC13	4	0.7	Low
79	Fosfomycin	J01XX01	4	0.7	Low
80	Furosemide	C03CA01	68	11.3	Medium
81	Gentamicin	J01GB03	9	1.3	Low
82	Glimepiride	A10BB12	10	1.7	Low
83	Glipizide	A10BB07	9	1.5	Low
84	Glyceryl trinitrite	C01DA02	9	1.5	Low
85	Haloperidol	N05 AD01	5	0.8	Low
86	Heparin	B01AB01	3	0.5	Low
87	Hydrocortisone	D07AA02	30	5.0	Low

Table 7 Description about the usage of all prescribed medicines *(Continued)*

88	Hydralline	C02DB02	15	2.5	Low
89	Hydralazine	C02DB02	6	1.0	Low
90	Ibuprofen	M01AE01	24	4.0	Low
91	Imipenem	J01DH51	3	0.5	Low
92	Imipramine	N06AA02	1	0.2	Low
93	Indacaterol	R03AC18	2	0.3	Low
94	Indomethacin	M01AB01	5	0.8	Low
95	Insulin	A10AB02	40	6.7	Low
96	Ipratropium	R01AX03	19	3.2	Low
97	Isoniazid	J04 AC01	23	3.8	Low
98	Isosorbide mononitrite	C01DA14	3	0.5	Low
99	Isosorbide dinitrite	C01DA08	2	0.3	Low
100	Ketorolac	M01AB15	43	7.2	Low
101	Lactulose	A06AD11	49	8.2	Low
102	Labetalol	C07AG01	3	0.5	Low
103	Leflunamide	L04AA13	3	0.5	Low
104	Leviteracetam	N03AX14	32	5.3	Low
105	Levodopa	N04BA01	4	0.7	Low
106	Levofloxacin	J01MA12	11	1.8	Low
107	Lisinopril	C09AA03	8	1.3	Low
108	Loperamide	A07DA03	5	0.8	Low
109	Losartan	C09CA01	3	0.5	Low
110	Lovastatin	C10AA02	2	0.3	Low
111	Lumefantrine	P01BF01	1	0.2	Low
112	Mannitol	B05BC01	27	4.5	Low
113	Mebeverine	A03AA04	3	0.5	Low
114	Mecobalamine	B03BA01	2	0.3	Low
115	Midazolam	N05CD08	3	0.5	Low
116	Mercaptopurine	L01BB02	1	0.2	Low
117	Meropenem	J01DH02	4	0.7	Low
118	Metformin	A10BA02	53	8.8	Low
119	Methotrexate	L01BA01	3	0.5	Low
120	Metoclopramide	A03FA01	86	14.3	Medium
121	Metoprolol	C07AB02	1	0.2	Low
122	Metaproterenol	R03AB03	1	0.2	Low
123	Metronidazole	A01AB17	119	19.8	Medium
124	Midazolam	N05CD08	15	2.5	Low
125	Mirtazapine	M06AX11	3	0.5	Low
126	Misoprostol	A02BB01	4	0.7	Low
127	Mg-hydroxide	A02AA04	5	0.8	Low
128	Montelukast sodium	R03DC03	16	2.7	Low
129	Morphine	N02AA01	3	0.5	Low
130	Moxifloxacin	J01MA14	23	3.8	Low
131	Nalbufine	N02AF02	13	2.2	Low
132	Naltrexone	V03AB30	6	1.0	Low

Table 7 Description about the usage of all prescribed medicines *(Continued)*

133	Natalizumab	L04AA23	1	0.2	Low
134	Nedocromil	R01AC07	3	0.5	Low
135	Nefazodone	N06AX06	1	0.2	Low
136	Nifedipine	C08CA05	2	0.3	Low
137	Nimodipine	C08CA06	11	1.8	Low
138	Nitroglycerine	C01DA02	6	1.0	Low
139	Nitropruside	C02DD01	1	0.2	Low
140	Nitrazepam	N05CD02	2	0.3	Low
141	Octreotide	H01CB02	30	5.0	Low
142	Omeprazole	A02BC01	308	51.3	High
143	Paracetamol	N02BE01	305	50.8	High
144	Paclitaxel	L01CD01	3	0.5	Low
145	Pantoprazole	A02BC02	1	0.2	Low
146	Phenelzine	N06AF03	2	0.3	Low
147	Phenytoin	N03AB02	2	0.3	Low
148	Pipracilline	J01CA12	1	0.2	Low
149	Prazosin	C02CA01	2	0.3	Low
150	Prednisone	H02AB07	1	0.2	Low
151	Prednisolone	H02AB06	1	0.2	Low
152	Probenecid	M04AB01	3	0.5	Low
153	Procainamide	C01BA02	1	0.2	Low
154	Propoxyphene	N02 AC04	2	0.3	Low
155	Propranolol	C07AA05	20	3.3	Low
156	Propylthiouracil	H03BA02	3	0.5	Low
157	Polymixin	J01XB02	2	0.3	Low
158	Pyrazinamide	J04AK01	23	3.8	Low
159	Pyridoxine	A11HA02	17	2.8	Low
160	Quinine	P01BC01	3	0.5	Low
161	Ranitidine	A02BA02	37	6.2	Low
162	Rifampicin	J04AB02	21	3.5	Low
163	Rifaxamin	D06AX11	5	0.8	Low
164	Reserpine	C02AA02	1	0.2	Low
165	Rituximab	L01XX21	1	0.2	Low
166	Rosuvastatin	C10AA07	17	2.8	Low
167	Salbutamol	R03AC02	43	7.2	Low
168	Sulbactum	J01CG01	11	1.8	Low
169	Salmeterol	R03AC12	22	3.7	Low
170	Simvastatin	C10AA01	63	10.5	Medium
171	Sitagliptin	A10BH01	4	0.7	Low
172	Selegiline	N04BD01	2	0.3	Low
173	Sertraline	N06AB06	1	0.2	Low
174	Somatostatin	H01CB01	1	0.2	Low
175	Solifenacin	G04BD08	1	0.2	Low
176	Spironolactone	C03DA01	7	1.2	Low
177	Streptomycin	J01GA01	4	0.7	Low

Table 7 Description about the usage of all prescribed medicines *(Continued)*

178	Sucralfate	A02BX02	9	1.5	Low
179	Sodium picosulfate	A06AB08	1	0.2	Low
180	Sulfasalazine	A07EC01	3	0.5	Low
181	Tamsulosin	G04CA02	2	0.3	Low
182	Tazobactum	J01CG02	19	3.2	Low
183	Theophylline	R03DA04	5	0.8	Low
184	Thioridazine	N05 AC02	1	0.2	Low
185	Thyroxin	H03AA01	4	0.7	Low
186	Tizinidine	M03BX02	1	0.2	Low
187	Terbutaline	R03AC03	4	0.7	Low
188	Tramadol	N02AX02	26	4.3	Low
189	Transemic acid	B02AA02	7	1.2	Low
190	Telmisartan	C09CA07	5	0.8	Low
191	Trustuzumab	L01XC03	2	0.3	Low
192	Vancomycin	J01XA01	23	3.8	Low
193	Venlafaxine	N06AX16	1	0.2	Low
194	Verapamil	C08DA01	7	1.2	Low
195	Vincristine	L01CA02	1	0.2	Low
196	Ziprasidone	N05AE04	1	0.2	Low
197	Zinc sulphate	A12CB01	1	0.2	Low

[a]Percentages given with respect to total sample size (n = 600)

Abbreviations
ADRs: Adverse Drug Reactions; ATC: Anatomical Therapeutic Chemical; ATDs: Alimentary Tract Disorders; BMI: Body Mass Index; CNS: Central Nervous System; CVDs: Cardiovascular Disorders; DDDs: Defined Daily Doses; LBP: Low Back Pain; SPSS: Statistical Package for Social Sciences; WHO: World Health Organization

Acknowledgements
None.

Funding
No funding was involved in the preparation of this article or in the decision to submit it for publication.

Authors' contributions
MRS and MAT conceptualized and designed the study. MAT is the research supervisor of MRS. SS, ZB, AS and MQZ also participated in design of the study. MRS collected, analyzed and interpreted the data. MRS, MQZ, ZB, SS, AS and MAT drafted the manuscript. SS made substantial contributions in preparing the revised manuscript. All authors read and approved final version of the manuscript.

Competing interests
The authors declare that they have no competing interests.

Author details
[1]Department of Pharmacy, The Islamia University of Bahawalpur, Bahawalpur, Pakistan. [2]School of Management, Massey University, Auckland, New Zealand. [3]Department of Pharmacy, University of Huddersfield, Huddersfield, UK.

References

1. Pappa E, et al. Prescribed-drug utilization and polypharmacy in a general population in Greece: association with sociodemographic, health needs, health-services utilization, and lifestyle factors. Eur J Clin Pharmacol. 2011; 67(2):185–92.
2. Haider SI, et al. Analysis of the association between polypharmacy and socioeconomic position among elderly aged≥ 77 years in Sweden. Clin Ther. 2008;30(2):419–27.
3. Haider SI, et al. The influence of educational level on Polypharmacy and inappropriate drug use: a register-based study of more than 600,000 older people. J Am Geriatr Soc. 2009;57(1):62–9.
4. Junius-Walker U, Theile G, Hummers-Pradier E. Prevalence and predictors of polypharmacy among older primary care patients in Germany. Fam Pract. 2007;24(1):14–9.
5. Little P, et al. Importance of patient pressure and perceived pressure and perceived medical need for investigations, referral, and prescribing in primary care: nested observational study. BMJ. 2004;328(7437):444.
6. Furu K, Straume B, Thelle D. Legal drug use in a general population: association with gender, morbidity, health care utilization, and lifestyle characteristics. J Clin Epidemiol. 1997;50(3):341–9.
7. Fillenbaum GG, et al. Factors predicting change in prescription and nonprescription drug use in a community-residing black and white elderly population. J Clin Epidemiol. 1996;49(5):587–93.
8. Milton JC, Hill-Smith I, Jackson SH. Prescribing for older people. BMJ. 2008; 336(7644):606–9.

9. Acurcio FdA, et al. Use of medications by elderly Brazilian retirees: 1-methodology and response rates of a multicenter survey. Cadernos de Saúde Pública. 2006;22(1):87–96.
10. Jalal S, Younis MZ. Aging and elderly in Pakistan. Ageing Int. 2014;39(1):4–12.
11. Zafar SN, et al. Health and needs assessment of geriatric patients: results of a survey at a teaching hospital in Karachi. J Pak Med Assoc. 2006;56(10):470.
12. Baksaas I, Lunde P. National drug policies: the need for drug utilization studies. Trends Pharmacol Sci. 1986;7:331–4.
13. Laporte J-R, Porta M, Capella D. Drug utilization studies: a tool for determining the effectiveness of drug use. Br J Clin Pharmacol. 1983;16(3):301–4.
14. Health Department. Health Services. 2016 [cited 2016 29 June]; Available from: http://health.punjab.gov.pk/Services_Package.
15. The News. Population shoots up by 47 percent since 1998, in the News. 2012. THE NEWS INTERNATIONAL.
16. Raosoft. Sample size calculator. 2015 [cited 2016 December 2015]; Available from: http://www.raosoft.com/samplesize.html.
17. World Health Organization. The anatomical therapeutic chemical classification system with defined daily doses (ATC/DDD). Oslo: WHO; 2006.
18. Field, A., Discovering statistics using SPSS. 2009 London. 2005, SAGE ISBN: 9781847879073.
19. Lovell RM, Ford AC. Global prevalence of and risk factors for irritable bowel syndrome: a meta-analysis. Clin Gastroenterol Hepatol. 2012;10(7):712–21. e4
20. Shaheen NJ, et al. The burden of gastrointestinal and liver diseases, 2006. Am J Gastroenterol. 2006;101(9):2128–38.
21. Russo MW, et al. Digestive and liver diseases statistics, 2004. Gastroenterol. 2004;126(5):1448–53.
22. Peery AF, et al. Burden of gastrointestinal disease in the United States: 2012 update. Gastroenterol. 2012;143(5):1179–87 e1-3.
23. Jyrkkä J, et al. Patterns of drug use and factors associated with polypharmacy and excessive polypharmacy in elderly persons. Drugs Aging. 2009;26(6):493–503.
24. Nobili A, et al. Drug utilization and polypharmacy in an Italian elderly population: the EPIFARM-elderly project. Pharmacoepidemiol Drug Saf. 2011;20(5):488–96.
25. Arcidiacono P, et al. Pharmaceutical followers. Int J Ind Organ. 2013;31(5): 538–53.
26. Targownik LE, et al. Use of proton pump inhibitors and risk of osteoporosis-related fractures. Can Med Assoc J. 2008;179(4):319–26.
27. Eusebi LH, et al. Proton pump inhibitors: risks of long-term use. J Gastroenterol Hepatol. 2017;32(7):1295-1302.
28. Heidelbaugh JJ, et al. Overutilization of proton-pump inhibitors: what the clinician needs to know. Ther Adv Gastroenterol. 2012;5(4):219–32.
29. Forsythe P, et al. Mood and gut feelings. Brain Behav Immun. 2010; 24(1):9–16.
30. Wittchen HU, et al. The size and burden of mental disorders and other disorders of the brain in Europe 2010. Eur Neuropsychopharmacol. 2011; 21(9):655–79.
31. Atif M, Azeem M, Sarwar MR. Potential problems and recommendations regarding substitution of generic antiepileptic drugs: a systematic review of literature. SpringerPlus. 2016;5(1):1.
32. Mirza I, Jenkins R. Risk factors, prevalence, and treatment of anxiety and depressive disorders in Pakistan: systematic review. BMJ. 2004;328(7443):794.
33. Jyrkkä J, et al. Increasing use of medicines in elderly persons: a five-year follow-up of the Kuopio 75+ study. Eur J Clin Pharmacol. 2006;62(2):151–8.
34. Linjakumpu T, et al. Use of medications and polypharmacy are increasing among the elderly. J Clin Epidemiol. 2002;55(8):809–17.
35. Jörgensen T, et al. Prescription drug use, diagnoses, and healthcare utilization among the elderly. Ann Pharmacother. 2001;35(9):1004–9.
36. Whiteford HA, et al. The global burden of mental, neurological and substance use disorders: an analysis from the global burden of disease study 2010. PLoS One. 2015;10(2):e0116820.
37. Andersson G. The epidemiology of spinal disorders. The adult spine: Principles and practice. 1997;
38. Phillips FM, et al. Lumbar spine fusion for chronic low back pain due to degenerative disc disease: a systematic review. Spine. 2013;38(7):E409–22.
39. Taimela S, et al. The prevalence of low back pain among children and adolescents: a nationwide, cohort-based questionnaire survey in finland. Spine. 1997;22(10):1132–6.
40. Vos T, et al. Years lived with disability (YLDs) for 1160 sequelae of 289 diseases and injuries 1990–2010: a systematic analysis for the global burden of disease study 2010. Lancet. 2013;380(9859):2163–96.
41. Guo HR, et al. Back pain prevalence in US industry and estimates of lost workdays. Am J Public Health. 1999;89(7):1029–35.
42. Rubin DI. Epidemiology and risk factors for spine pain. Neurol Clin. 2007; 25(2):353–71.
43. Naghavi M, et al. Global, regional, and national age-sex specific all-cause and cause-specific mortality for 240 causes of death, 1990-2013: a systematic analysis for the global burden of disease study 2013. Lancet. 2015;385(9963):117–71.
44. Atif M, et al. Rights and responsibilities of tuberculosis patients, and the Global Fund: a qualitative study. PLoS One. 2016;11(3):e0151321.
45. Reardon S. Antibiotic resistance sweeping developing world. Nature. 2014; 509(7499):141–2.
46. Van Boeckel TP, et al. Global antibiotic consumption 2000 to 2010: an analysis of national pharmaceutical sales data. Lancet Infect Dis. 2014; 14(8):742–50.
47. Mendis S, Puska P, Norrving B. Global atlas on cardiovascular disease prevention and control. Geneva: World Health Organization; 2011.
48. Go AS, et al. Heart disease and stroke statistics–2014 update: a report from the American Heart Association. Circulation. 2014;129(3):e28.
49. Go A, et al. Heart disease and stroke statistics-2013 update: a report from the American Heart Association. Circulation. 2013;127(1):e1–e240.
50. Williams MA, et al. Secondary prevention of coronary heart disease in the elderly (with emphasis on patients≥ 75 years of age) an American Heart Association scientific statement from the council on clinical cardiology subcommittee on exercise, cardiac rehabilitation, and prevention. Circulation. 2002;105(14):1735–43.
51. Freemantle N, et al. β blockade after myocardial infarction: systematic review and meta regression analysis. BMJ. 1999;318(7200):1730–7.
52. Taylor J. 2013 ESH/ESC guidelines for the management of arterial hypertension. Eur Heart J. 2013;34(28):2108–9.
53. Barat I, Andreasen F, Damsgaard EMS. The consumption of drugs by 75-year-old individuals living in their own homes. Eur J Clin Pharmacol. 2000; 56(6–7):501–9.
54. Arber S, Cooper H. Gender differences in health in later life: the new paradox? Soc Sci Med. 1999;48(1):61–76.
55. Marmot MG, et al. Contribution of job control and other risk factors to social variations in coronary heart disease incidence. Lancet. 1997; 350(9073):235–9.
56. Barnett RC, Hyde JS. Women, men, work, and family. An expansionist theory. Am Psychol. 2001;56(10):781–96.

Exploring the status of retail private drug shops in Bangladesh and action points for developing an accredited drug shop model

Syed Masud Ahmed[1*], Nahitun Naher[1], Tarek Hossain[1] and Lal Bahadur Rawal[2]

Abstract

Background: The private retail drug shops market in Bangladesh is largely unregulated and unaccountable, giving rise to irrational use of drugs and high Out-of-pocket expenditure on health. These shops are served by salespersons with meagre or no formal training in dispensing.

Method: This facility-based cross-sectional study was undertaken to investigate how the drug shops currently operate vis-a-vis the regulatory regime including dispensing practices of the salespersons, for identifying key action points to develop an accredited model for Bangladesh. About 90 rural and 21 urban retail drug shops from seven divisions were included in the survey. The salespersons were interviewed for relevant information, supplemented by qualitative data on perceptions of the catchment community as well as structured observation of client-provider interactions from a sub-sample.

Results: In 76% of the shops, the owner and the salesperson was the same person, and >90% of these were located within 30 min walking distance from a public sector health facility. The licensing process was perceived to be a cumbersome, lengthy, and costly process. Shop visit by drug inspectors were brief, wasn't structured, and not problem solving. Only 9% shops maintained a stock register and 10% a drug sales record. Overall, 65% clients visited drug shops without a prescription. Forty-nine percent of the salespersons had no formal training in dispensing and learned the trade through apprenticeship with fellow drug retailers (42%), relatives (18%), and village doctors (16%) etc. The catchment population of the drug shops mostly did not bother about dispensing training, drug shop licensing and buying drugs without prescription. Observed client-dispenser interactions were found to concentrate mainly on financial transaction, unless, the client pro-actively sought advice regarding the use of the drug.

Conclusions: Majority of the drug shops studied are run by salespersons who have informal 'training' through apprenticeship. Visiting drug shops without a prescription, and dispensing without counseling unless pro-actively sought by the client, was very common. The existing process is discouraging for the shop owners to seek license, and the shop inspection visits are irregular, unstructured and punitive. These facts should be considered while designing an accredited model of drug shop for Bangladesh.

Keywords: Informal sector, Retail drug shops, Drug shop salespersons, Irrational use of drugs, Bangladesh

* Correspondence: ahmed.sm@bracu.ac.bd
[1]Centre of Excellence for Universal Health Coverage, James P Grant School of Public Health, BRAC University, 5th Floor, (Level-6), icddr,b Building, 68 Shahid Tajuddin Ahmed Sharani, Mohakhali, Dhaka -1212, Bangladesh
Full list of author information is available at the end of the article

Background

Retail drug shops are often the first and only source of healthcare outside home for a majority of patients in developing countries such as Bangladesh [1, 2]. It has been found in Bangladesh that more than 80% of the population seeks care from untrained or poorly trained *Pallichikitsoks* (village doctors) and drug shop retailers [3]. Currently in Bangladesh, 1,06,919 licensed [4] and an estimated equal number of unlicensed retail drug shops are involved in selling all types of drugs beside the "over-the-counter (OTC)" drugs. The latter are 'medicines sold directly to a consumer without a prescription from a healthcare professional, as opposed to prescription drugs, which may only be sold to consumers possessing a valid prescription' [5]. These are usually safe if used at recommended doses and duration, but can also be abused like other prescription drugs e.g., Cough medicines (e.g. Dextromethorphan), Cold medicines (e.g. Pseudoephedrine), Motion sickness pills (e.g. Dimenhydrinate), and Pain relievers (e.g. Acetaminophen). Bangladesh has currently 39 allopathic medicines in the OTC drug list [6]. About 2/3rd of the total health expenditure is from out-of-pocket (OOP), and of this, 65% is spent at the private drug retail shops [7].

According to law, the person dispensing drugs at drug retail outlets i.e., drug shops (drug shop salespersons, drug sellers) should at least have a 'Grade C pharmacist' certificate for the dispenser. This certificate is given after a short training of 12 weeks duration covering the basics of dispensing practice without any hands on training and is being conducted by the Pharmacy Council of Bangladesh (PCB) since 1995, in association with the Chemist and Druggist Association (shop owners association) of Bangladesh (BCDA) [8]. Only when this criterion is fulfilled, the shop owner can apply to the Directorate General of Drug Administration (DGDA) for issuance of a drug (pharmacy) license [9]. However, most of the salespersons at these retail drug shops do not have training in dispensing drugs or in diagnosing and treating medical conditions, which are the tasks they frequently perform [10]. Because drug shop salespersons have no other channel of information from the formal sectors open to them, they fall easy prey to the aggressive marketing strategies of the pharmaceutical companies [11]. Overprescribing, polypharmacy, prescribing unnecessary and expensive brand drugs, dispensing drugs without prescription, and OTC sell of antibiotics and steroids have been found to be the most common problems with these retailers [12–15].

Experiences in other parts of the world have demonstrated that private-sector drug seller initiatives designed on the basis of an accreditation and regulation model are feasible, improve access to medicines, and can be scaled up [16, 17]. Given the importance of the informal sector and private retail drug shops in Bangladesh, better regulation of the sector offers an opportunity to provide better pharmaceutical services which is essential for reducing total health expenditure and achieving universal health coverage in the country. There is dearth of data for informing the design of an accredited model of drug shops in Bangladesh. This study was undertaken to fill in this knowledge gaps by collecting relevant data on drug shops including its interactions with the regulatory regime; education, training and dispensing characteristics of the salespersons; users' perceptions about the services provided by, and the technical knowledge of, the dispensers; and stakeholders' experiences and opinions regarding the feasibility of designing such a model for Bangladesh.

Methods

Study aim and design

This was a facility-based (drug shops) cross-sectional study, exploring the status, mode of operation, and regulatory practices of the retail drug shops in the private sector in Bangladesh. It included samples of retail drug shops from rural and urban areas in all seven administrative divisions of the country.

Settings

For the purpose of this study, the 'drug shops' were defined as private retail drug shops which are eligible for mandatory approval and registration from the DGDA under the Ministry of Health and Family Welfare of the Government of Bangladesh (MOHFW, GOB). This definition did not include facilities that sell Ayurveda, Homeopathy, and Unani remedies at retail shops.

A variety of methods was used to elicit relevant data: (a) document review (for data on policy and regulatory environment); (b) quantitative survey (for profiling retail drug shops, and gathering data on training and working experiences of the salespersons); (c) qualitative exploration (for eliciting perception of the catchment community and other stakeholders), and (d) structured observation in a subsample of the drug shops to document client-salesperson interactions in real time.

Respondents of the study included (a) the salesperson or the owner of each of the drug shops who was present at the time of the survey (in 12% of the cases where the owner was a different person, only the salespersons were interviewed); (b) a sample of respondents from the catchment areas of the shops who visited the nearest drug shop within past one month (for focus group discussions); (c) relevant stakeholders e.g., DGDA authorities at the district and central levels, and the representatives of drug related associations and experts (in-depth interview).

Sampling strategy and sample

Quantitative survey

The rural samples included drug shops in the neighborhood of the *upazila* (sub-district) health complex (UHC), market places, and key business hubs. Because of time and resource constraints, we conveniently limited the number of sampled *upazilas* to 30 that were randomly selected from the seven administrative divisions, the number of *upazilas* being proportionate to the size of the division. Again, only one *upazila* was selected conveniently from each district in a division: either a *upazila* situated distally in a central district of a division or a *upazila* situated centrally in a peripheral district of the division. Next, three retail drug shops were selected from each of the sampled *upazila* which fulfilled the following criteria:

1. Drug shop in the neighborhood of the UHC, or within three kilometer radius of the UHC
2. Drug shop on the basis of their distance from the UHC (one nearest to the UHC, one farthest from the UHC, and one at a distance in-between) as available
3. Drug shop that had substantial customer visits (based on spot assessment)

The urban sampling was relatively simpler, taken exclusively from the seven city corporation areas (out of a total of 11 city corporations), which are the divisional headquarters. From the central thana (a police district, also known as a kotwali thana) of each city corporation area, three drug shops were selected using the following criteria ($n = 21$):

- First drug shop was selected from the central area near the kotwali thana
- Second drug shop was selected 1 km away from the first one
- Third drug shop was selected from the border area of the city (peri-urban area)

Thus, a total of 111 drug shops (90 rural and 21 urban areas) from the seven administrative divisions were included in the survey (see flow chart, Fig. 1). The sampled sites from where the sample upazillas/urban thanas were selected are shown in Fig. 2.

Qualitative exploration

Focus group discussions (FGD) and key informant interviews (KII) For the FGDs, the catchment areas of a sub-sample of the surveyed shops at the divisional levels were selected. From these areas, a sample of patients/clients who have had visited the drug shops for buying medicines or other services within past 30 days from the day of survey were selected. In all, 16 such FGDs were conducted. Stakeholders from divisional head quarters (drug superintendants or drug inspectors working under the district DGDA) and high officials of the DGDA head quarter at Dhaka were conveniently selected for KI interviews ($n = 22$).

Structured observation Structured observations of interaction between the salesperson and the patient/client visiting the 111 drug shops surveyed were done to document the nature and contents of the interaction. These were carried out simultaneously by a team of two interviewers: one proceeded with the survey while the other took notes about such interactions occurring during the survey. To reduce Hawthorne effect, interviewers spent some time for rapport building before the actual data collection took place. The observations documented were not specific to any particular illness but any such interaction that occurred during the period of survey. A total of 345 such interactions (three two hours session at different times of the day to capture the diversity) were documented. The study methods for addressing particular objectives, sampling frame and sample size is shown in Table 1.

Tools development and training of data collectors Tools for data collection such as the survey questionnaires (adapted after contextualizing from tools used by similar study in Tanzania) [18], Focus Group Discussions (FGD) and Key Informant Interviews (KII) and structured observation guidelines were developed and pretested for consistency, culture sensitiveness and ease of administration in the field before finalization.

The field data collectors (field interviewers) recruited for this study were science graduates with experiences in conducting community surveys and qualitative interviews in health sector. They underwent five days of intense training which consisted of didactic lectures on the content of the instruments followed, mock interviews, and field-testing through repeated practice sessions outside the study areas. End-of-training debriefings and necessary feedback, suggestions, and guidance were provided by the research team. Seven teams were formed, each with four to five interviewers and a team leader.

Data collection and quality control The day-to-day field activities of the teams (total seven) were overseen by the team leaders and assigned supervisors. To ensure completeness of the survey, the field research team members cross-checked each other's filled-in questionnaires every day before leaving the survey sites under the supervision of the team leader. The whole survey activity was supervised and managed by the PIs and co-

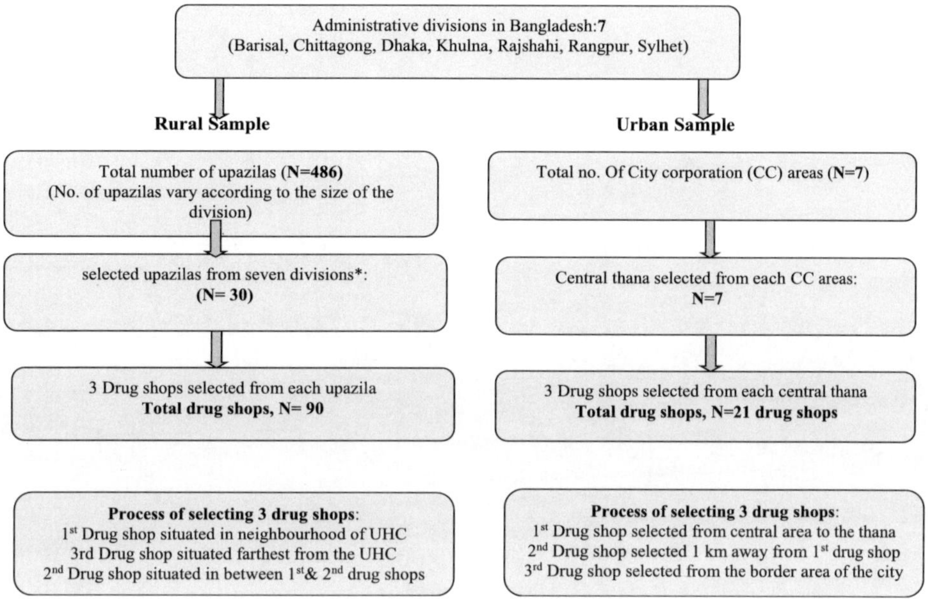

Fig. 1 Flow chart describing sampling of drug shops in the rural & urban areas. *no. of upazillas selected for study according to their proportion in the different divisions (30/486)

PIs, who made frequent field visits and provided assistance and guidance as and when needed.

An independent, mobile quality-control team also randomly checked 5%of the questionnaires completed the previous day in the working areas of each of the study teams. Such checks occurred in random spots in the field and feedbacks were provided to the team on any errors or gaps identified. Instructions for corrections were communicated to all the teams simultaneously to ensure standardization.

Again, the research team in the central office also cross-checked all questionnaires for inconsistencies not conforming to the instructions given at the time of training of the interviewers. If any such error was found, the questionnaire was discarded, and the survey was redone. This extensive process ensured the quality of data in a time of great political instability and difficulty of movement in the field between January and February 2015.

Data management and analysis The field activity and data entry work was completed within 45 working days. When the field activities were completed, data were entered using the statistical package for the social sciences (SPSS version no. 17) by a professional data management team. Of the total data, 5% was re-entered to control data-entry quality. During the data entry, the PIs and project manager supervised the data management team to ensure the quality and validity of the data, and the codebook developed by the research team was used for this purpose. When data entry was completed, the files were transferred into the SPSS for cleaning, consistency check, and cross-tabulation. The research team analyzed the final cleaned dataset using SPSS, following an analysis plan prepared beforehand.

For the qualitative data, content analysis was done with consolidation of relevant codes into sub-themes and themes. For example, some of the important themes included drug shop licensing (sub themes: licensing process, drug shop owners' perception of the process, informal payment for license, capacity of the regulatory authority etc.), dispensing practices (sub themes: capacity of the salespersons, selling non-OTC drugs without prescriptions, counseling etc.), and accredited drug shop model (sub themes: necessity and requirements, stakeholders' perceptions, services to offer etc.). Triangulation of data was done by eliciting information on a particular issue from different sources e.g., Observation data on shop visits by the clients without prescription was cross-checked in FGDs with community members in the catchment areas of the shops as well as stakeholders such as service providers and regulatory personnel.

Results

Findings from the quantitative survey

The quantitative survey involved 111 drug shops in total, 90 from rural areas and 21 from urban areas. Majority of the drug shops (45%) were running for more than 10 years, in greater proportion in the rural areas (Table 2).

Interestingly, more than 90% of the drug shops were physically located within 30 min walking distance of some health facilities, mostly in the public sector. Most (96%) of the shops reportedly possessed trade license, but a lesser proportion (83%) reported to have a drug

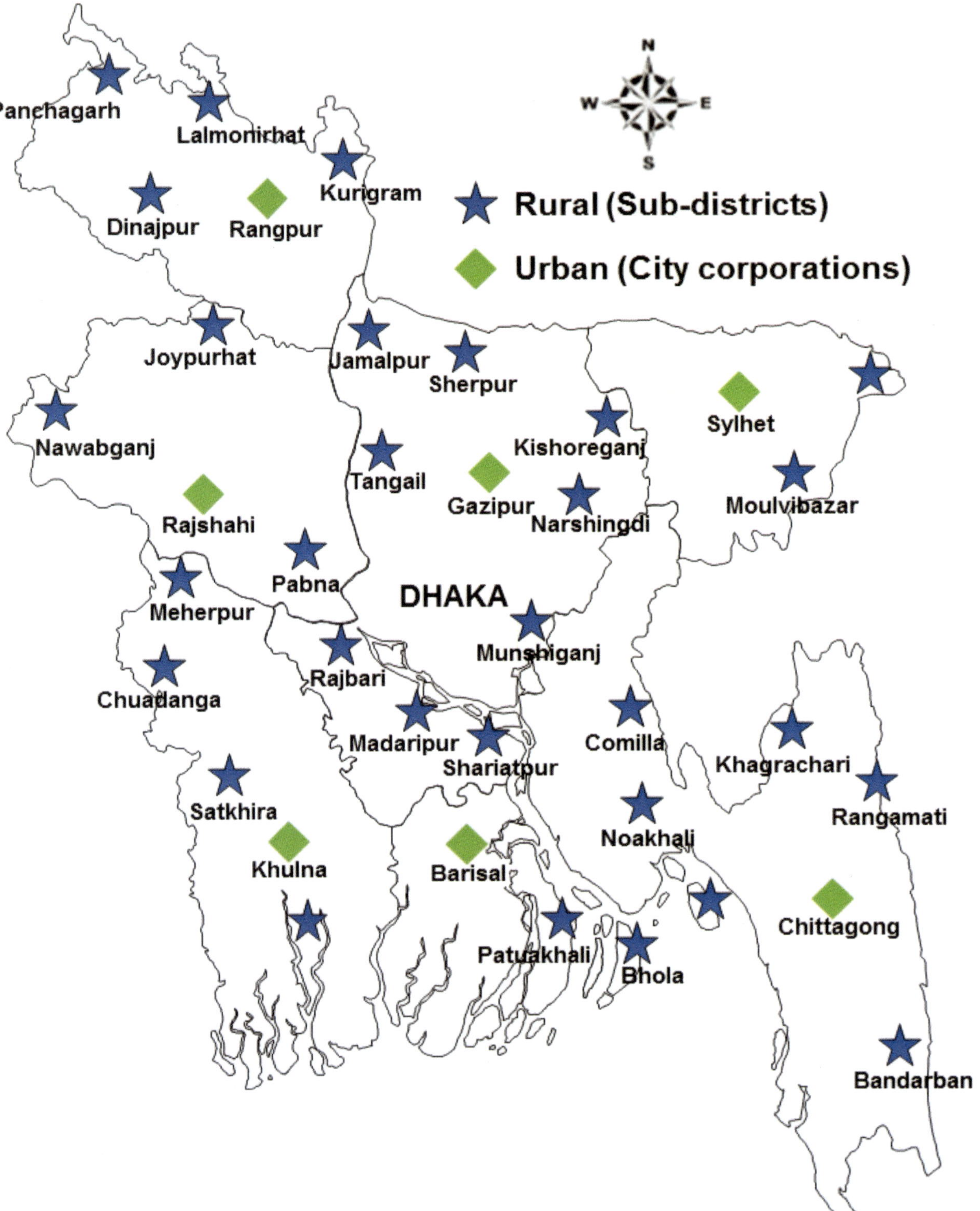

Fig. 2 Rural and urban sites from where the sample upazilas (rural) and thanas (city corporation areas) were drawn. (Source http://www.ngof.org/nrc/wdb/watsanmap.php)

Table 1 Study methods and objectives addressed, sample Size, and sampling frame

Methods (objectives addressed)	Sampling frame
Drug shop survey (characteristics of the drug shops, salespersons, and regulatory environment) ($n = 111$)	Salesperson or dispensers from sampled retail drug shops
Structured observation of interaction between salesperson and clients (dispensing practices) ($n = 345$)	Interactions between salesperson or dispensers and clients visiting sampled retail drug shops
Focus group discussion (client perception of salespersons and experiences of services received from the drug shops) ($n = 16$)	Community members visiting the sampled retail drug shops
Key informant interview (stakeholders' perceptions regarding current operation of drug shops and feasibility of designing an accredited model of drug shop fro Bangladesh) (For list, see appendix C)	i. Regulatory authority at district levels (drug superintendent or inspector) ii. National-level key stakeholders (from DGDA, BCDS,PCB)

DGDA Directorate General of Drug Administration, *BCDS* Bangladesh Chemist and Druggists Samity, *PCB* Pharmacy Council of Bangladesh

license. However, the validity of the drug licenses was not checked in this survey. Within past one year, 83% of the shops were reported to have been inspected at least once by a drug inspector from the local (district) DGDA office.

Sixty-five percent of the visiting clients (presumably, out of an average tentative number of clients visiting in a day) came to purchase drugs without a prescription (Table 2). The clients visited the shops mostly by self-referral which was more common in the urban shops (76%) compared to the rural shops (67%). Besides dispensing drugs, the shops also provided some additional services such as pushing injections (60%), some petty diagnostic services such as measuring blood pressure or testing for blood sugar (63%),

Table 2 Characteristics of the sampled drug shops %

	Rural ($n = 90$)	Urban ($n = 21$)	All ($N = 111$)
Drug shop has been in operation for_			
< 5 years	32	38	33
5–10 years	21	24	22
10+ years	47	38	45
Distance from nearest health facility is ≤30 min walk	90	95	91
Possess drug license (reported)	81	90	83
Possess trade license (reported)	96	100	96
The shop was reported to be inspected by a Drug Inspector			
Within past one year	84	79	83
Within past two years	16	21	17
Stock register maintained (reported)	8	14	9
Drug sales record maintained (reported)	8	19	10
Functional refrigerator available (checked)	31	33	31
Besides dispensing, additional services available (multiple response)			
Pushing injections	59	67	60
Diagnostic services (e.g., testing blood sugar, measuring blood pressure)	62	67	63
Vaccination services (e.g., TT, rabies vaccine)	30	38	31
Burn and wound treatment/dressing	66	52	63
Source of clients (multiple responses)			
Public health facilities/clinics/hospitals	34	19	31
Private health facilities/clinics/hospitals	10	19	12
Private chambers of doctors	7	5	6
Self-referral	67	76	68
Clients visiting daily without prescription[a]	69 ($n = 4511$)	64 ($n = 973$)	65 ($n = 5484$)

[a]average number of clients visiting a drug shop in a day as reported by the respondents

first-aid services such as wound and/or burn dressing (63%) etc. Only 9% of the shops reported to have maintaineda stock register while 10% maintained a record of drugs sold (Table 2). Around 1/3rd of the shops surveyed were found to have a functioning refrigerator.

In 76% of cases, the owner and the salesperson was the same person, more so in the urban shops (Table 3). Forty-nine percent of them had no formal training in pharmacy/dispensing and of those who had, the overwhelming majority (93%) had a three months training in a Grade C Certificate Course only. Majority of those receiving some ad-hoc training received it from the pharmaceutical companies (38%). The other group i.e., without any training whatsoever, learned the trade through apprenticeship with fellow drug retailer (42%), relatives (18%), village doctors (16%) and so on (Table 3).The respondents valued the necessity of training for a variety of reasons such as efficient dispensing (66%), gaining knowledge about rules and regulation of dispensing (84%), and developing good relation with clients and goodwill for business (21%).

Table 3 Characteristics of the salespersons attending the sampled drug shops

	Rural	Urban	All
	(*n* = 90)	(*n* = 21)	(*N* = 111)
Salesperson and owner is the same person	76	81	76
Educational status of the salespersons			
≤ 10 yrs. of schooling	4	—	4
10 completed years of schooling (SSC)	27	38	29
12 completed years of schooling (HSC)	32	38	33
Graduate	37	24	34
Involvement in any other occupation			
Farming	48	20	43
Self-employment	15	40	19
Others[a]	37	40	38
Pharmacy training status of the salespersons			
Have formal training	49	62	51
No formal/some ad-hoc training	51	38	49
Of those who have formal training,	(*n* = 44)	(*n* = 13)	(*n* = 57)
Category B pharmacist training (one year Diploma in pharmacy)	7	8	7
Category C pharmacist training (three months Certificate course in dispensing/pharmacy)	93	92	93
*Of those who have some ad-hoc training, training is provided by_*	(*n* = 46)	(*n* = 8)	(*n* = 54)
Government organization	36	—	31
Private organization	29	—	25
Pharmaceutical companies	28	100	38
NGOs	7	—	6
Of those receiving no training of any type, mode of informal learning (multiple responses)	(*n* = 32)	(*n* = 6)	(*n* = 38)
Fellow drug seller in other store(s)	44	33	42
MBBS doctor in the drug shop or pharmacy[a]	9	17	10
Pharmacist	3	—	3
Village doctor	16	17	16
Relatives	22	—	18
LMAF course	3	—	3
Pharmaceutical company	3	33	8

N all observations, *n* observation subset, — not applicable, *SSC* Secondary School Certificate, *HSC* Higher Secondary Certificate
[a]nursery, fishery, business, or student

Findings from qualitative exploration (presented by themes)

Drug shops, salespersons and dispensing practices

The drug shops were quite a familiar entity in the community life. As some of the drug shops were as old as 10 to 20 years, many remembered their interaction with the shops since their childhood. The salespersons of the drug shops were also a very common face to them as they mostly originated from the local community, were amiable and trustworthy, and well respected. Some clients (respondents from the catchment community who purchased drugs from the sampled shops within past one month) mentioned that they had a very good relation with the people at the drug shops.

The clients were aware that the salespersons may have some training on drug dispensing but in most instances, they did not bother much. Some even said that training was not necessary as they already have many years of experience. To quote one:

"He doesn't need training; he already has achieved vast knowledge on drug dispensing from his 30 years of work experience."
-A drug shop client from Dhaka

However, some emphasized the importance of education and training in dispensing:

"...if the drug seller does not know about drug dispensing, he cannot provide me proper medicine that I need..."

"...if the drug seller has educational and professional qualification, then he will be able to provide us a proper service..."
-A drug shop client from Khulna

The need of prescription for buying drugs other than the' Over-the-counter (OTC) drugs' was considered superfluous by the respondents as the salespersons were known to them. They explained that if a person required a drug, s/he would explain his/her illnesses to the salesperson, and get necessary drugs based on symptoms. Structured observation done on a number of 'client-salesperson interactions' at drug shops also corroborated this process. For example, in about one-third of such interactions in the urban areas, only 36% salespersons asked about the nature of illness, 27% about the symptoms of illness, and 26% about the duration of the illness. Sometimes, depending upon symptoms, the salesperson made a superficial, nonspecific physical examination such as feeling the client's pulse, checking for anemia, measuring temperature and blood pressure, auscultation of the chest with a stethoscope if there is cough, pressing the abdomen if there is a complaint of digestive disturbances etc.

Clients having chronic illnesses also didn't think it necessary to show the prescription when buying the particular drug. They usually used to bring old receipts or empty medicine packets to buy the same drug again. They were also complacent about receiving receipts against the cash paid for drugs, the transactions taking place based on mutual trust:

"The drug seller does not provide any money receipt and, as a consumer, I do not feel needs of collecting the money receipt because we both know each other and we are neighbors."
-A drug shop client from Chittagong

Most respondents said that the salespersons explained to them about the quantity, frequency, time and duration of intake, whether to take the medicines before or after a meal, and how to prepare syrup for kids and so forth. To quote:

"Sometimes the drug seller counsels us about the total doses that if you do not complete your dose ... you will not get effective result."
-A drug shop client from Khulna

If a prescribed drug is not available, the drug sellers often would substitute another brand, sometimes without informing the client. For situations which the drug seller could not manage after repeated attempts, patients are usually referred to a doctor or a nearby health facility. One respondent reported:

"If the patient's condition became worse than his previous condition, then the drug seller usually changes the medicine."
-A drug shop client from Rangpur

Regulatory processes

According to the law, the storage, display, and sale of drugs are punishable crimes without a license issued by the DGDA. At the time of the study, the DGDA had licensed 1,15,439 drug shops, but it was suspected that there are an approximately equal number of shops which are unlicensed. Because of a shortage of required personnel, the inspection and checking process of the drug shops appeared to be superficial, few and far between, and that process was not compliant with stipulated laws. One drug inspector summarized the field-level problems of inspection:

"We don't have our own office, no transport facilities, no protocol.There are around 3,000 shops in my area! Civil surgeon of the hospital... has car facilities; my work area is more, but I don't have that facility"
-A drug inspector

Interestingly, many respondents did not know that a license is required before opening a drug shop. To quote one respondent:

"I do not know the importance to have a license for a drug shop..."
-A drug shop client from Chittagong

Yet another emphasized its importance:

"...I think it is a good practice to have a license because if they have a valid license ...they will not be able to dispense harmful medicine."
-A drug shop client from Barisal

However, the respondents perceived the process of applying for and getting a drug license to be a cumbersome, lengthy, and costly process. Resentments were echoed uniformly by the owners/salespersons regarding both the licensing and the inspection process. All tiers of the regulators were of the opinion that the existing system is inadequate. One inspector observed:

"Once I observed that the drug seller shut down his shop, while the government authority came to inspect the drug shops of this area."
-A drug inspector from Rangpur

Key-informant interviews with field-level drug inspectors emphasized that the existing regulatory system needed to be improved in areas such as logistics, availability of trained personnel, adequate budget for regular and timely inspection visits, and reduction of lead time for issuing the license after application.

The numbers of unlicensed shops are large, and the Bangladesh Chemists and Druggists Samity (i.e., Association, BCDA)thought this situation to be due to problems with the regulatory authority's capacity to oversee the market. They complained that rules and regulations are frequently not enforced, resulting from corruption at the grassroots level. As BCDA does not have a monitoring role, the association informs the relevant DGDA authorities about irregularities that come to their notice. The BCDA informed that it has distributed about 200,000 informational leaflets to build awareness among the consumers. To address the severe shortage of trained dispensers, the BCDA, with technical help from the Pharmacy Council of Bangladesh (PCB) conducts a three-month long training course to award grade C certificate for dispensers working in the drug shops.

Feasibility of developing an accredited model of drug shops for Bangladesh

The regulators at the central and district levels were unanimous about the necessity of developing an accredited model of a drug shop (Accredited Drug Shops, ADS) in the country to improve the current chaotic situation. According to the regulators, this is all the more necessary because Bangladesh has a large illiterate semiliterate population who can't distinguish the good from the bad. Because a drug shop is the first contact with any kind of health care service for a majority of the people, especially those in the rural and remote areas, this accreditation is a must for maintaining standards and quality. The regulators at the DGDA preferred the model drug shops to be run by the registered pharmacists i.e., those who are graduates or have diplomas. As one respondent from the DGDA explained:

"Pharmacists should dispense medicine to patients as per doctor's prescription. If any doctor writes a wrong medicine, the pharmacist should consult with the doctor before giving the medicine to the patient. Pharmacists will counsel the patient how to take medicine and will explain this properly. A pharmacist will check the expiry dates of the medicines in the shop ... he will ensure whether the shop is well-organized, and the records are well-maintained."
-A regulatory authority from Barisal

However, in the short term, these could be run by at least a person certified in the practice of dispensing. They also suggested extensive review of the current course for content and pedagogy including recruitment of students from science background, inclusion of topics in the curricula such as Primary Health Care (PHC), first aid, legal and ethical aspects of dispensing, inter-personal communication with customers, pharmacist and customer relationship and rational use of drugs. In addition, they advised for some job placement or in-service training or practical experiences before the pharmacist certificate can be issued. A number of suggestions were put forward e.g., organizing a "Drug Day" or "Drug Week" campaigns and arranging a "Drug Fair" to generate awareness among the community and drug sellers/owners.

Discussion

This study provides necessary information for developing of an accredited model of drug shops in Bangladesh by focusing on (a) consumer perceptions about the drug shops and its salespersons, (b) regulatory regime, and (c) the challenges and opportunities for designing an accredited drug shop model for Bangladesh. The findings and its implications are discussed under these themes, and finally, some recommendations are made how to go forward with pilot testing such a model in near future.

Consumer perception about drug shops and salespersons

Most community members were not concerned about the educational and technical credentials of the drug sellers/dispensers and considered the salespersons/dispensers as a "friend in deed." This view is very common in low- and middle-income countries (LMICs), especially in the remote and hard-to-reach areas that do not have doctors or, for that matter, any formal health facilities or providers [12, 13, 16, 19–22]. Purchasing non-OTC drugs without a prescription is also common in Pakistan [23], India [24] and other LMICs [25] as it is in Bangladesh. When seeking treatment advice by the patients/clients by describing symptoms, the practice of arriving at a diagnosis by a brief history taking and nominal physical examination, is all too common with drug sellers in the LMICs [25].Lack of professional training of any kind, as observed in this study for nearly half of the respondents, is not uncommon in countries such as the Lao People's Democratic Republic, Pakistan, and Vietnam [12, 23, 26].

Regulatory regime

It appears that the lengthy and costly licensing process discouraged the drug shop owners from applying for a license. One reason identified by the shop owners is that the license application, after field inspection by the Drug Inspectors/Superintendent, has to be placed before the district drug committee for approval. Only then, it can be sent to DGDA office, Dhaka for approval. Further inquiry revealed that the district committee meetings are few and far between and this result in backlogs. Second, the alleged informal costs associated with getting a license over and above the required government fees discourage the unlicensed drug shops to get registered. Third, due to constraints in human and financial resources of the regulatory authority which is critical for regulation [27], the shop visits are not regular and systematic too. The resulting short time allocated to a visit allow the inspectors and superintendents to have a superficial inspection only which is not helpful for enforcing regulation, a common problem with enforcing regulation in general in the broader health system [28]. Thus, the creation of a user-friendly regulatory environment is essential for improving the pharmacy practices at the drug shops, including the unlicensed shops [25]. The critical role of Consumer Association of Bangladesh (CAB) and similar associations should be leveraged to promote the rational use of drugs.

Challenges and opportunities for developing an accredited drug shop model for Bangladesh

The Accredited Drug Shop (ADS) model of retail drug shops such as tested in Tanzania standardizes the drug shop's operation by staffing the shop with appropriately trained dispensers, strictly enforcing regulations, and providing supportive supervision [18]. The current state of drug shops in the private informal sector in Bangladesh justifies an adapted model for Bangladesh, and is feasible as revealed by different stakeholders in this sector. However, for the model's implementation, certain conditions have to be fulfilled as elicited from the regulators and other stakeholders using qualitative methods. These include, but are not restricted to (1) training a cadre of dispensers/community pharmacists using a revised and updated curriculum, (2) franchising the training of vast numbers of salespersons/attendants at drug retail outlets to registered training organisations/institutions as a stop gap measure, (3) expanding pharmacy services beyond dispensing drugs (e.g., first-aid services, measuring and monitoring blood pressure and blood sugar for diabetes, and provision of some basic curative services as provided by the Community Health Workers (CHWs), and (4) building community awareness on the importance of quality pharmacy services and rational use of drugs.

Study Limitations

Though the salespersons were asked whether their drug shop possessed drug and trade license but due to sensitive nature of the issue, these could not be physically verified. The sample size could have been expanded and made more representative to capture local level variations but was limited by time and resource constraints.

So, how to overcome the ground realities for designing an ADS model: Recommendations

To summarise, Bangladesh has now a large number of private drug shops where all kind of drugs are sold by salesperson with meagre or no training in dispensing whatsoever, under the supervision of a weak and poorly resourced regulatory body. To overcome this chaotic scenario, the following measures are suggested:

i. In the immediate, **short term (one to three years)**: To restore some discipline in the prevailing chaotic situation and bring the informal drug shops under some regulation, the drug licensing process should be made user-friendly, less time consuming, efficient, and inexpensive so that the shop owners are encouraged to become licensed after fulfilling the requirements. The inspection visits to drug shops should be regular, comprehensive, supervised (by district DGDA), and problem solving—not punitive. This would ensure enforcement of minimum regulatory requirements. Finally, some expedited measures ('crash programme') need to be in place to train the vast number of drug sellers/salespersons in unlicensed shops within as short a time as practically feasible. To accomplish this, public-private partnerships (PPPs) including non-profit Non-Government-Organization (NGOs) should be encouraged to play a significant role in franchising the above Grade C Certificate (course for dispensers) course.

ii. **In the long term**, three basic tasks should be prioritized. *First,* re-visiting the current curriculum and revising the contents, forms, and duration of the grade C certificate course for the dispensers, using modern pedagogic methods. It should also have an in-built internship programme where they would receive hands-on training by working under a qualified pharmacist for a fixed period of time. The curriculum may include basic PHC services (standard for CHWs) so that it can serve as the first health post in remote and hard-to-reach areas.

Second, all efforts should be made to increase the human and technical capacity of the DGDA (e.g., establish more drug-testing laboratories) to streamline regular inspection visits of the drug shops and discourage marketing of counterfeit, expired, and poor-quality drugs. Possibility for establishing the digital pharmaceuticals systems should also be explored mainly for the purpose of registration and renewal of drug shop licence, verifying the genuine drug products and facilitating effective monitoring systems.

Third, to regulate the unethical and aggressive marketing practices of the pharmaceutical companies and their medical representatives [11], and promote rational use of drugs, measures should be taken to enforce the 'Code of Pharmaceutical Marketing Practices' promulgated in 1994 [29]. Last but not the least, an extensive information, education, and communication (IEC) campaign to build awareness of the public and pharmacy stakeholders on the irrational use of drugs and their harmful effects (e.g., antimicrobial resistance, MDR TB, etc.) should be launched.

Conclusion

The private drug shop market in Bangladesh is now largely unregulated and unaccountable, and run by salespersons who are mostly trained informally through a process of 'apprenticeship'. Clients visiting drug shops without a prescription, and inadequate dispensing practice resulting in OTC sale of all forms of medicine was very common. The existing process is discouraging and time consuming for the shop owners to seek license, and the shop inspection visits are irregular, unstructured and punitive. Urgent measures such as a 'crash' programme to train the salespersons; making inspection visits regular, comprehensive, and problem solving; improving technical and human resource capacity of the regulatory authority and making the licensing process 'user-friendly' are needed to improve the current chaotic scenario and mainstream these shops into the existing PHC infrastructure. Besides, key action points for designing an accredited drug shop model for Bangladesh is discussed informed by these findings.

Abbreviations

ADS: Accredited Drug Shops; AHUB: Ayurveda, Homeopathy, and Unani Board; BCDA: Bangladesh Chemists and Druggists Samity; CHWs: Community Health Workers; DGDA: Directorate General of Drug Administration; FGD: Focus Group Discussions; GOB: Government of Bangladesh; HRH: Human Resource for Health; IEC: Information, Education and Communication; KII: Key Informant Interviews; LMICs: Low- and Middle-Income Countries; MDR TB: Multi-Drug-Resistant Tuberculosis; MOHFW: Ministry of Health and Family Welfare\; NGOs: Non-Governmental Organization; OOP: Out-Of-Pocke; OTC: Over-the-counter; PCB: Pharmacy Council of Bangladesh; PHC: Primary Health Care; PPPs: Public-Private Partnership; SPSS: Statistical Package for the Social Sciences; UHC: Upazila Health Complex

Acknowledgements

The authors gratefully acknowledge the insights provided by Prof. Sitesh C.Bachar of the Department of Pharmacy, Dhaka University on drug shops, and subsequent designing of the study. Thanks are also due to Dr. Tapash Roy and Dr.KaosarAfsana (BRAC Health, Population and Nutrition Programme, and adjunct faculty of the School) for encouraging us to do this study and connecting us to the people at the Manangement Sciences for Health (MSH) in Dhaka, and through them to Washington head office. Dr. Edmund Rutta and Emily Delmotte were instrumental for the study by providing essential training and technical assistance throughout the study period. Thanks are also due to Dr.Sanaul Bashar, FazleKarim and Dr. Afsana Khan from MSH Dhaka office for helping us with the design of the study, and to Dr.Zubayer Hussain of the MSH head office for his constant encouragement to conduct the study.

Funding

This work was supported by the US Agency for International Development (USAID), under the terms of cooperative agreement number [AID-OAA-A-11-00021].

Authors' contributions

SMA and LBR conceptualized and designed the study. NN and TH organized field data collection and data analysis. SMA, NN and TH analysed and interpreted the data and SMA drafted the first version of the manuscript. All authors participated in critical revision of the manuscript and contributed to its intellectual improvement. Final draft was prepared by SMA. All authors went through the final draft and approved it for submission.

Competing interests

The authors declare that they have no competing interests.

Author details

[1]Centre of Excellence for Universal Health Coverage, James P Grant School of Public Health, BRAC University, 5th Floor, (Level-6), icddr,b Building, 68 Shahid Tajuddin Ahmed Sharani, Mohakhali, Dhaka -1212, Bangladesh. [2]Health Systems and Population Studies Division, icddr,b, Dhaka 1212, Bangladesh.

References

1. Ahmed SM, Hossain MA, Chowdhury MR. Informal sector providers in Bangladesh: how equipped are they to provide rational health care? Health Policy Plan. 2009;24(6):467–78.
2. Ahmed SM, Hossain MA, Chowdhury AMR, Bhuiya AU. The health workforce crisis in Bangladesh: shortage, inappropriate skill-mix, and inequitable distribution. Hum Resour Health. 2011;9:3.

3. Ahmed SM, Hossain MA. Knowledge and practice of unqualified and semi-qualified allopathic providers in rural Bangladesh: implications for the HRH problem. Health Policy. 2007;84(2–3):332–43.
4. Directorate General of Drug Administration DGDA website. http://www.dgda.gov.bd/. Accessed 8 June 2017.
5. Over-the-counter drugs. https://en.wikipedia.org/wiki/Over-the-counter_drug. Accessed 7 June 2017.
6. List of allopathic OTC drugs. http://dgda.gov.bd/index.php/laws-and-policies/204-national-drug-policy-2016-including-essential-drug-list-and-otc-list/file Accessed 7 June 2017.
7. Ministry of Health and Family Welfare, Government of Bangladesh (MoHFW, GoB). Bangladesh National Health Accounts 1997–2012. Dhaka: Health Economics Unit, MoHFW, GoB; 2015.
8. Mazid MA, Rashid MA. Pharmacy education and carrier opportunities for pharmacists in Bangladesh. Bangladesh Pharm J. 2011;14(1):1-9.
9. Ministry of Law, Government of Bangladesh. The Pharmacy Ordinance 1976 (Ordinance No. XIII of 1976). http://bdlaws.minlaw.gov.bd/print_sections_all.php?id=513. Accessed 8 June 2017.
10. Amzad R. To explore the knowledge and practices of the drug shop attendants regarding dispensing and prescribing (disease specific) medicines and the difference, if any, between the 'grade C' pharmacy certificate holders and the other (those who don't have grace C certificate) in these aspects. In: MPH Dissertation. Dhaka: James P Grant School of Public Health, BRAC University; 2012.
11. Mohiuddin M, Rashid SF, Shuvro MI, Naher N, Ahmed SM. Qualitative insights into promotion of pharmaceutical products in Bangladesh: how ethical are the practices? BMC Medial Ethics. 2015;16:80.
12. Chuc N. Towards good pharmacy practice in hanoi: a multi-intervention study in private sector, PhD thesis. Karolinska Institutet: Stockholm; 2002.
13. Chalker JC. Interventions for improved prescribing and dispensing in Nepal, Thailand, and Vietnam, PhD thesis. Stockholm: Karolinska Institutet; 2003.
14. Chowdhury PM. An overview of the pharmaceutical sector in Bangladesh. Dhaka: BRAC EPL Stock Brokerage LTD; 2010.
15. Bloom G, Wilkinson A, Tomson G, et al. Addressing resistance to antibiotics in pluralistic health systems. In: STEPS Working Paper. Brighton, STEPS Centre; 2015. p. 84.
16. Goodman C, Brieger W, Unwin A, et al. Medicine sellers and malaria treatment in sub-Saharan Africa: what do they do and how can their practice be improved? Am J Trop Med Hyg. 2007;77(Suppl 6):203–18.
17. Drug Seller Initiatives (DSI). Sustainable drug seller initiatives .2014. http://www.drugsellerinitiatives.org/about/projects/. Accessed 10 Sept. 2015.
18. Rutta E, Liana J, Johnson K, et al. Erratum to: Accrediting retail drug shops to strengthen Tanzania's public health system: an ADDO case study. BMC J Pharm Policy Practice. 2015;20158:29.
19. Kamat VR, Nichter M. Pharmacies, self-medication, and pharmaceutical marketing in Bombay. India Soc Sci Med. 1998;47(6):779–94.
20. Kafle KK, Madden JM, Shreshta AD, et al. Can Licensed Drug Sellers Contribute to Safe Motherhood? A Survey of the Treatment of Pregnancy-Related Anaemia in Nepal. Soc Sci Med. 1999;42(11):1,577–88.
21. Stanback J, Otterness C, Bekita M, et al. Injected with controversy: sales and administration of injectable contraceptives in drug shops in Uganda. Int Perspect Sex Reprod Health. 2011;37(1):24–9.
22. Wafula FN, Miriti EM, Goodman CA. Examining characteristics, knowledge, and regulatory practices of specialized drug shops in sub-saharan africa: a systematic review of the literature. BMC Health Serv Res. 2012;12:223. doi:10.1186/1472-6963-12-223.
23. Rabbani F, Cheema FH, Talati NS, et al. Behind the counter: pharmacies and dispensing patterns of pharmacy attendants in Karachi. J Pakistan Med Assoc. 2001;51(4):149–53.
24. Sabde YD, Diwan V, Saraf VS, et al. Mapping private pharmacies and their characteristics in Ujjain District, Central India. BMC Health Serv Res. 2011;11:351. doi:10.1186/1472-6963-11-351.
25. Miller R, Goodman C. Performance of retail pharmacies in low- and middle-income Asian settings: a systematic review. Health Policy Plan. 2016;012016:1–14.
26. Stenson B, Syhakhang L, Eriksson B, Tomson G. Real world pharmacy: assessing the quality of private pharmacy practice in the Lao People's Democratic Republic. Soc Sci Med. 2001;52(3):393–404.
27. Sauwakon R, Wondemagegnehu E. Effective drug regulation. A multicountry study. World Health Organization. 2002.
28. Garimella S, Sheikh K. Workforce governance: reflections on the role of postings and transfers at the primary health care level. BMJ Open. 2015; 5 (Suppl 1):A1-53.
29. Code of Pharmaceutical Marketing Practices. Ministry of Health and Family Welfare. Government of Peoples Republic of Bangladesh. http://www.dgda.gov.bd/index.php/2013-03-31-05-16-29/forms/77-code-of-pharamaceutical-marketion-practices/file. Accessed 8 June 2017.

13

Evaluating insulin information provided on discharge summaries in a secondary care hospital in the United Kingdom

Amie Bain[1*], Lois Nettleship[1], Sallianne Kavanagh[2] and Zaheer-Ud-Din Babar[1,3]

Abstract

Background: Prescribing errors at the time of hospital discharge are common and could potentially lead to avoidable patient harm, especially when they involve insulin, a high-risk medicine widely used for the treatment of diabetes mellitus. When information regarding insulin therapy is not sufficiently communicated to a patient's primary care provider, continuity of care for patients with diabetes may be compromised. The objectives of this study were to investigate the nature and prevalence of insulin-related medication discrepancies contained in hospital discharge summaries for patients with diabetes. A further objective was to examine the timeliness and completeness of relevant information regarding insulin therapy provided on discharge summaries.

Methods: The study was undertaken at a large foundation trust hospital in the North of England, UK. A retrospective analysis of discharge summaries of all patients who were being treated with insulin and were included in the 2016 National Inpatient Diabetes Audit was conducted. Insulin regimen information provided on discharge summaries was scrutinised in light of available medical records pertaining to the admission and current national recommendations.

Results: Thirty-three (79%) out of the 42 patients included in the study had changes made to their insulin regimen during hospital admission. Eighteen (43%) patients were identified as having an error or discrepancy relating to insulin on their discharge summary. A total of 27 insulin errors or discrepancies were identified on discharge, most commonly involving non-communication of an insulin dose change ($n = 8$) and wrong insulin device ($n = 7$). Seventeen issues relating to completeness of insulin information were identified, including the omission of the prescribed time of insulin administration ($n = 10$) and unexplained insulin dose change ($n = 4$). Two patients who had insulin-related errors identified on their discharge summaries were readmitted to hospital within 30 days of discharge due to poor diabetic control.

Conclusions: This small-scale study demonstrates that errors and discrepancies regarding insulin therapy on discharge persist despite current insulin safety initiatives. Poorly communicated information regarding insulin therapy may jeopardise optimal glycaemic control and continuity of patient care. Insulin-related information should be comprehensively documented at the point of discharge. This is to improve communication across the interface and to minimise risks to patient safety.

Keywords: Insulin, Patient discharge summaries, Medication errors, Diabetes mellitus

* Correspondence: a.bain@hud.ac.uk
[1]School of Applied Sciences, University of Huddersfield, Queensgate, Huddersfield HD1 3DH, United Kingdom
Full list of author information is available at the end of the article

Background

Discharge summary information

A quality discharge process is vital to ensuing patient safety and continuity of care in the community. On discharge from hospital it is important that general practitioners (GPs, primary care physicians) receive accurate and timely communication with respect to patients' medications. This is important in the context to prevent potentially harmful medication-related errors that could result in further hospitalisation [1]. Medication errors at the point of discharge have previously been reported as 'common' [2, 3] and can include unintended omission of medication, continuation/re-prescribing of an intentionally stopped medication, or an error in medication dose, frequency or formulation [3–5]. Such errors have been found to persist post-discharge and pose a greater risk to patient care than those on identified on admission, [6] potentially leading to readmission [7, 8]. A United Kingdom (UK) government report highlighted the need for hospitals to improve the information provided about medications on discharge following findings suggesting that the majority of medication information on discharge summaries was incomplete or inaccurate [9]. In 2008, the UK National Prescribing Centre (NPC), specified a minimum dataset of information to be communicated at all transitions of patient care. This was to maintain patient safety [10]. Despite this, one study found that these requirements were consistently not being met in sampled discharge summaries, with 71.7% adhering to the total NPC minimum dataset, 67.2% adhering to medicine information requirements and less than half (48.9%) adhering to therapy change information requirements, with rationale for medication change amongst the most frequent omissions [11]. Similar rates (65.5–68%) of poor documentation of medication changes on electronic discharge summaries have been identified in other studies conducted in England by Cresswell et al. [12] and in Ireland by Grimes et al. [13], with higher rates (80.5%) being reported in Australia by Lehnbom et al. [14]. Callen et al. [4], found similar rates of medication error between handwritten and electronic discharge summaries when using systems similar to those reported in this study. The authors of these studies suggest that input from clinical pharmacy teams and junior doctor training may hold the potential to reduce discharge medication errors, as well as the use of integrated systems within a complete electronic health record [4, 12–14].

Insulin therapy and hospital discharge

The importance of communicating sufficient information pertaining to discharge medication is even more pertinent when high-risk drugs, capable of causing patient harm, are involved. Insulin is a high-risk, critical medicine widely used in the treatment of diabetes mellitus [15], where inappropriate use can lead to poor glycaemic control, patient harm or even death [16, 17]. Anecdotal evidence reported by Leech et al. [18] describes incidences where GPs were unsure of what dose of insulin to prescribe after patients were discharged from hospital because *"patients tell [them] completely different doses to the [discharge] letter"* and where district nurses find it *"really difficult getting details [regarding insulin therapy after discharge] and patients can be very uncertain."* Upon discharge from hospital the communication must ensure that not only the correct insulin is prescribed, but that this is supported with sufficient additional information to prevent consequential patient harm. Medication errors involving insulin have been previously reported as occurring at various points throughout the patient hospital stay, including at the point of discharge [19, 20]. A large audit of 54 National Health Service (NHS) trusts found that insulin-related medication errors were common at the point of prescribing in hospital. The most common error reported was 'unclear or missing administration device', which the authors comment is particularly problematic at care interfaces, such as discharge from hospital [21].

In 2015, A Canadian study reported improvements in the quality and value of information communicated across the interface for patients with diabetes with the use of a specialised discharge letter template [22]. During the same year, the Joint British Diabetes Society (JBDS) released guidelines to help healthcare professionals in secondary care to plan the safe and effective discharge of adult inpatients with diabetes. Recommendations included the use of a comprehensive checklist to ensure that adequate information is transferred between care providers. Data from the 2016 National Inpatient Diabetes Audit (NaDIA) of England and Wales indicated, however, only 11.5% of sites currently implement these guidelines, and that the prevalence of insulin-related medication errors has not decreased since 2011 [23].

There is a paucity in the literature regarding the nature and prevalence of insulin-related prescribing errors at the point of discharge. Also there is lack of quality of insulin information being communicated in hospital discharge summaries, particularly relating to insulin devices and dose changes [18, 21], and a poor uptake of the JDBS discharge guidelines [23]. In this context, this study was planned.

Aims and objectives

The aim of the study was to investigate the nature of insulin-related prescribing errors and to evaluate the completeness of relevant information provided on the discharge summaries of insulin-treated patients with diabetes. The objectives of this study included:

- To classify the nature of insulin-related prescribing errors or discrepancies on discharge summaries from the hospital.
- To determine the prevalence of insulin-related prescribing errors or discrepancies on discharge in the study population.
- To examine the timeliness and completeness of information related to insulin therapy communicated to general practitioners on discharge summaries.

To determine if any of the study population affected by a prescription error or information discrepancy had a diabetes- related emergency hospital readmission within 30 days of discharge.

Methods

Study context

The study was undertaken over a 6-week period during January and February 2017 at a large NHS Foundation Trust in South Yorkshire, UK, providing local secondary and specialist tertiary diabetes care. The study site does not currently employ the use of an integrated electronic patient record and inpatient prescribing system. Inpatient medical notes, including prescriptions, are documented on paper and retrospectively uploaded to an electronic patient record after discharge. All information communicated on discharge, including the discharge medication prescription, is however, manually entered into to an electronic discharge template by prescribers (via transcription from paper inpatient prescription charts). Then it is sent to primary care providers (e.g. GPs) via an online integrated clinical environment (ICE) system, which is used throughout the local area. This electronic discharge template contains mandatory fields that need to be populated before allowing prescribers to complete the discharge summary, for example 'follow-up plans for hospital/community'. An optional section regarding "medication changes", where prescribers are requested to document any intentional changes to medication made since admission to hospital, is also included. After the prescriber completes an individual discharge summary, a clinical pharmacist will electronically verify the prescription and then the nurse will finalise the process by completing and printing the discharge summary (for the patient and their medical records). The system then automatically sends the document electronically to the respective GP. Completion of all the processes is indicated via an icon change on the computer screen.

Data collection

A retrospective analysis was conducted that included all patients with insulin-treated diabetes who were receiving care as inpatients at the study hospital during the 29th September 2016, who were eligible for inclusion in the National Diabetes Inpatient Audit (NaDIA) and whose data was collected for the NaDIA. Patients who were excluded from the NaDIA (e.g. paediatric patients, patients on mental health wards, in the emergency department, day case wards, short-stay units or palliative care units) or whose data was unable to be retrieved during the NaDIA (e.g. due to unavailability of patient records) were therefore not included.

Patients' medical records were examined by a single reviewer for the entire inpatient episode that included the NaDIA collection date (29th September 2016). This included admission documentation, prescription charts and electronic discharge summaries. Patients who had unavailable medical records or who had died during their inpatient stay were not included in the final analysis. The data collection sheet was designed to capture in free-form any noted discrepancies or errors relating to insulin information and prescription, as well as the extent of adherence to medication-related discharge recommendations specified by both the NPC and JBDS (see Table 1). Where ambiguities in interpretation of information contained in medical records arose, a single clinical pharmacist was consulted to clarify and confirm information at the point of data collection.

Changes to a patient's insulin regimen were identified by recording insulin prescription information. This information included preparation, device, frequency of administration, time of administration and number of units used. These changes were documented on three occasions throughout the patient stay. These were on admission, the handwritten prescription on the day of discharge and on the electronic discharge summary. The electronic discharge summary's status was also recorded in order to indicate if it had been provided to the patient and sent to the patient's GP in line with local and national recommendations.

All data collected as part of the study was anonymised in order to maintain patient confidentiality. The study design and data collection method was reviewed and

Table 1 Medicines-related information to be communicated in discharge summaries according to JBDS and NPC criteria (adapted from 24,10)

A list of all medicine prescribed for the patient on discharge from hospital (and not just those dispensed at the time of discharge)
Dose, frequency, formulation and route of all the medicines listed
Medicine stopped and started, with reasons
Details of increasing, or decreasing dose regimens
This information should be clear, unambiguous and legible and should be available to the GP as soon as possible.
Patients should be given a copy of their discharge summary (JBDS 2015)

endorsed by a specialist panel as part of the hospital's clinical effectiveness unit.

Insulin prescription errors, discrepancies and completeness of information issues

In order to investigate and classify the nature of insulin-related errors or discrepancies, data was collected regarding any changes that have been made to the insulin regimen during the inpatient stay, whether an error or discrepancy had occurred at the point of discharge and the nature of any such errors or discrepancies. For the purposes of this study, an error was defined as erroneous or incomplete documentation of insulin preparation, device, route, dose (number of units) or frequency transcribed onto the discharge summary when compared with the inpatient prescription on the day of discharge [19]. A discrepancy was defined as a failure to communicate any changes made to insulin therapy in the designated "medication changes" section of the discharge prescription (e.g. where an insulin dose had changed since admission but no indication of the intention of this was documented) [24, 25]. A lack of explicit documentation of insulin regimen changes could cause confusion and uncertainty regarding the accuracy of the discharge information in primary care, and could result in consequential prescribing errors or suboptimal glycaemic control in primary care.

Examination of completeness of information provided on discharge summaries involved studying the whole discharge summary in order to identify any omissions of relevant insulin information to be communicated to the GP. A 'completeness of information issue' was identified when an important piece of insulin information was omitted from the discharge summary. This may include, for example, failure to record a time for insulin administration (e.g. stating 'daily' rather than 'every morning') or an explanation for any intentional change in insulin regimen (e.g. dose decreased due to persistent hypoglycaemia). Although these issues are arguably less likely to cause direct harm to a patient (e.g. compared to a prescription error), they may lead to interface issues and difficulties in providing continuity of care to patients in the community. For example, in the case of missing or unclear information provision, primary care providers may need to contact the hospital in order to clarify important information pertaining to a patient's insulin therapy.

Data analysis

Information regarding patients' insulin regimens and any errors, discrepancies or issues was collected in free-form. Errors, discrepancies and completeness of information issues were then classified during thematic analysis. Data analysis was carried out using Microsoft Excel 2016 and IBM SPSS Statistics v22. Data for patients who had died during inpatient stay, or those for whom a complete set of medical notes could not be obtained, were removed before final analysis.

Results

Study population

A total of 72 patients who were prescribed insulin for a diabetes diagnosis were included in the National Diabetes Inpatient Audit data collection at the trust, and were therefore eligible for inclusion in the study. Six patients had died during their inpatient stay and a further 24 patients were excluded due to a lack of availability of medical notes during data collection. A total of 42 patients were therefore included in the final study. Of the included patients; 64% (n = 27) had type 2 diabetes, 29% (n = 12) had type 1 diabetes and 7% (n = 3) had cystic fibrosis-related diabetes. An average of 1.1 insulin preparations were prescribed per patient both on admission and discharge. Table 2 shows the proportion of patients who were prescribed different numbers of insulin preparations on admission and discharge, illustrating that most patients included in the study were using a single insulin preparation.

Thirty-eight (90%) of patients had undergone a medicines reconciliation process on admission to hospital by a pharmacy team member. Thirty-three out of 42 patients (79%) had changes to their insulin regimen made during their inpatient stay. This included the initiation and/or discontinuation of insulin therapy, insulin dose changes and insulin preparation/brand.

The majority of patients were inpatients in care of the elderly (COTE) wards (23.8%), followed by; admissions wards (19%), surgical (16.7%), cardiology (14.3%), diabetes and endocrine (11.9%), cystic fibrosis (7.1%), orthopaedics (4.8%) and respiratory (2.4%) wards.

The length of inpatient stay ranged from 3 to 228 days, with the mean duration of stay being 36 days (SD = 40).

Nature and prevalence of insulin-related prescribing errors or discrepancies on discharge

Eighteen (43%) patients had an error or discrepancy relating to insulin on their discharge summary, 11 (61%) of whom had type 2 diabetes, 6 (33%) had type 1 diabetes and 1 (6%) had cystic fibrosis-related diabetes. All

Table 2 Numbers of insulin preparations per patient on admission and discharge

Number of insulin preparations prescribed per patient	Numbers of patients on admission	Numbers of patients on discharge
$n = 0$	6 (14%)	5 (12%)
$n = 1$	27 (64%)	29 (69%)
$n = 2$	9 (21%)	8 (19%)

patients who had a change made to their insulin during admission had at least one error, discrepancy or completeness of information issue identified on their discharge prescription. A total of 27 errors or discrepancies were identified across the 42 patients included in the study, giving a frequency of 0.6 per patient. The most frequent error or discrepancy identified was the failure to communicate an intentional insulin dose change in the "medication changes" section (Fig. 1). The greatest number of errors or discrepancies identified for one patient was 4, which included the failure to document the discontinuation of one insulin preparation, the initiation of another insulin preparation and the dose change for another insulin preparation under the "medication changes" section, and not including the dose of an insulin preparation on the discharge prescription.

Most errors had occurred on discharge from COTE (26%, n = 7) and surgical wards (26%, n = 7), followed by; cardiology (19%, n = 5), diabetes and endocrine (15%, n = 4), admissions (7%, n = 2) and cystic fibrosis (7%, n = 2) wards.

Timeliness and completeness of information communicated to general practitioners

All discharge summaries analysed (100%) were of the same electronic format and had been marked as sent to the GP via the ICE interface. As the system automatically prints a copy of the discharge summary for the patient upon transmission to the GP, it can be assumed that 100% of patients also received a paper copy of the same discharge summary as per hospital procedure, although this could not be determined definitively from this study.

A total of 17 (40%) patients had discharge summaries containing incomplete insulin information (henceforth referred to as 'completeness of information issues'). A total of 17 completeness of information issues were identified in total, giving a frequency of 0.4 per patient. The nature and prevalence of these issues is shown in Fig. 2, with failure to specify a time for insulin administration being the most prevalent.

Completeness of information issues had occurred on three occasions on discharge summaries produced from COTE, cardiology, admissions and diabetes and endocrine wards (18% each); on two occasions by both orthopaedic and cystic fibrosis wards (12% each) and once from surgical wards (6%).

Readmission

Twelve (29%) patients were readmitted back to the hospital trust within 30 days of the recorded discharge date with an emergency, of which three (25%) were due to a diabetes-related reason. Two (66%) of these three patients had a discrepancy identified on the discharge summary written prior to readmission. The first patient was readmitted due to 'poor diabetic control' who did not have their insulin dose change explicitly written on their discharge summary from a COTE ward. The second patient was readmitted for hyperglycaemia, who also did not have their insulin dose change explicitly communicated on their last discharge summary from a diabetes and endocrine ward.

Discussion

This study provides a unique insight into the current situation regarding the quality and accuracy of insulin-related information documented for patients with diabetes who are being discharged from hospital. Initial results may help inform quality improvement initiatives to reduce the risk to patients and improve the safe usage

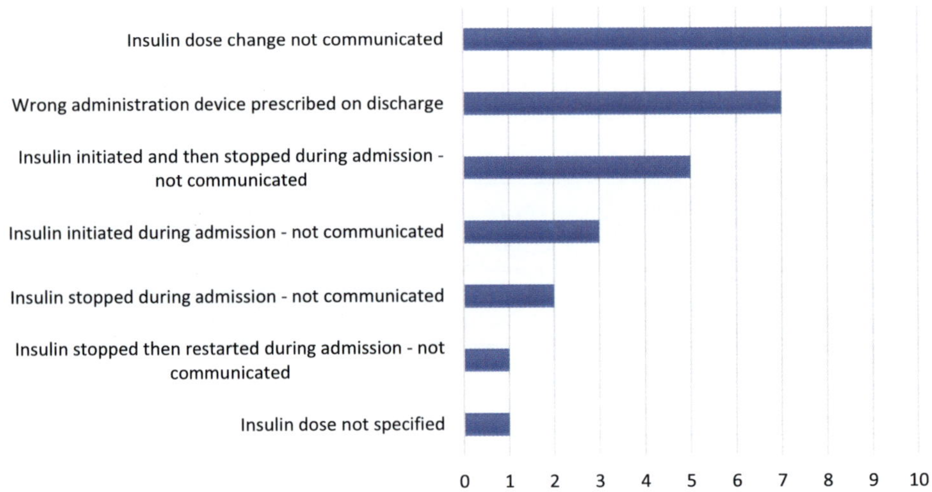

Fig. 1 The nature and prevalence of insulin errors or discrepancies identified at discharge

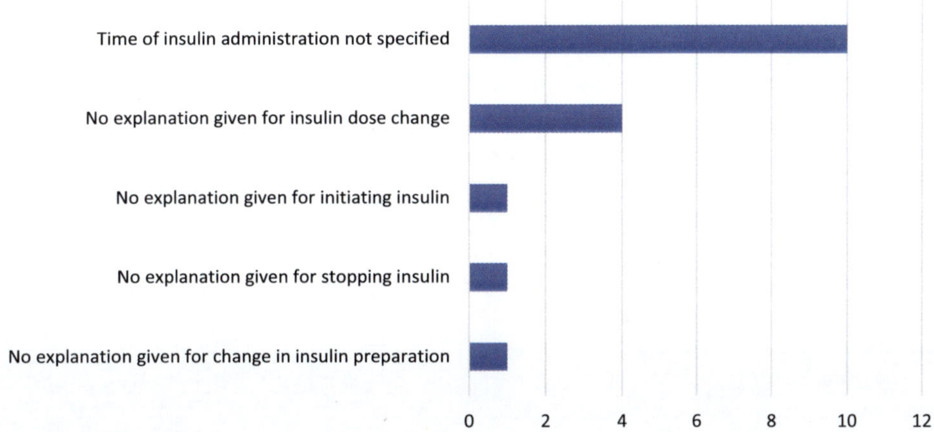

Fig. 2 The nature and prevalence of completeness of information issues identified on discharge summaries

of insulin. Findings suggest that electronic discharge summaries can provide timely information to primary care providers and patients. Important information contained in discharge summaries is, however, often incomplete and sometimes erroneous, with the potential implication for compromised continuity of care and patient safety.

Nature and prevalence of insulin-related prescribing errors or discrepancies on discharge

The majority of patients had changes made to their insulin therapy during hospital stay. All patients with changes had an error or discrepancy identified on their discharge summary. This suggests that further progress is required to ensure consistent quality of communication on discharge for patients with insulin-treated diabetes, with particular care being paid to those where a change has occurred. The proportion of total patient discharge summaries with identified insulin-related prescribing errors is similar to that found for inpatients by the hospital trust's NaDIA in 2016 [23], suggesting that errors can easily be continued through to discharge at similar rates during inpatient stay.

The most common type of insulin error or discrepancy identified on discharge was a failure to communicate an insulin dose change. This result differs from studies that cite drug omission from discharge prescriptions as the most frequent error type [3–5]. These studies do not focus on patients with insulin-treated diabetes specifically, however, and due to the high-risk and critical nature of insulin, it could be less likely to be omitted altogether from the discharge prescription (especially when medicines reconciliation are completed on admission was the case for the majority of patients in this study) compared to other medication. The results, do, however, support the findings of studies that report a high proportion of discharge summaries excluding medication changes [11, 12]. Failure to explain or confirm an insulin dose change on discharge may not be as serious as a dosing prescribing error, but the lack of clarity in communication can risk the patient, carer or primary care provider administering an erroneous dose (e.g. that prescribed before or during admission) and therefore risk optimal glycaemic control. The need for GPs or other community healthcare professionals to clarify any changes made may result in a disruption to continuity of care and risk patient safety (especially when a dose change cannot be promptly clarified, e.g. by a carer administering insulin to patients in their home immediately after discharge). This can also result in inefficiencies due to an avoidable increased workload. Recommendations for future policy and practice could include prescriber review of insulin therapy at the point of discharge prescription writing (e.g. by comparison with medicines reconciliation documentation), ensuring that details of any intentional changes being made are explained on the discharge summary.

The second most frequent insulin error or discrepancy identified at discharge was prescription of the wrong administration device on the discharge summary. Other studies have found that increasing diversity in the types of insulin and variety of devices available in the UK may cause confusion when prescribing insulin and may result in the incorrect device being prescribed [26]. This finding reflects the results of a large audit conducted by East and South East England Specialist Pharmacy Services [21], which found the most common inpatient insulin prescribing error was selection of the wrong administration device. The input of clinical pharmacy services throughout admission and again on discharge may account for the decreased prevalence of this error identified in this study, which looked at discharge summaries after pharmacist review. Interestingly, the NaDIA [23] does not include administration device error as a medication error, despite the potentially harmful consequences of prescribing and dispensing the wrong device, which could result in patients being unable to administer their insulin. For example, erroneously prescribing and dispensing insulin cartridges instead of a disposable pen or a vial could lead to an inability to administer insulin. Another example is dangerous administration practices such as drawing insulin out of a cartridge with a syringe [16, 27].

The majority of insulin errors or discrepancies were in patients discharged from care of the elderly (COTE) and surgical wards. The result for COTE wards was expected as they contained the majority of patients. Patients on surgical wards, however, were more likely to experience an insulin-related error or discrepancy. Furthermore, the surgical wards included in this study had the greatest range of insulin errors or discrepancies identified on discharge. The higher frequency of insulin-related errors on discharge summaries from surgical specialities somewhat contrasts national data that shows no difference between insulin-related errors on medical and surgical wards, despite a higher incidence of medicines management and general diabetes medication prescribing errors [23]. Patients with diabetes discharged from surgical wards are possibly less likely to have a diabetes-related admission, with a consequential decrease in likelihood of any specialist diabetes team involvement in their care, and are also more likely to have their discharge summaries written by doctors working in surgical specialists who may have less prescribing support from senior colleagues [28].

Timeliness and completeness of information communicated to general practitioners

As all 42 discharge summaries were marked as sent to the general practitioner and patient, this study reports 100% adherence to the recommendation that "information should be made available to the GP as soon as possible" [10] and "patients should be given a copy of their discharge summary" [24] – see Table 1. The use of an electronic system to ensure discharge summaries are promptly sent to general practitioners and provided for patients has previously been shown to aid the timeliness of communication to GPs compared with other methods, such as postal or manual delivery of paper documents [29, 30]. It is therefore very likely that the electronic discharge template contributed to the 100% compliance with this standard found in this study. Timeliness of information communication regarding medication is particularly important when critical medicines such as insulin are involved, especially when a third party is responsible for the administration of insulin to patients (e.g. where patients rely on domiciliary carers to administer insulin doses) [25].

Completeness of information issues were fewer in number than prescribing errors or discrepancies, but may also lead to lack of clarity and problem development at the interface of care. The most common completeness of information issue identified was non-specification of the time of insulin dose. This finding supports that of the North-East RISK project, which established that many of discharge prescriptions did not contain information relating to the time of insulin administration [18]. This particular completeness of information issue was found to have been distributed fairly evenly across the clinical areas included in the study. As the inclusion of details regarding time of insulin dose is not a mandatory requirement on the electronic discharge system at the study hospital, the relative prevalence of this issue may be explained. Introduction of electronic prescribing systems with details of administration time could aid this issue in future by pre-populating the prescription with this information.

Readmission

Emergency hospital readmission within 30 days of discharge is widely used as a quality indicator for the success of hospitals in helping people to recover [31]. Hospital readmission can lead to the increased expenditure of secondary care providers and have a negative impact on patient health [32]. The readmission of the two patients in this study for a diabetes-related problem and with insulin-related discrepancies on their discharge summary could not be definitively attributed to the insulin issues in question, due to the complexities and contributing factors pertaining to hospital readmission. This is reinforced by a study conducted by Rubin in 2015, which concluded that factors such as socio-economic status, race and ethnicity also influenced the incidence of readmission [32]. Although a definitive link cannot be established between discharge summary quality and readmission in this study, other studies have reported that communication gaps with respect to medication changes may contribute to preventable hospital readmissions [33].

Strengths and limitations

This study describes an accessible means of obtaining meaningful data with respect to discharge summary information for patients who use insulin to manage their diabetes. The results provide an insight into the nature and prevalence of insulin-related prescribing errors and discrepancies as well as the completeness of information provided on transfer of care from hospital to community sectors. Use of the NaDIA data collected by the trust enabled a wide-variety of patient information to be analysed and offered a convenient sampling method that could be replicated in other hospitals elsewhere in the UK, or further afield by use of similar national audit data collections. Limitations of the study included the small sample size and the large proportion of patients who were not included on account of unavailable patient medication records at the time of data collection. We anticipate that complete data capture would be less problematic for hospital trusts who make use of a fully integrated electronic patient medical record and prescribing system, unlike the study hospital who still employ the use of paper documentation for inpatient medical records and prescriptions.

Although timeliness of transfer of discharge summaries could be studied from the hospital, we did not measure the time lapse in GP receipt and processing of discharge summaries in primary care. Further work that examined primary care healthcare professionals' perceptions of timeliness and completeness of information would further complement this study's findings.

Furthermore, as data was collected retrospectively, clinical pharmacy intervention at the point of verification of discharge prescriptions was not examined. This meant that only discharge summaries that had been authorised by a pharmacist, and therefore transferred to the general practitioner, were studied. Although this provides an accurate reflection of the quality of documentation transferred to the GP, prospective examination of discharge summaries before clinical pharmacy intervention may provide a more accurate, less conservative, picture of prescriber error and information discrepancy rate on discharge.

Conclusions

This study highlights the current status with respect to quality of insulin-related information communicated at the point of discharge, and the types of problems that may occur on the interface for patients with insulin-treated diabetes. We conclude that the use of electronic discharge templates can provide a timely method for communicating important insulin information to GPs when transferred locally via an integrated system. The study concludes that the insulin information provided on discharge summaries is however are often incomplete and sometimes erroneous, particularly in relation to insulin administration device, details of dose changes and time of administration. Such errors and omissions in information have the potential to contribute to continued insulin-related medication errors in the community and possibly even readmission to hospital.

Further research

Further research into this area is required to develop evidence-based initiatives both locally and nationally that incorporate both NPC and JBDS guidelines for this particular patient group. Triangulation of data with qualitative studies concerning discharge summary generation, content, verification and processing (e.g. in primary care) for this particular patient group would further enable strategies to be developed to improve patient safety and continuity of care for patients with diabetes using insulin.

Abbreviations

COTE: Care of the Elderly (clinical speciality); GP: General Practitioner (primary care physician); ICE: Integrated Clinical Environment; JBDS: Joint British Diabetes Societies; NaDIA: National Diabetes Inpatient Audit; NHS: National Health Service; NPC: National Prescribing Centre; UK: United Kingdom

Acknowledgements

The authors would like to thank Dr. Neil Hamilton for his valuable support throughout this study.

Funding

This research received no specific grant from any funding agency in the public, commercial or not-for-profit sectors.

Authors' contributions

AB and SAK designed the study. LN contributed to study design, collected and analysed the data. AB advised on and contributed to data collection and prepared the first draft of the manuscript. ZB and SAK reviewed the manuscript. All authors had access to the study data that support the publication and revised and approved the final manuscript.

Competing interests

The authors declare that they have no competing interests.

Author details

[1]School of Applied Sciences, University of Huddersfield, Queensgate, Huddersfield HD1 3DH, United Kingdom. [2]Pharmacy Department, Sheffield Teaching Hospital NHS Foundation Trust, Herries Road, Sheffield S5 7AU, United Kingdom. [3]School of Pharmacy, Faculty of Medical and Health Sciences, University of Auckland, Private Mail Bag, Auckland 92019, New Zealand.

References

1. WHO Collaborating Centre for Patient Safety Solutions. Assuring Medication Accuracy at Transitions in Care. [Internet]. 2007 [cited 2017 May 5];1(6) Available from: http://www.who.int/patientsafety/solutions/patientsafety/PS-Solution6.pdf
2. Vira T. Reconcilable differences: correcting medication errors at hospital admission and discharge. Qual Saf Heal Care. 2006;15(2):122–6.
3. Riordan CO, Delaney T, Grimes T. Exploring discharge prescribing errors and their propagation post-discharge: an observational study. Int J Clin Pharm. 2016;38(5):1172–81.
4. Callen J, McIntosh J, Li J. Accuracy of medication documentation in hospital discharge summaries: a retrospective analysis of medication transcription errors in manual and electronic discharge summaries. Int J Med Inform. 2010 Jan;79(1):58–64.
5. Herrero-Herrero J-I, García-Aparicio J, Porsius AJ, De BA, Cortes T, et al. Medication discrepancies at discharge from an internal medicine service. Eur J Intern Med. 2011 Feb;22(1):43–8.

6. Pippins JR, Gandhi TK, Hamann C, Ndumele CD, Labonville SA, Diedrichsen EK, et al. Classifying and predicting errors of inpatient medication reconciliation. J Gen Intern Med. 2008 Sep 19;23(9):1414–22.
7. Amori R, Pittas A, Siegel R, Kumar S, Chen J, Karnam S, et al. Inpatient medical errors involving glucose-lowering medications and their impact on patients: review of 2,598 incidents from a voluntary electronic error-reporting database. Endocr Pract. 2008 Jul;14(5):535–42.
8. c Van W, Seth R, Austin PC, Laupacis A. Effect of discharge summary availability during post-discharge visits on hospital readmission. J Gen Intern Med. 2002;17(3):186.
9. Quality Commission C. Managing patients' medicines after discharge from hospital. 2009 [cited. May 5. 2017; Available from: http://webarchive.nationalarchives.gov.uk/20101201001009/http:/www.cqc.org.uk/_db/_documents/Managing_patients_medicines_after_discharge_from_hospital.pdf
10. National Prescribing Centre. Medicines Reconciliation: A Guide to Implementation. [Internet]. 2008 [cited 2017 Jun 26] Available from: https://www.nicpld.org/courses/fp/assets/MM/NPCMedicinesRecGuideImplementation.pdf
11. Hammad EA, Wright DJ, Walton C, Nunney I, Bhattacharya D. Adherence to UK national guidance for discharge information: an audit in primary care. Br J Clin Pharmacol. 2014/07/22 ed. 2014;78(6):1453–64.
12. Cresswell A, Hart M, Suchanek O, Young T, Leaver L, Hibbs S. Mind the gap: Improving discharge communication between secondary and primary care. BMJ Qual Improv Reports. 2015 Sep 2;4(1):u207936.w3197.
13. Grimes T, Delaney T, Duggan C, Kelly JG, Graham IM. Survey of medication documentation at hospital discharge: implications for patient safety and continuity of care. Ir J Med Sci. 2008 Jun 15;177(2):93–7.
14. Lehnbom EC, Raban MZ, Walter SR, Richardson K, Westbrook JI. Do electronic discharge summaries contain more complete medication information? A retrospective analysis of paper versus electronic discharge summaries. Heal Inf Manag J. 2014;43(3):4–12.
15. Institute of Safe Medication Practices. ISMP List of High-Alert Medications in Acute Care Settings. Inst Safe Medicat Pract [Internet]. 2011; Available from: https://www.ismp.org/Tools/institutionalhighAlert.asp
16. National Patient Safety Agency. Safer administration of insulin. NHS. 2010. p. 14410.
17. Smith WD, Winterstein AG, Johns T, Rosenberg E, Sauer BC. Causes of hyperglycemia and hypoglycemia in adult inpatients. Am J Heal Pharm. 2005;62(7):714–9.
18. Leech NJ, Johnson G, Nayar R, Nunez E, Macleod J. Tackling insulin safety using a multifaceted multidisciplinary regional approach first report from the north east regional insulin safety and knowledge (RISK) project. Heal Found. 2013;
19. Cousins D, Rosario C, Scarpello J. Insulin, hospitals and harm: a review of patient safety incidents reported to the National Patient Safety Agency, vol. 11. Clinical Medicine: Journal of the Royal College of Physicians of London; 2011. p. 28–30
20. Rousseau M-P, Beauchesne M-F, Naud A-S, Leblond J, Cossette B, Lanthier L, et al. An Interprofessional qualitative study of barriers and potential solutions for the safe use of insulin in the hospital setting. Can J Diabetes. 2014 Apr;38(2):85–9.
21. East & South East England Specialist Pharmacy Services. Pharmacy contribution to patient safety: Results of collaborative insulin baseline audit. 2010 [cited. Jun 6. 2017; Available from: https://www.sps.nhs.uk/wp-content/uploads/2010/11/Report_Collaborative_Insulin_Baseline_Audit_20Aug10_v4_CL.pdf
22. Doyle MA, Malcolm JC, Liu D, Maranger J, Ooi TC, Keely E. Using a structured discharge letter template to improve communication during the transition from a specialized outpatient diabetes clinic to a primary care physician. Can J Diabetes. 2015;39(6):457–66.
23. NaDIA advisory group. National Diabetes Inpatient Audit England and Wales, 2016 [Internet]. 2016 [cited 2017 Jun 6]. p. 1–123. Available from: http://www.content.digital.nhs.uk/catalogue/PUB23539/nati-diab-inp-audi-16-rep.pdf.
24. Cornish W. Safe and appropriate use of insulin and other antihyperglycemic agents in hospital. Vol. 38, Canadian Journal of Diabetes. 2014. p. 94–100.
25. C. Jairam EW. Discharge planning for adult inpatients with diabetes [Internet]. 2015 [cited 2017 Jun 6] Available from: http://www.diabetologists-abcd.org.uk/JBDS/JBDS_Discharge_Planning_Final_2015.pdf
26. Staff PE. Insulin use: preventable errors. Prescrire Int. 2014 Jan;23(145):14–7.
27. NHS Improvement. Risk of severe harm and death due to withdrawing insulin from pen devices. Patient Saf Alert [Internet]. 2016 [cited 2017 May 22]; Available from: https://improvement.nhs.uk/uploads/documents/Patient_Safety_Alert_-_Withdrawing_insulin_from_pen_devices.pdf
28. Dornan T, Investigator P, Ashcroft D, Lewis P, Miles J, Taylor D, et al. An in depth investigation into causes of prescribing errors by foundation trainees in relation to their medical education. EQUIP study. Vol. 44, Methods. 2010.
29. Pocklington C, Al-Dhahir L. A Comparison of Methods of Producing a Discharge Summary: handwritten vs. electronic documentation. Br J Med Pract BJMP.org BJMP. 2011;44(33).
30. Barr R, Chin KY, Yeong K. Improving patient discharge process using electronic medication input tool and on-line guide to arranging follow-ups. BMJ Qual Improv Rep. 2013/01/01 ed. 2013;2(1).
31. Clinical Indicators Team, Health and Social Care Information Centre. Indicator Quality Statement: Emergency readmissions within 30 days of discharge from hospital. NHS Outcomes Framew 3b [Internet]. 2014 [cited 2017 Jun 14]; Available from: https://indicators.hscic.gov.uk/download/Outcomes%20Framework/Specification/NHSOF_3b_I00712_Q.pdf.
32. Rubin DJ. Hospital Readmission of Patients with Diabetes. Curr Diab Rep. 2015;15(4).
33. Witherington EMA, Pirzada OM, Avery AJ. Communication gaps and readmissions to hospital for patients aged 75 years and older: observational study. Qual Saf Heal Care. 2008 Feb 1;17(1):71–5.

14

Hypnotics use in children 0–18 months: moderate agreement between mother-reported survey data and prescription registry data

Ingvild Holdø[1], Jørgen G. Bramness[2], Marte Handal[3], Leila Torgersen[3], Ted Reichborn-Kjennerud[3,4], Eivind Ystrøm[3,5,6], Hedvig Nordeng[3,5] and Svetlana Skurtveit[1,3*]

Abstract

Background: Different methods in pharmacoepidemiology can be used to study hypnotic use in children. But neither questionnaire-based data nor prescription records can be considered a "gold standard". This study aimed to investigate the agreement between mother-reported questionnaire-based data and prescription record data for hypnotic drugs in children aged 0–18 months. The agreement was compared to the agreement for a group of antiepileptic drugs.

Methods: Prescription record data were collected from the Norwegian prescription database for 47,413 children also surveyed in the Norwegian mother and child cohort between 2005 and 2009. Agreement between in the two data sources was calculated using Cohens Kappa. Multinomial logistic regression was used to calculate the effect of sociodemographic variables on discrepancies in data sources.

Results: The agreement between mother-reported and dispensed hypnotics was less than 50% for all hypnotics. Sensitivity of reporting increased with number of filled prescriptions. The agreement of antiepileptic drugs was 92.9% in the same population. Of several sociodemographic factors only paternal educational level and maternal work situation was significantly related to agreement between prescription record and survey data.

Conclusion: There was a moderate agreement between reported use and dispensed hypnotic drugs for infants and toddlers. Results indicate that sociodemographic factors play only a minor role in explaining discrepancy.

Keywords: MoBa, Hypnotics and sedatives, Agreement, Child, Prescriptions

Background

Prescribing sleep-inducing medication for otherwise healthy infants and toddlers is a controversial subject. Different countries have different therapeutic traditions, but pharmacological treatment of sleep problems in the youngest children is frequent in many countries [1–4]. For infants and toddlers antihistamines, α_2-agonists or chloral hydrate are most often the drugs of choice, while melatonin, benzodiazepines and the benzodiazepine like z-hypnotics (i.e. zolpidem, zopiclone) are mainly prescribed for older children and teen-agers [3, 4]. In Norway, the antihistamine alimemazine (an aliphatic phenothiazine) is the most used sleep inducing drug in infants and toddlers, despite not being approved for the age group less than 2 years of age [1, 3, 5–9].

There is a lack of evidence of effect and safety for sleep inducing drugs to small children. This is especially true for the older drugs introduced in a time where drugs testing was less regulated. To compensate for this, observational studies of real life use in children can be useful. There are many types of data

* Correspondence: svetlana.skurtveit@fhi.no
[1]Norwegian Centre of Addiction Research (SERAF), University of Oslo, Oslo, Norway
[3]Domain of Mental and Physical health, Norwegian Institute of Public Health, Oslo, Norway
Full list of author information is available at the end of the article

sources for such studies and all will have their strengths and limitations, but few studies have estimated the quality of different data sources on the use of prescription drugs in young children. Two such data sources may be survey data and prescription data. However both sources have their limitations and none of them can be considered the "gold standard" [10]. One prior study, comparing the Norwegian Prescription Database (NorPD) with maternal report of prescribed anti-asthma drugs for children aged 7 years in the Norwegian Mother and child cohort study (MoBa) showed high agreement with maternal report [11]. However, little is known about other drugs.

The aim of this study was to investigate the agreement between maternal-report on sleep inducing drug use by 0–18 month's old children in the Norwegian Mother and Child Cohort with information on dispensed hypnotic drugs from pharmacies in the Norwegian Prescription Database. The results were compared with the agreement for antiepileptic drugs that should be taken more regularly for a chronic somatic disease, thus theoretically representing a drug with an expected higher agreement between the two data sources. Since alimemazine traditionally is used in Norway as a hypnotic drug to young children, we finally estimated the extent to which sociodemographic background variables and the number of prescriptions of alimemazine could account for possible discrepancies.

Methods

MoBa

The Norwegian Mother and Child cohort study (MoBa) is a prospective population-based pregnancy cohort study conducted by the Norwegian Institute of Public Health and aims to study causes of disease [12, 13]. Women were invited to join after attending routine ultrasound appointment in pregnancy week 18. From one participating hospital in one region in 1999 the study gradually included more hospitals. In the period 2005–2008 almost all Norwegian women were invited to participate. Overall in the period 1999 to 2008 approximately 41% of the invited consented to participation. The last birth into the cohort was in June 2009. The MoBa study collected questionnaires at specific time points; our study uses questionnaires from baseline and at child's age 6 and 18 months [14]. The personal identification numbers [15] assigned to all individual in Norway allow for linking of MoBa data with other registries and studies. In this study, MoBa data was linked to data from the Norwegian Prescription Database.

Norwegian prescription record (NorPD)

NorPD holds a complete record of all dispensed prescription drugs since 2004 [16]. Pharmacies are obliged to register prescriptions electronically and submit information every month. NorPD includes both prescriptions made to individuals and institutions, but prescriptions in institutions are not registered at a person level [17]. For each prescription drug specific information, patient data and prescriber information are registered. In the present study we only studied prescriptions made to children in the MoBa study. We used information on patient ID, drug name, date of dispensing, and reimbursement code.

Sample

To ensure that information was available from both data sources, we only included children in MoBa when the 6 month questionnaire was filled after 1. January 2005. Both the 6 months and the 18 months questionnaire had to be filled in for the child to be included in our study. The study population thus consisted of 47,310 children (see Fig. 1).

From baseline questionnaires we used the following information: parents' age, family income, parents' education, if the pregnancy was planned or not, maternal marital status, maternal parity and maternal employment status. From the 6 and 18 months questionnaires we used reported drug use (Additional file 1). Trained personnel interpreted and converted drug names from the questionnaires to ATC codes when entering data.

Drugs included in the study

For the present study information on all anxiolytics, hypnotics and sedatives, dexchlorpheniramine, alimemazine and promethazine was used (Table 1). As comparison we also included a group of antiepileptic drugs recommended as first choices for treatment of childhood

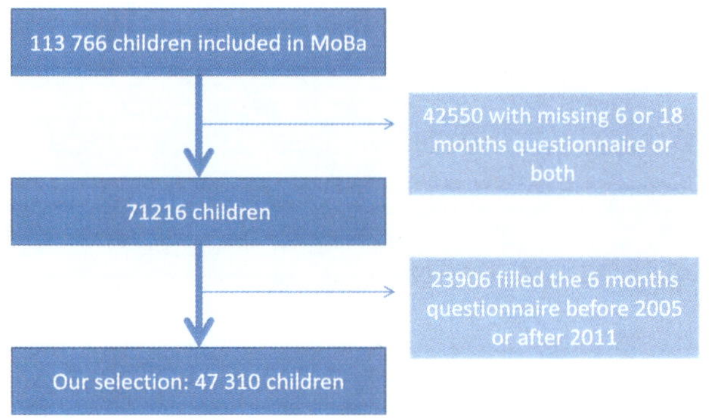

Fig. 1 Inclusion in study based on participants in the Norwegian Mother and child cohort study

Table 1 Drug name and number of prescriptions for all sedative drugs from birth until 18 months of age[a] in our selection of children in the MoBa cohort, 3071 children with unique IDs

Drug name	Atc code	N° of prescriptions	Main reimbursed diagnosis	Reimbursement (%)
clonazepam	N03AE01	23	epilepsy	69.57%
diazepam	N05BA01	399	epilepsy	14.79%
clobazam	N05BA09	7	epilepsy	42.86%
hydroxyzine	N05BB01	3	allergy	66.67%
nitrazepam	N05CD02	41	epilepsy	68.29%
midazolam	N05CD08	14	epilepsy	57.14%
melatonin	N05CH01	33	(no reimbursement)	0.00%
deksklopheniramin	R06AB02	3038	allergy	42.59%
alimemazine	R06AD01	993	allergy	2.72%
sum		4551		31.58%

[a]Date of filling of 18 months questionnaire used as cut off

epilepsy [18]; Carbamazepine, oxcarbazepine, lamotrigine, topiramate, and valproate.

From NorPD we included hypnotics and antiepileptics dispensed to the child from birth until the date the mother filled the 18 months questionnaire.

Analysis strategy and statistics

a) Reported (yes/no) and dispensed prescriptions (yes/no) for all hypnotic drugs and the control group of antiepileptic drugs were cross-tabulated. We used Cohen's Kappa with Fleiss' subdivision to determine agreement between reported use and registry data (Table 1) [19].
b) Prescriptions for alimemazine were subdivided into categories based on number of prescriptions (0, 1, 2 and 3 or more) and we compared this to information on reported alimemazine use from the questionnaires(yes/no). Setting prescription record data as reference standard, we measured sensitivity of reporting by number of prescriptions (Table 2).
c) Mother-reported sociodemographic data was used to characterize the children with discrepancy between reported use and dispensed prescriptions of alimemazine. We compared three groups: 1) Only mother-reported alimemazine use in MoBa, 2) Only dispensed alimemazine in the NorPD prescription record and 3) Both mother-reported use and dispensed prescriptions for alimemazine. The groups were compared using the Chi-square test (Table 3). The sociodemographic variables showing significance ($p < 0.1$) in Table 3 were included in a multinomial logistic regression analysis. The outcome measure was the relative risk (RR) with confidence intervals, using the category both mother-reported use and dispensed prescriptions for alimemazine as reference category.

Statistical analyses were conducted using SPSS version 22 for Windows.

Ethics

Informed consent was obtained from mothers before inclusion in MoBa. The Regional Committees for Medical and Health Research Ethics and the Norwegian Data Protection Authority approved the linkage of NorPD and MoBa.

Results

Prevalence of hypnotic use

The prevalence of hypnotic drug use was lower in the mother-reported MoBa study than in the prescription database NorPD for all groups of medications except promethazine (Table 2). Alimemazine and dexchlorpheniramine were the two substances most frequently reported used and dispensed. Alimemazine was reported used by 367 (0.8%) children, but was dispensed to 746 (1.6%) children under the age of 18 months. Dexchlorpheniramine was reported used by 1131 (2.4%) children in MoBa, but 2103 (4.4%) had filled a prescription according to NorPD.

Agreement between mother-reported use (MoBa) and dispensed (NorPD) hypnotic drugs.

The agreement between the two data sources was lower than 50% for all the hypnotic drugs. It was best for alimemazine (46.3%) and poorest for anxiolytics (19.1%). The agreement was, however, excellent for the group of antiepileptic's recommended for childhood epilepsy (92.9%) (Table 2).

The sensitivity of the mother-reported alimemazine use increased by numbers of prescriptions filled. Sensitivity was 30.3% when the children had received only one prescription, increasing to 48.1% for children receiving two prescriptions and to 66.7% for those receiving 3 prescriptions or more (Table 3).

Table 2 Agreement between at least one-time mother reported use of hypnotics and at least one dispensed prescription for a hypnotic drug to children aged 0–18 months

	Maternal report (MoBa)			Dispensed drugs (NorPD)			Neither	Only MoBa	Only NorPD	Both		Agreement[d]
Drug category (ATC code)	n	%	95% CI	n	%	95% CI	n	n	n	n	total	
Alimemazine (R06AD01)	367	0.78%	0.70–0.86%	745	1.58%	1.47–1.69%	46,459	106	484	261	47,310	46.3
Promethazine (R06AD02)	14	0.03%	0.02–0.05%	0			47,297	14	0	0	47,310	0
Dexchlorpheniramine (R06AB02)	1131	2.39%	2.26–2.53%	2101	4.44%	4.26–4.64%	44,811	398	1368	733	47,310	43.6
Hypnotics and sedatives (N05C)[a]	39	0.08%	0.06–0.11%	38	0.08%	0.06–0.11%	47,249	23	22	16	47,310	41.0
Anxiolytics (N05B)[b]	62	0.14%	0.11–0.17%	351	0.74%	0.67–0.82%	46,935	24	311	40	47,310	19.1
Recommended antiepileptic's (from ATC N03A)[c]	49	0.10%	0.08–0.14%	50	0.11%	0.08–0.14%	47,257	3	4	46	47,310	92.9

[a]includes nitrazepam, midazolam and melatonin

[b]includes diazepam, clobazam and hydroxyzine

[c]First choice drugs for treatment of childhood epilepsy. Includes carbamazepine N03AF01, oxcarbazepine N03AF02, lamotrigine N03AX09, topiramat N03AX11, and valproate N03AG01. Recommended by the Norwegian Society of Paediatricians

[d]Calculated using Cohen's Kappa

Table 3 Validity of maternal report on use of compared to number of dispensed prescriptions of alimemazine

	Neither	MoBa	NorPD	Both	
Alimemazine R06AD01	*n*	*n*	*n*	*n*	Sensitivity[b]
Total[a]	46,462	106	485	261	34.99%
1 prescription	–	–	415	180	30.25%
2 prescriptions	–	–	55	51	48.11%
3 or more prescriptions	–	–	15	30	66.67%

[a]total number of children included is 47,314
[b]dispensed prescriptions is reference standard for sensitivity analysis

Sociodemographic background variables

The differences of sociodemographic characteristics between mother-reported use and prescription record data of alimemazine use are shown in Table 4. The adjusted multinomial logistic regression analysis showed that when fathers had higher education the risk of children's alimemazine use being only mother-reported was 2.3 times higher (95% Confidence interval [95% CI] 1.3–3.9) than having consistent data in both mother-reported MoBa and prescription record NorPD. Mothers being unemployed increased the risk of children being in the prescription record group only, 1.9 times (95%CI 1.0–3.4) as opposed to the group with consistent data in both sources(data not shown).

Discussion

The agreement between mother-reported hypnotic drug use by their child and data on dispensed prescriptions was found to be moderate to poor for hypnotic drugs. For alimemazine, agreement increased with increasing numbers of dispensed prescriptions. With the exception of paternal education and mothers work situation, no differences in social factors between reported use and dispensed alimemazine were seen.

Mother-reported drug use was generally lower than prescriptions would imply. Some of the dispensed drugs were probably not taken as the questionnaires asked for *use* of medication not received prescriptions. Theoretically, using filled prescriptions as opposed to prescribed prescriptions

Table 4 Sociodemographic characteristics of alimemazine use categorized in three groups: reported use in MoBa but no prescriptions in NorPD, no reported use in MoBa but prescription in NorPD and reported use in MoBa and prescription in NorPD

		Only in MoBa[a] (*N* = 106)		Only in NorPD[b](*N* = 485)		Both MoBa & NorPD[c] (*N* = 261)		*P*-value****
Socioeconomic variables		n	%	n	%	n	%	
Mothers education (*n* = 822)	low (≤12)	30	29.41%	170	36.48%	106	41.73%	
	high (≥13)	72	70.59%	296	63.52%	148	58.27%	0.083
Fathers education (*n* = 766)	low (≤ 12)	35	38.46%	245	56.71%	145	59.67%	
	high (≥13)	56	61.54%	187	43.29%	98	40.33%	0.002
Planned pregnancy (*n* = 837)	no	17	16.50%	101	21.26%	48	18.53%	
	yes	86	83.50%	374	78.74%	211	81.47%	0.448
Maternal employment situation (*N* = 839)	not working	4	3.88%	53	11.13%	17	6.56%	
	working	99	96.12%	423	88.87%	242	93.44%	0.019
Family income (*N* = 818)	low	22	21.57%	126	27.21%	72	28.46%	
	medium	64	62.75%	288	62.20%	161	63.64%	
	high	16	15.69%	49	10.58%	20	7.91%	0.227
Maternal marital status (*N* = 851)	married/cohabiting	101	95.28%	471	97.31%	249	95.40%	
	other	5	4.72%	13	2.69%	12	4.60%	0.312
Parity (*N* = 851)	0	44	41.51%	211	43.60%	122	46.74%	
	1	47	44.34%	168	34.71%	83	31.80%	
	≥2	15	14.15%	105	21.69%	56	21.46%	0.164
Age mother (years) (N = 851)	≤29	41	38.68%	185	38.22%	122	46.74%	
	≥30	65	61.32%	299	61.78%	139	53.26%	0.069
Age father (years) (N = 851)	≤29	26	24.53%	126	26.03%	77	29.50%	
	≥30	80	75.47%	358	73.97%	184	70.50%	0.5

****Chi-square test
[a]Only reported use in MoBa. No prescription in NorPD
[b]Only filled prescription in NorPD. No reported use in MoBa
[c]Both reported use in MoBa and filled prescription in NorPD

should increase the adherence, as we at least know that the drugs were in the patient's possession. However, when using data on dispensed medication we still do not know if the medication was actually taken or subject to so called secondary non-compliance. Many patients are not adherent to prescribed drug therapy [20]. A Canadian study of non-adherence found that sedative- hypnotics had a 35% frequency of non-adherence among the general population [21]. The lower frequency of mother-reported drug use could in this sense be closer to reality than dispensed prescriptions.

Reporting -no use of a hypnotic drug even when a prescription had been filled can also be due to lack of memory. It's more difficult to remember drug use happening a long time ago [10, 22], drugs taken as needed [23–25] and drug use when asked open-ended questions [26]. Hypnotic drugs for small children is controversial and thus might be afflicted with feelings of shame and guilt by the mother, which in turn could have caused lower agreement. Others studies have shown larger discrepancies between prescribed and reported use when the drugs are afflicted with stigma [24, 27]. In MoBa the mothers were asked open questions about their child's drug use up to a year earlier. On the other hand, the high agreement we found for chronically used antiepileptic drugs indicates that the long time periods and open-ended questions was not a problem. A study validating the same data sources in children aged 7 years but with specific asthma questions found higher agreement [11]. The agreements we found for systemic antihistamines and for antiepileptic drugs were similar to those found among pregnant women reporting on their own use of drugs in an Italian study [28].

Perhaps more surprising is the large number of mothers who reported use of alimemazine even if no prescription was filled. Possible explanations could be that the drugs had been prescribed for someone else, purchased abroad or even been given to the child while in hospital, such use would not be captured in the prescription database. Alimemazine is frequently used as sleep inducer for children in hospitals [16].

A large proportion of prescriptions to the age group 0–2 years had missing identification numbers in the years 2006–2007 due to a problem with assignment of these numbers to new-borns (personal communication Olaug Sveinsgjerd Fenne). However, the high agreement for antiepiletics might indicate that this problem was not dominant in our selection.

We did not find any substantial systematic differences of sociodemographic variables on discrepancy between mother-reported information and data on dispensed medication. Family income, marital status, parity, mothers age, if the pregnancy was planned or not and mother's education were all similar between the groups. Non-working mothers had a higher percentage of drug only reported in the prescription record whereas families with college educated fathers had more use only reported in the cohort study. But considering that other similar variables like family income and maternal education level did not influence the outcome this might not be clinically relevant findings. Results from other studies indicate that the effect of sociodemographic variables on recall is conflicting. Some find no effect of sociodemographic variables [29, 30] whereas age and education level have been shown to affect recall, but in different directions [10, 28, 31–34].

The Norwegian Mother and Child cohort study included more than 100,000 pregnancies and continues to follow the children through life. Of the included women 87% completed the 6 months questionnaire and 77% completed the 18 months questionnaire [35]. Compared with the average pregnant woman the participants were more often living with a partner, less likely to smoke, more likely to be compliant to health advice, older and less likely to have more than two children, despite of this the bivariate associations between exposure and outcome variables for eight different conditions were not statistically different from those of the general population [12, 35]. In MoBa mothers are asked to remember drugs use up to 1 year prior. Large longitudinal studies like MoBa must make a trade-off between amount of information and the burden placed on the participants. The scope of this study was to evaluate existing sources of drug use information with the limitation they have.

This study is one of very few studies comparing mother-reported survey data with prescription data for hypnotic use among infants and toddlers. Reliable sources of information on medication use are important in clinical and epidemiological research. In the paediatric field there are still many unanswered questions about drug use and drug safety and evaluating data sources in this field is thus especially interesting. Like former studies performed on adults and adolescents this study on children shows that generally agreement between different sources of drug use is better for prescription drugs used chronic than drugs taken as needed [36, 37].

Conclusion

There was a moderate agreement between reported use and dispensed hypnotic drugs for infants and toddlers. There were, however, few differences between the two sources of data when considering sociodemographic variables. This might indicate that there are not systematic differences between the group who has been dispensed an hypnotic drug and those who report to have used it.

Abbreviations
MoBa: Norwegian mother and child cohort study; NorPD: Norwegian prescription database

Acknowledgements
Thank you to the group responsible for the project 2012/570 *Sleep medication in younger children* for allowing this paper to be a part of their project. Thank you to administrative staff and coworkers at both Norwegian Institute of Public Health and University of Oslo for supporting the authors, answering questions and helping with both technical and content related questions. Thank you to the Norwegian Prescription Database and the Norwegian Mother and Child Cohort Study for providing the data for this publication. The Norwegian Mother and Child Cohort Study are supported by the Norwegian Ministry of Health and Care Services and the Ministry of Education and Research, NIH/NIEHS (contract no N01-ES-75558), NIH/NINDS (grant no.1 UO1 NS 047537-01 and grant no.2 UO1 NS 047537-06A1). We are grateful to all the participating families in Norway who take part in this on--going cohort study.

Funding
This research did not receive any specific grant from funding agencies in the public, commercial, or not-for-profit sectors. Funded by internal sources from Norwegian Centre for Addiction Research only.

Authors' contributions
IH had the day-to-day responsibility of the article, did the analysis, wrote the first manuscript and coordinated the editing of the article. JGB contributed in designing the study and choosing analysis and participated in writing the manuscript. Reviewed and revised the manuscript. MH contributed in designing the study and in choosing analysis, reviewed and revised the manuscript and participated in writing the manuscript. LT contributed in designing the study and in choosing analysis, reviewed and revised the manuscript. TR contributed in designing the study and in choosing analysis, reviewed and revised the manuscript. EY contributed to the interpretation of data, revising the manuscript. HN contributed in discussing the analytical approach, reviewed and revised the manuscript. SS contributed in designing the study and participated in analysing and choosing, statistics. Reviewed and revised the manuscript. She approved the final draft before submitting. All authors read and approved the final manuscript.

Competing interests
The authors declare that they have no competing interests.

Author details
[1]Norwegian Centre of Addiction Research (SERAF), University of Oslo, Oslo, Norway. [2]Norwegian National Advisory Unit on Concurrent Substance Abuse and Mental Health Disorders, Ottestad, Norway. [3]Domain of Mental and Physical health, Norwegian Institute of Public Health, Oslo, Norway. [4]Institute of Clinical Medicine, University of Oslo, Oslo, Norway. [5]PharmacoEpidemiology and Drug Safety Research Group, School of Pharmacy, University of Oslo, Oslo, Norway. [6]Section of Health, Developmental and Personality Psychology, Department of Psychology, University of Oslo, Oslo, Norway.

References
1. Hartz I, Furu K, Bratlid T, Handal M, Skurtveit S. Hypnotic drug use among 0-17 year olds during 2004-2011: a nationwide prescription database study. Scand J Public Health. 2012;40(8):704–11.
2. Stojanovski SD, Rasu RS, Balkrishnan R, Nahata MC. Trends in medication prescribing for pediatric sleep difficulties in US outpatient settings. Sleep. 2007;30(8):1013–7.
3. Heussler H, Chan P, Price AM, Waters K, Davey MJ, Hiscock H. Pharmacological and non-pharmacological management of sleep disturbance in children: an Australian paediatric research network survey. Sleep Med. 2013;14(2):189–94.
4. Owens JA, Rosen CL, Mindell JA. Medication use in the treatment of pediatric insomnia: results of a survey of community-based pediatricians. Pediatrics. 2003;111(5 Pt 1):e628–35.
5. Sorensen E. Sleep disorders in children and adolescents. Tidsskr Nor Laegeforen. 2009;129(19):2000–3.
6. Holdo I, Handal M, Skurtveit S, Bramness JG. Association between prescribing hypnotics for parents and children in Norway. Arch Dis Child. 2013;98(9):732–6.
7. Slordal L, Bramness JG. Is alimemazine a suitable sleeping agent for children? Tidsskr Nor Laegeforen. 2008;128(19):2194–6.
8. Sanz EJ. Drug prescribing for children in general practice. Acta Paediatr. 1998;87(5):489–90.
9. Lissauer T, Clayden G. Illustrated textbook of paediatrics, vol. 2nd ed. Edinburgh: Mosby; 2001.
10. West SL, Savitz DA, Koch G, Strom BL, Guess HA, Hartzema A. Recall accuracy for prescription medications: self-report compared with database information. Am J Epidemiol. 1995;142(10):1103–12.
11. Furu K, Karlstad O, Skurtveit S, Haberg SE, Nafstad P, London SJ, Nystad W. High validity of mother-reported use of antiasthmatics among children: a comparison with a population-based prescription database. J Clin Epidemiol. 2011;64(8):878–84.
12. Magnus P, Irgens LM, Haug K, Nystad W, Skjaerven R, Stoltenberg C. Cohort profile: the Norwegian mother and child cohort study (MoBa). Int J Epidemiol. 2006;35(5):1146–50.
13. Magnus P, Birke C, Vejrup K, Haugan A, Alsaker E, Daltveit AK, Handal M, Haugen M, Hoiseth G, Knudsen GP, et al. Cohort profile update: the Norwegian mother and child cohort study (MoBa). Int J Epidemiol. 2016; 45(2):382–8.
14. Questionnaires from MoBa [https://www.fhi.no/en/studies/moba/for-forskere-artikler/questionnaires-from-moba/]. Accessed 13 June 2016.
15. Irgens LM. The medical birth registry of Norway. Epidemiological research and surveillance throughout 30 years. Acta Obstet Gynecol Scand. 2000;79(6):435–9.
16. Furu K. Establishment of the nationwide Norwegian prescription database (NorPD) - new opportunities for research in pharmacoepidemiology in Norway. Nor Epidemiol. 2008;18(2):129–36.
17. Rønning M, Berg C, Furu K, Litleskare I, Sakshaug S, Selmer R, Skurtveit S, Strøm H. Reseptregisteret 2005-2009. Tema: Vanedannende legemidler, Folkehelseinstituttet. Statistikk 2010. ISBN: 978-82-8082-409-7, ISBN (elektronisk): 978-82-8082-408-0, ISSN: 1890-9647.
18. Generell veileder i pediatri [http://www.helsebiblioteket.no/retningslinjer/pediatri/forside]. Accessed 01 Aug 2015.
19. Fleiss JL. Statistical methods for rates and proportions. 2nd ed. New York: Wiley; 1981.
20. Sabaté E. Adherence to long-term therapies : evidence for action. Geneva: World Health Organization; 2003.
21. Bulloch AG, Patten SB. Non-adherence with psychotropic medications in the general population. Soc Psychiatry Psychiatr Epidemiol. 2010;45(1):47–56.
22. West SL, Ritchey ME, Poole C. Validity of Pharmacoepidemiologic drug and diagnosis data. In: Pharmacoepidemiology. Oxford: Wiley-Blackwell; 2012. p. 757–94.
23. Stephansson O, Granath F, Svensson T, Haglund B, Ekbom A, Kieler H. Drug use during pregnancy in Sweden - assessed by the prescribed drug register and the medical birth register. Clin Epidemiol. 2011;3:43–50.
24. Nielsen MW, Sondergaard B, Kjoller M, Hansen EH. Agreement between self-reported data on medicine use and prescription records vary according to method of analysis and therapeutic group. J Clin Epidemiol. 2008;61(9):919–24.

25. Monster TB, Janssen WM, de Jong PE, de Jong-van den Berg LT. Pharmacy data in epidemiological studies: an easy to obtain and reliable tool. Pharmacoepidemiol Drug Saf. 2002;11(5):379–84.
26. Mitchell AA, Cottler LB, Shapiro S. Effect of questionnaire design on recall of drug exposure in pregnancy. Am J Epidemiol. 1986;123(4):670–6.
27. Skurtveit S, Selmer R, Tverdal A, Furu K. The validity of self-reported prescription medication use among adolescents varied by therapeutic class. J Clin Epidemiol. 2008;61(7):714–7.
28. Pisa FE, Casetta A, Clagnan E, Michelesio E, Vecchi Brumatti L, Barbone F. Medication use during pregnancy, gestational age and date of delivery: agreement between maternal self-reports and health database information in a cohort. BMC Pregnancy Childbirth. 2015;15:310.
29. Grimaldi-Bensouda L, Rossignol M, Aubrun E, El Kerri N, Benichou J, Abenhaim L. Agreement between patients' self-report and physicians' prescriptions on cardiovascular drug exposure: the PGRx database experience. Pharmacoepidemiol Drug Saf. 2010;19(6):591–5.
30. Sarangarm P, Young B, Rayburn W, Jaiswal P, Dodd M, Phelan S, Bakhireva L. Agreement between self-report and prescription data in medical records for pregnant women. Birth Defects Res A Clin Mol Teratol. 2012;94(3):153–61.
31. West SL, Savitz DA, Koch G, Sheff KL, Strom BL, Guess HA, Hartzema AG. Demographics, health behaviors, and past drug use as predictors of recall accuracy for previous prescription medication use. J Clin Epidemiol. 1997;50(8):975–80.
32. Stolley PD, Tonascia JA, Sartwell PE, Tockman MS, Tonascia S, Rutledge A, Schinnar R. Agreement rates between oral contraceptive users and prescribers in relation to drug use histories. Am J Epidemiol. 1978;107(3):226–35.
33. Rockenbauer M, Olsen J, Czeizel AE, Pedersen L, Sorensen HT. Recall bias in a case-control surveillance system on the use of medicine during pregnancy. Epidemiology. 2001;12(4):461–6.
34. Radin RG, Mitchell AA, Werler MM. Predictors of recall certainty of dates of analgesic medication use in pregnancy. Pharmacoepidemiol Drug Saf. 2013;22(1):25–32.
35. Nilsen RM, Vollset SE, Gjessing HK, Skjaerven R, Melve KK, Schreuder P, Alsaker ER, Haug K, Daltveit AK, Magnus P. Self-selection and bias in a large prospective pregnancy cohort in Norway. Paediatr Perinat Epidemiol. 2009;23(6):597–608.
36. Skurtveit S, Selmer R, Odsbu I, Handal M. Self-reported data on medicine use in the Norwegian mother and child cohort study compared to data from the Norwegian prescription database. Nor Epidemiol. 2014;24(1–2): 209–16.
37. Furu KSS, Rosvold EO. Drug use questions in Norwegian health surveys – response rate and agreement between specific and open-ended questions. Nor Epidemiol. 2003;13(1):147–54.

Evaluating treatment outcomes and durations among cases of smear-positive pulmonary tuberculosis in Yemen

Ammar Ali Saleh Jaber[1,2*], Amer Hayat Khan[1*] and Syed Azhar Syed Sulaiman[1]

Abstract

Background: Evaluating outcomes after tuberculosis (TB) treatment can help identify the primary reasons for treatment success or failure. However, Yemen has a treatment success rate that remains below the World Health Organization's target. This study aimed to identify factors that were associated with unsuccessful treatment and prolonged treatment (>1 year).

Method: Newly diagnosed cases of smear-positive pulmonary TB were prospectively followed at two centers (Taiz and Alhodidah, Yemen) between April 2014 and March 2015. Standardized forms were used to obtain information from the patients regarding their socio-demographic and clinical characteristics, treatment duration, and TB-related information. Multivariate logistic regression analyses were performed to identify factors that were associated with unsuccessful treatment and prolonged treatment (>1 year).

Results: The study included data from 273 cases of newly diagnosed TB, with treatment being successful in 227 cases (83.1%) and unsuccessful in 46 cases (16.9%). Among the 46 patients with unsuccessful treatment, 29 patients (10.6%) stopped treatment, 6 patients (2.2%) transferred to another facility, 6 patients (2.2%) experienced treatment failure, and 5 patients (1.8%) died. The multivariate logistic regression analyses revealed that unsuccessful treatment was associated with female sex, illiterate status, and the presence of comorbidities. Prolonged treatment durations were associated with living in a rural area, smoking, chewing khat, a cough that lasted for >3 weeks at the beginning of treatment, and bilateral cavities during radiography.

Conclusion: These results confirm that the treatment success rate in Yemen is lower than the World Health Organization's target for smear-positive pulmonary tuberculosis. Targeting the risk factors that we identified may help improve treatment outcomes. Furthermore, it may not be prudent to re-treat patients using first-line TB drugs after an initial treatment failure.

Keywords: Khat, Yemen, Tuberculosis, Comorbidities, United Nations Children's emergency fund (UNESCO), Treatment duration, Treatment success

* Correspondence: amarali20142015@gmail.com; dramer2006@gmail.com; dramer@usm.my
[1]School of Pharmaceutical Sciences, Universiti Sains Malaysia, Penang, Malaysia
Full list of author information is available at the end of the article

Background

The World Health Organization (WHO) estimates that >30% of the global population has latent or active tuberculosis (TB), and approximately 8 million new cases are detected every year [1]. In addition, TB is considered a deadly infection that causes 1.5 million deaths per year worldwide [2–4]. Furthermore, studies from the pre-chemotherapy era had revealed that approximately 70% of people with sputum smear-positive pulmonary TB died within 10 years. Thus, evaluating treatment outcomes among patients with newly diagnosed smear-positive TB can help determine the success of national TB control programs (NTCPs) [2]. Furthermore, NTCP data can be used to identify treatment weaknesses and related risk factors, which can be targeted to improve the programs' overall performance [5, 6].

Yemen has a relatively low treatment success rate, compared to the WHO's target of 90% [4]. In addition, TB is the fourth leading cause of death in Yemen and is considered a major priority by the Ministry of Health [5]. Thus, prospective evaluation of treatment outcomes can be used to identify risk factors that are associated with TB treatment outcomes and predictors of TB treatment success [6]. Furthermore, the WHO recommends analyzing smear-positive and smear-negative pulmonary and extrapulmonary TB as separate cohorts, and no studies have evaluated the risk factors for unsuccessful treatment of newly diagnosed smear-positive TB in Yemen. Moreover, treatment duration is an important consideration, as a duration of >6 months can significantly affect the quality of life and clinical outcomes of patients with TB [7]. Therefore, the present study evaluated newly diagnosed cases of smear-positive TB at two centers in Yemen, and evaluated factors for associations with unsuccessful treatment outcomes and prolonged treatment durations.

Methods

Study setting

This prospective follow-up study was performed at two major TB centers that are located in the cities of Taiz and Alhodidah in Yemen. These centers have central laboratories for diagnosing TB (i.e., they perform sputum testing and isolation cultures), are used as both research and surveillance centers [5], and employ >60 health workers, including physicians, laboratory technicians, officers, and pharmacists.

All patients with confirmed smear-positive pulmonary TB are advised to take anti-TB drugs daily during the intensive phase of treatment and weekly during the continued phase [6]. These treatments are administered as oral tablets that contain isoniazid, rifampicin, pyrazinamide, and ethambutol, with doses that are determined based on the patient's body weight. The intensive phase involves 2 months of treatment using isoniazid, rifampicin, pyrazinamide, and ethambutol, while the continued phase involves 4 months of treatment using only isoniazid and rifampicin [5]. Patients undergo monitoring and sputum smear testing at the end of the intensive phase, after 5 months, and during the last week of their treatment. If patients have a negative smear result at the end of the intensive phase, the treatment is continued as planned until the end of the program. If patients have a positive smear result, the treatment is extended for 1 month and the smear test is repeated at the end of the third month. If a negative smear result is subsequently observed at the end of the third month, the treatment is continued as planned. If positive results are observed after 3 months or 5 months, culturing and susceptibility testing is repeated. A positive smear result after 5 months is considered treatment failure.

In Yemen, the main tools for diagnosing smear-positive pulmonary TB are a direct sputum smear test using acid-fast bacillus microscopy, radiography, and the physician's clinical discretion. Sputum testing is also used to evaluate the outcomes of pulmonary TB. Other centers may perform additional testing for high-risk cases, such as testing for HIV, liver function, kidney function, and fasting blood glucose.

Study design and data collection

Between April 2014 and March 2015, 353 patients with newly diagnosed smear-positive pulmonary TB were registered in the two centers. However, we only included data from 273 patients who fulfilled the following criteria: age of ≥15 years, newly diagnosed smear-positive pulmonary TB, and willing to participate in the study [8]. Patients were excluded if they had unconfirmed TB, retreatment, multi-drug resistant TB, relapse, cancer, severe comorbid conditions (e.g., end-stage renal failure and advance heart disease), were pregnant, or were unwilling to participate. All patients were followed during their treatment until an outcome was recorded (treatment success, treatment failure, stopped treatment, transferred to another facility, or death).

A standardized data collection form was used to obtain the patients' demographic and clinical characteristics, such as age, sex, marital status, chewing khat, smoking, side effects of treatment, comorbidities, body mass index, residential area, level of education, laboratory results, clinical findings, and treatment outcomes. The participants also completed a questionnaire at their diagnosis regarding their TB-related knowledge and experiences. A medical chart and standardized form for all TB patients were created at their diagnosis and maintained until the end of their treatment period. A few sociodemographic factors were obtained directly from the patients, such as BCG test results, family history of TB, income, and level of education [3, 8].

The questionnaires contained 6 knowledge-related questions, 2 stigma-related questions, and 2 treatment-related questions. The stigma questions were scored on a scale of 0–2, with single-question scores of 1–2 being considered indicative of stigmatization. The knowledge questions were scored on a scale of 1–3, with good scores being defined as a total score of 4–6 and poor scores being defined as a total score of 1–3 [9]. The original questionnaire was sent to four international TB experts, as well as NTCP physicians in Yemen, and their comments were used to create the final version of the questionnaire. A pilot study was performed to evaluate the questionnaire's reliability and validity, and 30 patients with TB completed the questionnaires at the participating centers after providing informed consent. The patients were asked to evaluate the questionnaire's simplicity, and their comments were also considered when creating the final version. Reliability testing revealed that the questionnaire had a Cronbach's alpha value of 0.7. The final questionnaire was translated from Arabic into English for evaluation, and then back-translated into Arabic at Sana'a University (an English-language university). These translations were validated at the UNESCO office in Sana'a and by language experts from Sana'a University. In addition, approval for the study's protocol was obtained from the Ministry of Public Health in Yemen and the national tuberculosis control program.

Six trained pharmacists and nurses (three in each city) collected the data from the patients' TB cards and medical records. Treatment outcomes were reported based on the 6-month target from the WHO guidelines [10].

Definitions of terms

New case

Patients who had never received treatment for TB or who had received anti-TB drugs for <1 month.

Successfully treated

Patients who completed treatment or who were cured.

Stigma

An undesirable or discrediting attribute that an individual possesses, which reduces their social status.

Khat

An evergreen shrub of the Celastraceous family (*Catha edulis*) that grows in parts of the Middle East and eastern Africa. Its leaves are chewed for their stimulating effect [11].

Prolonged duration

A course of treatment that was >6 months.

Statistical analysis

All data were analyzed using PASW software (version 22; IBM Corp, Armonk, NY). Categorical variables were reported as number and percentage, and TB treatment outcomes were categorized as successful outcomes (cured or completed treatment) or unsuccessful outcomes (treatment failure, stopped treatment, transferred to another facility, and death) [3]. Univariate logistic regression analyses were used to evaluate the associations of the patients' characteristics with unsuccessful treatment outcomes and prolonged treatment durations. Multivariate logistic regression analyses were used to evaluate the characteristics' independent associations with these outcomes. The results were reported as odds ratios (OR), 95% confidence intervals (CIs), and standard error. Differences with a p-value of <0.05 were considered statistically significant.

Ethical considerations

All participants provided written informed consent before being included in this study. Ethical approval for this study was obtained from the National Committee of Health (Ministry of Health-Sana'a/Yemen) and the NTCP, which issued a collaboration letter to the two participating TB centers. All patient data were anonymized prior to the analyses.

Results

A total of 353 patients with smear-positive pulmonary TB were registered in the cities of Taiz and Alhodidah, although only 273 patients fulfilled the inclusion criteria and their demographic characteristics are shown in Table 1. Most patients were male (54.9%), 40.3% were 16–25 years old, 77.7% were of reproductive age (<45 years old), and 52.7% had a body mass index (BMI) of <18.5 kg/m^2. Although the study was performed in urban areas, approximately 31.5% of the patients came from rural areas and 67% were living under the poverty line (monthly income: <$50 dollars or <10,000 rial). Moreover, 55.3% of the patients were married and 58.6% were unemployed. Illiteracy was common (44.7%), and most illiterate patients were from Al Hudaydah (56.6%). Smoking was common (70%, with 71.8% of smokers smoking <20 cigarettes/day), and 64.5% of the patients chewed khat. We observed that 32.6% of the patients had a family history of TB, and that 18.3% underwent BCG vaccination. Comorbid conditions were observed in 161 patients.

Table 2 shows the patients' clinical characteristics. Approximately 47.3% of the patients had ≥5 clinical symptoms at the start of treatment, and 83.5% had a > 3-week history of coughing. Chest radiography revealed that unilateral lesions in 61.2% of the patients and single-lung cavities in 41.8% of the patients. The

Table 1 Socio-demographic characteristics of 273 smear-positive tuberculosis cases that were registered between April 2014 and March 2015

	City		Patients with tuberculosis n (%)
	Taiz, n (%)	Alhodidah, n (%)	
Sex			
Male	72 (48)	78 (52)	150 (54.9)
Female	73 (59.3)	50 (40.7)	123 (45.1)
Age (years)			
16–25	69 (62.7)	41 (37.3)	110 (40.3)
26–35	37 (52.9)	33 (47.1)	70 (25.6)
36–45	18 (56.3)	14 (43.8)	32 (11.7)
46–55	13 (40.6)	19 (59.4)	32 (11.7)
56–65	4 (22.2)	14 (43.8)	18 (6.6)
≥ 66	4 (36.4)	7 (63.3)	11 (4)
Weight (kg)			
≤ 30	2 (18.2)	9 (81.8)	11 (4)
31–40	43 (61.4)	27 (38.6)	70 (25.6)
41–50	69 (52.7)	62 (47.3)	131 (48)
51–60	19 (47.5)	21 (52.5)	40 (14.7)
61–70	8 (53.3)	7 (46.7)	15 (5.5)
> 70	4 (66.7)	2 (33.3)	6 (2.2)
BMI (kg/m^2)			
< 18.5	80 (55.6)	64 (44.4)	144 (52.7)
≥ 18.5	65 (50.4)	64 (49.6)	129 (47.3)
Area			
Urban	91 (48.7)	96 (51.3)	187 (68.5)
Rural	54 (62.8)	32 (37.2)	86 (31.5)
Level of education			
Illiterate	53 (43.4)	69 (56.6)	122 (44.7)
Primary	34 (54.8)	28 (45.2)	62 (22.7)
Pre-secondary	23 (82.1)	5 (17.9)	28 (10.3)
Secondary	25 (53.2)	22 (46.8)	47 (17.2)
University	10 (71.4)	4 (28.6)	14 (5.1)
Marital status			
Single	49 (45.8)	58 (54.2)	107 (39.2)
Divorced	2 (50)	2 (50)	4 (1.5)
Widow	6 (54.5)	5 (45.5)	11 (4)
Married	88 (58.3)	63 (41.7)	151 (55.3)
Employment status			
Employed	57 (50.4)	56 (49.6)	113 (41.4)
Unemployed	88 (55)	72 (45)	160 (58.6)
Smoking habit			
Yes	110 (57.6)	81 (42.4)	191 (70)
No	35 (42.7)	47 (57.3)	82 (30)
Chewing khat [a]			
Yes	90 (51.1)	86 (48.9)	176 (64.5)
No	55 (56.7)	42 (43.3)	97 (35)
Monthly income (rial[b])			
≤ 10,000	98 (53.6)	85 (46.4)	183 (67)
> 10,000	47 (52.2)	43 (47.8)	90 (33)
Stigma			
Yes	49 (41.2)	70 (58.8)	119 (43.6)
No	96 (62.3)	58 (54.7)	154 (56.4)
Knowledge			
Poor (1–3)	23 (59)	16 (41)	39 (14.3)
Good (4–6)	122 (52.1)	112 (47.9)	234 (85.7)
Family history of tuberculosis			
Yes	61 (68.5)	28 (31.5)	89 (32.6)
No	84 (45.7)	100 (54.3)	184 (67.4)
BCG vaccination			
Yes	42 (84)	8 (16)	50 (18.3)
No	103 (46.2)	120 (53.8)	223 (81.7)

BMI body mass index, *BCG* Bacillus Calmette–Guerin
[a]khat: a shrub that grows in parts of East Africa and Yemen, [b] rial: one dollar is approximately equivalent to 215 rial

outcomes were cure for 186 patients (68.1%), completed treatment for 41 patients (15%), treatment failure for 6 patients (2.2%), stopped treatment for 6 patients (2.2%), transfer to another facility for 29 patients (10.6%), and death for 5 patients (1.8%) (Table 3).

Risk factors associated with unsuccessful treatment outcomes

The results of the univariate analyses revealed that female sex, illiterate status, unemployment, smoking, an income of <10,000 rials/month, and comorbidities were associated with unsuccessful treatment outcomes. The significant univariate factors were entered into the multivariate analyses, which revealed that female sex, illiterate status, and comorbidities were independently associated with unsuccessful treatment outcomes (Table 4).

Risk factors associated with prolonged treatment duration

A total of 200 patients had an intensive phase that lasted for >2 months and 78 patients had a continued phase that lasted for >4 months. Among the 273 patients, 266 patients completed the intensive phase and 227 patients completed the continued phase (Table 5).

The univariate risk factors for prolonged treatment duration were entered into the multivariate analyses. These analyses revealed that prolonged treatment duration was independently associated with living in a rural area (adjusted odds ratio [AOR]: 2.358, 95% CI: 0.658–4.00), smoking (AOR: 0.054, 95% CI: 0.987–4.112),

Table 2 Clinical characteristics of the 273 patients with smear-positive tuberculosis

	City		Patients with tuberculosis, n (%)
	Taiz, n (%)	Alhodidah, n (%)	
Number of clinical symptoms			
≤ 2	29 (53.7)	25 (46.3)	54 (19.8)
3–4	50 (55.6)	40 (44.4)	90 (33)
≥ 5	66 (51.2)	63 (48.8)	129 (47.3)
Cough history			
< 3 weeks	37 (82.2)	8 (17.8)	45 (16.2)
≥ 3 weeks	108 (47.4)	120 (52.6)	228 (83.5)
Radiography lesions			
Unilateral	92 (55.1)	75 (44.9)	167 (61.2)
Bilateral	52 (53.1)	46 (46.9)	98 (35.9)
No test performed	1 (12.5)	7 (87.5)	8 (2.9)
Lung cavitation			
No cavities	42 (72.4)	16 (27.6)	58 (21.2)
One	57 (50)	57 (50)	114 (41.8)
Two	34 (48.6)	36 (51.4)	70 (25.6)
Three or more	11 (47.8)	12 (52.2)	23 (8.4)
No test performed	1 (12.5)	7 (87.5)	8 (2.9)
Comorbidity			
Yes	19 (43.2)	25 (56.8)	44 (16.1)
No	126 (55)	103 (45)	229 (83.9)

chewing khat (AOR: 2.615, 95% CI: 1.201–5.691), having a cough for >3 weeks at the start of treatment (AOR: 2.672, 95% CI: 1.053–6.782), and bilateral lesions during radiography (AOR: 2.134, 95% CI: 1.147–3.972) (Table 6).

Discussion

Our study obtained the risk factors associated with unsuccessful outcome and prolongs treatment duration for all smear positive tuberculosis patients. The present study had a relatively low inclusion rate (77% of potentially eligible individuals), which is likely related to several factors. First, approximately 6% of the individuals were excluded because they did not fulfill the inclusion criteria, and 17% of the individuals refused to participate despite being otherwise eligible. A similar WHO study in Yemen has also revealed unwillingness to participate in research among patients with TB [9]. Furthermore, the present study revealed a treatment success rate of 83%, and the latest WHO report has also detailed success rates of <85% among cases of smear-positive pulmonary TB [1]. Other developing countries also have success rates that are below the WHO target, such as India, Malaysia, Ethiopia, Pakistan, and Nigeria [12–17]. The low success rate in the present study may be related to the proportion of patients who did not complete treatment (10.6%), as most patients who experienced unsuccessful treatment outcomes were from poor areas and had an income of <10,000 rial/month, which could interfere with their ability to complete treatment. For example, a South African study revealed that difficulties in travelling from villages to cities could significantly affect the ability of patients with TB to complete their treatment [18]. Another study revealed that 29% of patients with TB only receive intermittent treatment doses from clinical centers [19]. In addition, health services are difficult to access in rural areas, and 31.5% of the participants were from rural areas and would have encountered difficulty in travelling to urban TB centers for treatment. A WHO study in Yemen [20] revealed that only 30–32% of patients with TB have access to nearby health services, and >50% of patients must travel for >1 h to the nearest TB center. Moreover, failure to complete treatment could be related to low satisfaction with the provided healthcare, which is commonly observed among patients during TB treatment [8]. Therefore, improving health services in rural areas, and decreasing the travel-related burden borne by patients with TB, may help reduce the rate of patients who fail to complete treatment.

Table 3 Treatment outcomes for patients with prolonged tuberculosis based on the WHO/IUALTLD criteria

Treatment outcome	Patients, n (%)	Groups, n (%)
Successful		
Cure	186 (68.1)	227 (83.1)
Completed treatment	41 (15.0)	
Unsuccessful		
Treatment failure	6 (2.2)	46 (16.9)
Died	5 (1.8)	
Stopped treatment	29 (10.6)	
Transferred to another facility	6 (2.2)	
Total	273 (100)	273 (100)

The present study revealed a treatment failure rate of 2.2%, although the latest WHO report revealed zero cases of treatment failure in Yemen [1]. Similar studies have revealed failure rates of 2.9% and 5% in Ethiopia and Nigeria, respectively [21, 22], although a different study revealed that no patients were lost to follow-up during TB treatment [12]. In this context, patients with smear-positive pulmonary TB are defined as experiencing treatment failure if a positive smear result is detected after 2 months or 5 months of treatment [5]. Similar studies in Hamburg and south India have revealed treatment failure rates of 2.3% and 2%, respectively [13, 23], while higher values have been reported in Russia and Turkey (8%) [24, 25] and lower values have

Table 4 Independent risk factors for unsuccessful treatment outcomes

		Treatment outcome n (%)	Univariate OR (95% CI)	Multivariate AOR (95% CI)	
		Successful	Unsuccessful		
Sex	Male	114 (76)	36 (24)	Ref	
	Female	113 (91.9)	10 (8.1)	0.470 (0.281–0.787)	0.248 (0.239–0.874)
Age, years	≤ 45	177 (83.5)	35 (16.5)	Ref	
	>45	50 (82)	11 (18)	1.210 (0.678–2.161)	
Area	Urban	152 (81.3)	35 (18.7)	Ref	
	Rural	75 (87.2)	11 (12.8)	1.054 (0.630–1.763)	
Education level	Literate	127 (82.5)	27 (17.5)	Ref	
	Illiterate	100 (84)	19 (16)	2.155 (1.22–3.801)	2.294 (1.272–4.137)
Occupation	Employed	90 (79.6)	23 (20.4)	Ref	
	Unemployed	137 (85.6)	23 (14.4)	1.591 (0.982–2.575)	0.980 (0.379–2.573)
BCG vaccination	Yes	46 (92)	4 (8)	Ref	
	No	181 (81.2)	42 (18.8)	1.651 (0.849–3.211)	
Marital status	Married	128 (84.8)	23 (15.2)	Ref	
	Unmarried	99 (81.1)	23 (18.9)	0.822 (0.506–1.334)	
Smoking habit	No	164 (85.9)	27 (14.1)	Ref	
	Yes	63 (76.8)	19 (23.2)	1.570 (0.943–2.613)	1.474 (0.867–2.578)
Chewing khat [a]	No	84 (86.6)	13 (13.4)	Ref	
	Yes	143 (81.3)	33 (18.8)	1.397 (0.840–2.322)	
Income (rial[b])	>10,000	73 (81.1)	17 (18.9)	Ref	
	≤10,000	154 (84.2)	29 (15.8)	0.651 (0.397–1.068)	
Stigma	No	127 (82.5)	27 (17.5)	Ref	
	Yes	100 (84)	19 (16)	0.683 (0.413–1.131)	
Knowledge	Good (4–6)	193 (82.5)	41 (17.5)	Ref	
	Poor (1–3)	34 (87.2)	5 (12.8)	0.831 (0.401–1.725)	
BMI, kg/m^2	<18.5	120 (83.3)	24 (16.7)	Ref	
	≥18.5	107 (82.9)	22 (17.1)	1.043 (0.646–1.685)	
Comorbid	No	197 (86)	32 (14)	Ref	
	Yes	30 (68.2)	14 (31.8)	1.730 (0.981–3.044)	1.995 (1.108–3.590)
Family history of tuberculosis	No	150 (81.5)	34 (18.5)	Ref	
	Yes	77 (86.5)	12 (13.5)	0.890 (0.525–1.509)	

Ref reference group, *BMI* body mass index, *BCG* Bacillus Calmette–Guerin, *AOR* adjusted odds ratio, *CI* confidence interval
[a]khat: a shrub that grows in parts of East Africa and Yemen, [b] rial: one dollar is approximately equivalent to 215 rial

been reported in Ethiopia (0.4%) and Switzerland (0.8%) [26, 27]. Interestingly, we observed that patients who experienced treatment failure had been re-treated using the same first-line anti-TB drugs, which could worsen their health and outcomes, as well as lead to drug resistance [2]. Moreover, we observed that approximately 2.2% of the participants were transferred to other TB centers, and these individuals were generally from rural

Table 5 Treatment durations for cases of smear-positive pulmonary tuberculosis

Duration of treatment	Patients, n (%)
End of the intensive phase	
≤ 2 months	66 (24.2)
> 2 months	200 (73.2)
Total	266 (100)
End of the continuation phase	
≤ 4 months	149 (56)
> 4 months	78 (29.3)
Total	227 (100)

areas. Thus, the economic costs (e.g., transportation, time off work) may have led patients to seek treatment closer to their homes, rather than in urban centers [17]. A recent study in Yemen revealed that 47% of patients who received treatment for TB in Sana'a were actually from rural areas [17], and similar transfer rates have been observed in Nigeria (3%) and Russia (1%) [24, 28]. A lower transfer rate has been reported in Taiwan (0.2%) [24].

The present study revealed a relatively low mortality rate (1.8%), although it is possible that this rate is underestimated based on patients who were lost to follow-up. For example, a European systematic review has indicated that proper follow-up of patients who fail to complete treatment may reveal a larger proportion of patients who have died despite receiving treatment for TB [25]. The present study also revealed a cure rate of approximately 68%, based on patients who completed treatment and had at least two negative smear results. Nevertheless, it may be difficult for the patient to produce sputum after treatment [3], and it is possible that our cure rate was overestimated, as the participating centers did not have access to advanced sputum collection methods (e.g., an ultrasonic nebulizer, gastric aspiration, or bronchoalveolar lavage) [6, 29].

Risk factors associated with unsuccessful treatment outcomes

The multiple logistic regression analyses revealed that unsuccessful treatment outcomes were independently associated with male sex, illiterate status, and comorbidities. Illiteracy was associated with a 2.3-fold higher risk of unsuccessful treatment, and approximately 41.2% of the participants were considered illiterate. A national report regarding education in Yemen also revealed that approximately 45% of the population is illiterate, and that most illiterate individuals are women [27]. Another study of adults in Yemen (2008–2012) revealed that the literacy rate was 65% [30], and those findings are generally in agreement with our findings. Illiteracy may be an important risk factor for unsuccessful treatment, as individuals could be less aware of TB and its routes of transmission [28]. For example, a prospective study in Yemen revealed that illiterate individuals had a 3-fold higher risk of developing TB, compared to literate individuals [31]. Other studies in India [32] and Rajasthan [28] have revealed large proportions of individuals who were illiterate and who had an elevated risk of poor treatment outcomes.

Comorbidities were associated with a 1.9-fold higher risk of unsuccessful treatment, and this result highlights the need to identify, monitor, and address comorbidities among patients who are receiving TB treatment [33]. For example, comorbidities can affect treatment outcomes by influencing the patient's weight [34] and increasing the risk of death. Our results indicate that 18.9% of the participants had comorbidities, and it is possible that routine health checkups might have identified further comorbidities. Thus, we recommend frequent monitoring for comorbid conditions.

Male sex was also a risk factor for unsuccessful treatment outcome, and similar results were observed in studies that were performed in Malaysia, Finland, Nigeria, Kenya, and Saudi Arabia [3, 29, 35–37]. Men in Yemen frequently have high-risk behaviors, such as chewing khat and smoking, which may also affect their treatment outcomes [3, 8].

Risk factors associated with prolonged treatment duration

Prolonged treatment duration was associated with living in a rural area, smoking, chewing khat, bilateral cavities during radiography, and a cough that lasted for >3 weeks at the start of treatment. It is important to identify risk factors for prolonged treatment duration, as it can lead to drug resistance and multidrug-resistant TB [38]. In the present study, bilateral cavities were associated with a 2.13-fold higher risk of prolonged treatment (vs. unilateral cavities), and previous studies have also revealed an association between lung cavities and prolonged treatment duration, based on the increased sputum conversion rate. Patients with TB who smoke have increased global rates of morbidity and mortality [39], as well as a 70% greater risk of unsuccessful treatment outcomes, compared to nonsmokers [39]. Furthermore, previous studies have revealed that prolonged treatment duration is associated with smoking habits [40], which may be related to the lower likelihood of smear conversion during the treatment [41]. Moreover, smoking destroys the lungs and weakens the immune system, which can lead to a prolonged treatment duration [41], as well as an increased risk of developing pulmonary TB.

The present study also revealed that chewing khat was associated with prolonged treatment duration (AOR:

Table 6 Independent risk factors for prolonged treatment duration

		Treatment duration		Univariate OR (95% CI)	Multivariate AOR (95% CI)
		≤6 months	>6 months		
Sex	Male	34 (29.8)	80 (70.2)	Ref	
	Female	23 (20.4)	90 (79.6)	0.539 (0.309–0.940)	1.623 (0.658–4.002)
Age, years	≤ 45	44 (24.9)	133 (75.1)	Ref	
	>45	13 (26)	37 (74)	0.873 (0.447–1.705)	
Area	Urban	38 (25)	114 (75)	Ref	
	Rural	19 (25.3)	56 (74.7)	2.636 (1.48–4.695)	2.358 (1.250–4.433)
Education level	Literate	34 (26.8)	93 (93.2)	Ref	
	Illiterate	23 (23)	77 (77)	0.972 (0.560–1.688)	
Occupation	Employed	25 (27.8)	65 (72.2)	Ref	
	Unemployed	32 (23.4)	105 (76.6)	0.442 (0.252–0.775)	0.633 (0.176–2.282)
BCG	Yes	12 (26.1)	34 (73.9)	Ref	
	No	45 (24.9)	136 (75.1)	1.103 (0.554–2.196)	
Marital status	Married	28 (21.9)	100 (78.1)	Ref	
	Unmarried	29 (29.3)	70 (70.7)	0.786 (0.450–1.370)	
Smoking habit	No	44 (26.8)	120 (73.2)	Ref	
	Yes	13 (20.6)	50 (79.4)	2.648 (1.453–4.82)	2.015 (0.987–4.114)
Chewing khat [a]	No	20 (23.8)	64 (76.2)	Ref	
	Yes	37 (25.9)	106 (74.1)	3.253 (1.720–6.152)	2.615 (1.201–5.691)
Monthly income (rial[b])	>10,000	19 (26)	54 (74)	Ref	
	≤10,000	38 (24.7)	116 (75.3)	0.421 (0.236–0.750)	0.744 (0.231–2.404)
Knowledge	Good	51 (26.4)	142 (73.6)	Ref	
	Poor	6 (17.6)	28 (82.4)	1.411 (0.669–2.975)	
Stigma	No	31 (24.4)	96 (75.6)	Ref	
	Yes	26 (26)	74 (74)	1.232 (0.710–2.136)	
Comorbidities	No	50 (25.4)	147 (74.6)	Ref	
	Yes	7 (23.2)	23 (76.7)	1.323 (0.602–2.910)	
Family history of TB	No	42 (28)	108 (72)	Ref	
	Yes	15 (19.5)	62 (80.5)	0.297 (0.667–1.214)	
Number of TB symptoms	3–4	3 (40)	7 (70)	Ref	
	≥5	54 (24.9)	163 (75.1)	2.156 (0.447–10.41)	
History of cough	< 3 weeks	12 (30)	28 (70)	Ref	
	≥3 weeks	45 (24.1)	142 (75.9)	2.393	2.672

Table 6 Independent risk factors for prolonged treatment duration *(Continued)*

		Treatment duration		Univariate OR (95% CI)	Multivariate AOR (95% CI)
		≤6 months	>6 months		
				(1.04–5.485)	(1.053–6.782)
Radiography lesions	Unilateral	41 (28.5)	103 (71.5)	Ref	
	Bilateral	16 (19.3)	67 (80.7)	2.021 (1.149–3.553)	2.134 (1.147–3.971
Lung cavitation	No	0 (0)	50 (100)	Ref	
	Yes	57 (32.2)	120 (67.8)	1.652 (0.819–3.333)	
BMI, kg/m^2	<18.5	38 (31.7)	88 (82.2)	Ref	
	≥18.5	19 (17.8)	88 (82.2)	1.345 (0.775–2.337)	

Ref reference group, *BMI* body mass index, *BCG* Bacillus Calmette–Guerin, *AOR* adjusted odds ratio, *CI* confidence interval
[a]khat: a shrub that grows in parts of East Africa and Yemen, [b] rial: one dollar is approximately equivalent to 215 rial

2.7). This may be related to the amphetamine and cathinone in khat suppressing the immune system, which could increase the likelihood of TB and prolonged treatment [42, 43]. Further studies are needed to evaluate the effects of khat on the clinical outcomes of TB treatment.

The present study also revealed that living in a rural area was associated with prolonged treatment (AOR: 2.3), which may be related to the greater transportation costs and unavailability of TB treatment in rural areas [10]. It is also possible that living in a rural area may delay the diagnosis of TB [44], which could increase the risk of prolonged treatment. For example, 83% of our participants had a cough at the start of their treatment, and patients with a cough that lasted for >3 weeks had an increased risk of prolonged treatment. A previous study has also revealed that having a cough for >3 weeks was associated with prolonged treatment during the intensive phase of treatment [45].

Study limitations

The present study has two important limitations. First, we only evaluated cases of smear-positive pulmonary TB, and further studies are needed to explore the risk factors for all forms of TB. Second, we only evaluated centers in two cities, based on the WHO's recommendation to evaluate cohorts at the district, city, or state level [2], and further studies are needed to evaluate patients with TB in all cities of Yemen.

Conclusion

The present study revealed a treatment success rate in Yemen that was below the WHO's target. Failure to complete treatment may be responsible for the low success rate, and it would be prudent to address factors that affect patients' ability to complete their treatment. Moreover, we conclude that monitoring and addressing the risk factors that were associated with treatment outcomes and duration may help improve the likelihood of achieving favorable outcomes among cases of smear-positive pulmonary TB in Yemen.

Acknowledgements
We would like to thanks all health workers in Taiz and Alhoudidah centers for given us the chance to conduct the study. we also appreciate Univeristi Sains Malaysia for the chance to conduct the study. we also thanks Yemen Health Ministry and National Tuberculosis Control Program (NTCP) to approve our work and collaborate with us. Finally, we would like to thank our supervisors for their constructive comments throughout our overall research activities.

Funding
No fund was given to our study.

Authors' contributions
Prof Syed and Dr. Amer wrote the proposal and follow up the stages of data collection and writing. Ammar Ali participated in data collection and analyzed the data and drafted the paper. All authors read and approved the final manuscript.

Competing interests
The authors declare that they have no competing interests.

Author details
[1]School of Pharmaceutical Sciences, Universiti Sains Malaysia, Penang, Malaysia. [2]School of Pharmacy, Lebanese International University, Taiz, Yemen.

References

1. World Health Organization. WHO Global tuberculosis report 2015. 2015;1:1689–99.
2. World Health Organization. Treatment of tuberculosis guideline. 2010.
3. Atif M, Sulaiman SAS, Shafie AA, Ali I, Asif M, Babar Z-U-D. Treatment outcome of new smear positive pulmonary tuberculosis patients in Penang. Malaysia BMC Infect Dis. 2014;14:1–8. https://doi.org/10.1186/1471-2334-14-399.

4. World Health Organization. Global tuberculosis report 2016. 2016.
5. World Health Organization. Treatment of tuberculosis: guidelines. 2010.
6. National Tuberculosis Control Program. Republic of Yemen Ministry of Public Health and population; 2010. p. 1–56.
7. Liew SM, Khoo EM, Ho BK, Lee YK, Mimi O, Fazlina MY, et al. Tuberculosis in Malaysia : predictors of treatment outcomes in a national registry. Int J Tuberc Lung Dis. 2014;2015(19):1–12.
8. Jaber AAS. PLOS Medicine Evaluation of Health-Related Quality of Life among Tuberculosis Patients in Two Cities in Yemen. PLoS One. 2016;:1–19.
9. World Health Organization. Diagnostic and treatment delay in tuberculosis. World Heal Organ. 2006; WHO-EM/TDR/009/E.
10. Jaber AAS, Khan AH, Sulaiman SAS, Ahmad N, Anaam MS. Evaluation of health-related quality of life among tuberculosis patients in two cities in Yemen. PLoS One. 2016.
11. Anaam MS, Mohamed Ibrahim MI, Al Serouri AW, Aldobhani A. Factors affecting patients' compliance to anti-tuberculosis treatment in Yemen. J Pharm Heal Serv Res. 2013;4:115–22.
12. World Health Organization. Definitions and reporting framework for tuberculosis – 2013 revision. 2013. papers2://publication/uuid/E6143945-51F7-485A-8C89-FAB2C7DF4F43.
13. Lukandu OM, Costea DE, Dimba EA, Neppelberg E, Bredholt T, Gjertsen BT, et al. Khat induces G1-phase arrest and increased expression of stress-sensitive p53 and p16 proteins in normal human oral keratinocytes and fibroblasts. Eur J Oral Sci. 2008;116:23–30. https://doi.org/10.1111/j.1600-0722.2007.00508.x.
14. Woldeyohannes D, Sisay S, Mengistu B, Kassa H. Directly observed treatment short-course (DOTS) for treatment of new tuberculosis cases in Somali regional state, Eastern Ethiopia: ten years retrospective study. BMC Res Notes. 2015;8:357. https://doi.org/10.1186/s13104-015-1325-3.
15. Chennaveerappa PK, Siddharam SM, Halesha BR, Vittal BG, Jayashree N. Treatment outcome of tuberculosis patients registered at DOTS centre in a teaching hospital, South India. Int J Biol Med Res. 2011;2:487–9. https://doi.org/10.1016/j.ijid.2014.03.953.
16. Khan AH, Syed Sulaiman SA, Abdul Muttalif AR, Hassali MA, Ahmad N. Tuberculosis treatment outcomes in four states of Malaysia. Value Heal. 2012;15:A387–8. https://doi.org/10.1016/j.jval.2012.08.1084.
17. Da Costa AL, Keny SJ, Lawande D. Treatment outcome of pulmonary and extra pulmonary tuberculosis patients in TB and chest disease hospital DOT Centre , Goa , India. Int J Curr Microbiol Appl Sci. 2016;5:437–41.
18. Khan MA, Basit A, Ullah Z, Javaid A. Outcome of tuberculosis patients registered during 2007 in major teaching hospitals of Peshawar. JPMI - J Postgrad Med Inst. 2009;23:358–62.
19. Ukwaja KN, Oshi SN, Alobu I, Oshi DC. Profile and determinants of unsuccessful tuberculosis outcome in rural Nigeria: implications for tuberculosis control. World J Methodol. 2016;6:118. https://doi.org/10.5662/wjm.v6.i1.118.
20. Peltzer K, Louw JS. Prevalence and associated factors of tuberculosis treatment outcome among hazardous or harmful alcohol users in public primary health care in South Africa. Afr Health Sci. 2014;14:157–66.
21. Shargie EB, Lindtjørn B. Determinants of treatment adherence among smear-positive pulmonary tuberculosis patients in southern Ethiopia. PLoS Med. 2007;4:0280–7.
22. Tafess K, Mengistu B, Woldeyohannes D, Sisay S. Determining treatment outcome of smear-positive pulmonary tuberculosis cases in Afar Regional State, Ethiopia: A retrospective facility based study. Int J Mycobacteriology. 2016;:1–6. doi:https://doi.org/10.1016/j.ijmyco.2016.02.003.
23. Nabi Koul A, Ahmad Wagay H, Bashir Rather A, Nabi Dhobi G, Ahmad Bhat F, Rafiq BM. Demography and clinical outcome of pulmonary tuberculosis in Kashmir; 2 year prospective study. Egypt J Chest Dis Tuberc. 2016;65:455–60. https://doi.org/10.1016/j.ejcdt.2015.12.015.
24. Diel R, Niemann S. Outcome of tuberculosis treatment in Hamburg: a survey, 1997-2001. Int J Tuberc Lung Dis. 2003;7:124–31.
25. Kherosheva T, Thorpe LE, Kiryanova E, Rybka L, Gerasichev V, Shulgina M, et al. Encouraging outcomes in the first year of a TB control demonstration program: Orel oblast, Russia. Int J Tuberc Lung Dis. 2003;7:1045–51.
26. Babalik A, Kilicaslan Z, Kiziltas S, Gencer S, Ongen G. A retrospective case-control study, factors affecting treatment outcomes for pulmonary tuberculosis in İstanbul, Turkey. Balkan Med J. 2013;30:204–10. https://doi.org/10.5152/balkanmedj.2013.005.
27. Getahun B, Ameni G, Medhin G, Biadgilign S. Treatment outcome of tuberculosis patients under directly observed treatment in Addis Ababa, Ethiopia. Braz J Infect Dis. 2013;17:521–8. https://doi.org/10.1016/j.bjid.2012.12.010.
28. Kherad O, Herrmann FR, Zellweger J-P, Rochat T, Janssens J-P. Clinical presentation, demographics and outcome of tuberculosis (TB) in a low incidence area: a 4-year study in Geneva, Switzerland. BMC Infect Dis. 2009;9:217.
29. Anderson De Cuevas RM, Al-Sonboli N, Al-Aghbari N, Yassin MA, Cuevas LE, Theobald SJ. Barriers to completing TB diagnosis in Yemen: Services should respond to patients' needs. PLoS One 2014;9.
30. Sunday O. Treatment outcome of tuberculosis patients registered at DOTs centre in a tertiary care hospital. Int J Infect Dis. 2014;21:256. http://ovidsp.ovid.com/ovidweb.cgi?T=JS&CSC=Y&NEWS=N&PAGE=fulltext&D=emed12&AN=71634290
31. Yen YF, Yen MY, Shih HC, Deng CY. Risk factors for unfavorable outcome of pulmonary tuberculosis in adults in Taipei, Taiwan. Trans R Soc Trop Med Hyg. 2012;106:303–8. https://doi.org/10.1016/j.trstmh.2012.01.011.
32. van Hest N a. H, Kodmon C, Verver S, Erkens CGM, Straetemans M, Manissero D, et al. Tuberculosis treatment outcome monitoring in European Union countries: systematic review. Eur Respir J 2012;41:635–643.
33. Al-Aghbari N, Al-Sonboli N, M a Y, JBS C, Atef Z, Al-Eryani A, et al. Multiple sampling in one day to optimize smear microscopy in children with tuberculosis in Yemen. PLoS One. 2009;4:2–5.
34. Ministry of Education Y. Adult Education Programs in the Republic of Yemen for The Sixth International Conference on Adult Education. In: UNESCO. 2009. p. 1–30.
35. UNICEF. Statistics Yemen. 2010. http://www.unicef.org/infobycountry/yemen_statistics.html. Accessed 8 Mar 2016.
36. Yadav SP, Mathur ML, Dixit AK. Knowledge and attitude towards tuberculosis among sandstone quarry workers in desert parts of Rajasthan. Indian J Med Res 2006;3.
37. Shamiry AAA-, Al-haddad AM. Co-existing diseases of patients with pulmonary tuberculosis in Yemen. J Trop Nephro-Urology. 2011;10:46–57.
38. Kaur G, Goel NK, Kumar D, Janmeja a,K, Swami HM, Kalia M. Treatment outcomes of patients placed on treatment under directly observed therapy short-course (dots). Lung India. 2008;25:75–7.
39. World Health Organization. The global plan to stop TB 2011-2015. 2011.
40. Hoa NB, Lauritsen JM, Rieder HL. Changes in body weight and tuberculosis treatment outcome in Viet Nam. Int J Tuberc Lung Dis. 2013;17:61–6. https://doi.org/10.5588/ijtld.12.0369.
41. Vasankari T, Holmström P, Ollgren J, Liippo K, Kokki M, Ruutu P. Risk factors for poor tuberculosis treatment outcome in Finland: a cohort study. BMC Public Health. 2007;7:291. https://doi.org/10.1186/1471-2458-7-291.
42. Fatiregun AA, Ojo AS, Bamgboye AE. Treatment outcomes among pulmonary tuberculosis patients at treatment centers in Ibadan, Nigeria. Ann Afr Med. 2009;8:100–4. http://www.ncbi.nlm.nih.gov/pubmed/19805940
43. Muture BN, Keraka MN, Kimuu PK, Kabiru EW, Ombeka VO, Oguya F. Factors associated with default from treatment among tuberculosis patients in Nairobi province, Kenya: a case control study. BMC Public Health. 2011;11:696. https://doi.org/10.1186/1471-2458-11-696.
44. Abouzeid MS. Al Hakeem RF, Memish Z a. Mortality among tuberculosis patients in Saudi Arabia (2001-2010). Ann Saudi Med. 2013;33:247–52.
45. Hijazi M, Jentsch H, Al-Sanabani J, Tawfik M, Remmerbach TW. Clinical and cytological study of the oral mucosa of smoking and non-smoking qat chewers in Yemen. Clin Oral Investig 2015. doi:https://doi.org/10.1007/s00784-015-1569-2.

Exploring the extended role of the community pharmacist in improving blood pressure control among hypertensive patients in a developing setting

Afia Frimpomaa Asare Marfo* and Frances Thelma Owusu-Daaku

Abstract

Background: In most developing countries including Ghana, there is scant literature on the involvement of the community pharmacist in the care of patients with chronic conditions such as hypertension and blood pressure control. The objective of the study was to evaluate the effect of a pharmaceutical care model on blood pressure control and adherence among hypertensive patients.

Methods: This was a quasi experimental design and the primary outcome measure was a change in systolic and diastolic blood pressure. One hundred and eighty hypertensive patients were recruited for the study: 90 in the intervention group and 90 in the control group. The intervention, consisting of health education, adherence counselling and medicine use review; was offered monthly for six months.

Results: At baseline there was no significant difference in demographic and clinical characteristics between the intervention and control group. Pharmaceutical care issues identified among the intervention group during the 6 months period were non effectiveness of therapy ($n = 23$), experience of side effects ($n = 20$) and nonadherence to therapy ($n = 40$). The mean diastolic blood pressure difference between the intervention group and the control group was statistically significant ($p = 0.001$). The mean adherence difference between the two groups was also statistically significant at the end of the study. (p = 0.001).

Conclusions: The pharmaceutical care intervention offered by the pharmacist led to the resolution of some pharmaceutical care issues, improvement in diastolic blood pressure and adherence among hypertensive patients. Guidelines and polices to streamline these services are needed if they are to be made available in community pharmacies in developing countries.

Keywords: Hypertension, Pharmacist, Pharmaceutical care, Blood pressure, Pharmacy

Background

Hypertension is currently on the rise in most developing countries including Ghana [1]. The crude prevalence of hypertension in rural and urban Ghana ranges from 19.3% to 54.6% and it was among the first five commonest cause of outpatient morbidity in most regions in the country [2, 3]. The lack of awareness and inadequate treatment of hypertensive patients are factors contributing to the high burden of hypertension in Ghana [4]. The typical doctor's review period for a Ghanaian hypertensive patient is every three months and yet blood pressure control is not adequate and patients lack information about their medicines and life style modifications [5]. There is therefore the need for services that would improve blood pressure control and prevent complications among patients with hypertension.

Community pharmacies in Ghana are privately owned and licensed by the Pharmacy Council with a mandate to promote rational use of medicines [6]. According to the Health Professionals Regulatory Bodies Act, a pharmacist can provide medical care as first aid during an

* Correspondence: afamarfo@gmail.com; afamarfo.pharm@knust.edu.gh
Faculty of Pharmacy and Pharmaceutical Sciences, Kumasi, Ghana

accident and also provide treatment for illness of common occurrence when consultation with a medical practitioner or dentist is not reasonably practicable [6]. It has, however, been observed that community pharmacies in most low income settings are often underutilized and the standard of care and services tend to be suboptimal [7]. Currently, community pharmacists in Ghana do not normally follow up and monitor patients with chronic diseases as these often visit the pharmacies only for prescription refills.

Although studies on how the community pharmacist can assist hypertensive patients control their blood pressure have been conducted with largely positive outcomes in some developed countries such as England, United States of America and Canada, not much has been done in the developing setting [8–11]. Moreover the interventions studied and the number of times pharmaceutical care was offered to hypertensive patients by the community pharmacist varied within these studies and not all pharmaceutical care issues were reported. Duplicating similar services in Ghana would therefore require evaluating a pharmaceutical care intervention suitable for the Ghanaian community pharmacy. The information obtained would be essential for the purposes of policy initiation and planning with regard to the extended roles of community pharmacists in caring for patient with chronic diseases.

This study was carried out to evaluate the effect of a pharmaceutical care intervention on blood pressure control, adherence and adoption of healthy lifestyle practices among hypertensive patients. In addition we sought to determine the pharmaceutical care issues that are common among hypertensive patients and the level of satisfaction among hypertensive patients to whom the intervention was offered.

Method

Study design and setting

This non-randomised controlled study was conducted in five community pharmacies, in or near the Kumasi metropolis in the Ashanti region. The design involved the generation of two comparison groups because it was not feasible to randomise individuals into treatment and control groups due to lack of logistics. The intervention was offered in three community pharmacies (the intervention group), Charma situated at Aputugya, Kama at Bomso and Bandy at Adum. The control group comprised Marrita pharmacy, situated at Dompoase-Aprabo and Royal Avenue pharmacy at Manhyia. The major activities in these pharmacies included dispensing prescription and non-prescription drugs, treating illnesses of common occurrence, counselling and drug information dissemination.

Purposive sampling to select the five pharmacies was based on the following criteria. The pharmacist should be available during pharmacy opening hours, have at least one year experience in community pharmacy practice and should be easily available for training.

Description of the intervention

The intervention offered was based on the pharmaceutical care model proposed by the American College of Clinical Pharmacists [12]. This model consists of three principal components; identifying actual and potential medication related problems, resolving actual medication related problems and preventing potential medication related problems. Drug therapy issues were categorized into four groups. These are indication, effectiveness, safety and adherence. Based on the pharmaceutical care model, the intervention offered by the community pharmacist was monthly medicines use review, health education and adherence counselling.

Medicine use review

The objective of the review was to identify and resolve drug related problems, focusing on improper drug selection, sub therapeutic doses, over dosage, adverse drug reactions, nonadherence to therapy, drug interactions and medicines use with no indication. In resolving drug therapy problems a care plan was developed via the SOAPO model [Subjective data, Objective data, Analysis, Plan and Outcome]. The subjective data was any signs and symptoms reported by the patient. The main objective data considered was the blood pressure and body mass index measurements. Based on the objective and subjective data; and medication history, an assessment of the medication related problem was made. The plan mainly consisted of recommended therapy, goals of therapy; counselling and monitoring. Patients and other health workers were involved in these plans. Patients were informed about all the necessary actions in the care plan and recommendations for medication regimen change; and elevated blood pressure was communicated to a doctor. In hypertensive patients without diabetes the targeted blood pressure was less than or equal to 140/90. In diabetic hypertensive patients the targeted blood pressure level was less than 130/80.

Health education

A concordant approach was used in educating the patient; thus patients' views and suggestions was considered before conclusions were drawn. Patients were also educated on the common side effects of their antihypertensive medication, precautionary measures associated with taking their medicines, individualized healthy life style practices that would help in controlling their blood pressure and consequences of not adhering to their therapy. Life style practices discussed included physical activity, diet (in particular sodium reduction and a diet rich in fruits and vegetables and less fat), weight loss management, reducing alcohol intake and smoke cessation.

Adherence counselling

Two strategies were used in improving patient adherence. Dissemination of knowledge (making sure that the patient was aware of the name, dosage, side effects and purpose of their medicines) and simplifying dosage regimen.

Training

A two day taught and practical training programme was given to the three pharmacists in the intervention group. The topics covered included pathophysiology, prevalence, risk factors, causes, diagnosis, and complication of hypertension. Goals of therapy, pharmacological methods available for managing hypertension, factors to be considered when choosing an appropriate therapy, and medicines available for the management of hypertension. Development of pharmaceutical care plans (SOAPO model), description of the pharmacist led hypertension pharmaceutical care service and procedures and protocols used in the project were also taught. Pharmacists in the control group were taught only the study procedures in the recruitment of subjects, and measurement of blood pressure and body mass index.

Inclusion/exclusion criteria

Hypertensive patients diagnosed for at least six months with a review period of at least two months were included in the study. The only co-morbid condition included was diabetes. Other hypertensive patients with comorbid conditions such as heart failure, stroke, and ischaemic heart disease, renal and liver diseases were excluded from the study. Furthermore pregnant women, patients with no contact numbers and patients who would not be able to return to the pharmacy for a scheduled visit were excluded from the study.

Sample size & sampling

The formula proposed by Charan & Bisawa, for calculating sample for size interventional studies [13, 14] yielded a sample of 180 hypertensive patients. Purposive sampling was used to select the first 180 patients who were within the inclusion criteria. Ninety patients were recruited into the control group: 45 patients from each of the two pharmacies; and ninety patients into the intervention Group. (IG): 30 from each of the three community pharmacies.

Identification & recruitment

Eligible hypertensive patients were identified when they visited the pharmacy with a refill prescription that had a diagnosis of hypertension. The blood pressure was measured at the pharmacy with an automated Sphygmomanometer to ensure that about 50% of the total study sample in both the intervention and control group had blood pressure levels above 140/90. When recruited the purpose and design of the study were also explained to the patient by the pharmacist. Patients then appended their signature or thumb print to a consent form if they agreed to be part of the study.

Outcome measures

The following outcomes were assessed at baseline and at the end of the study in both groups. However outcome 7 and 9 were assessed in only the intervention group (Table 1).

Data collection

Data were collected at baseline and then after 6 months for the control group. In the intervention group, the pharmacist initially interacted with the patient and offered the pharmaceutical care services described above. Information documented at baseline for both groups were: demographic characteristics, medication history (current medicines for the management of hypertension and other Over The Counter drugs and alternative medicines), life style practices (smoking status, frequency of exercise, alcohol use, consumption of salt), awareness of the name, dosage, frequency, side effect and purpose of antihypertensive prescribed and awareness of healthy lifestyle modification for managing blood pressure. Other information documented were blood pressure, body mass index measurement and level of adherence to antihypertensive medication. Additional information documented for the intervention group were pharmaceutical care issues and solutions offered. Follow up dates for subsequent visits were agreed with the patients and SMS messages were sent to remind patients of these dates. If patients failed to show up, a call was made to ascertain why the appointment was missed and a new follow up date was agreed. Patients with drug therapy related problems that needed change in therapy were referred to their normal review clinic.

During the intervention group's monthly visits, the pharmacist had a 10–30 min face-to-face consultation with the patient. In the consultation the pharmacist measured the patients' blood pressure and BMI. Identified drug related problems were discussed with the patient and a concordant solution sought. After the sixth month the same information documented at baseline was determined in the two groups.

For the patient satisfaction survey, a semi structured questionnaire was used to conduct a face to face interview among the 75 hypertensive patients in the intervention group after the sixth month. The questionnaire captured data on patient satisfaction with the medication use review service, health education and adherence counselling. Questions on client's satisfaction with the overall services provided by the pharmacist and if pharmacist should be paid for offering the service were open ended questions. All other question where closed ended.

Pharmacists who offered the intervention were remunerated over the study period.

Data analysis

Descriptive statistics in SPSS Version 16 were used to analyse baseline demographic and clinical data. Patients who did not exercise or patients who exercised less than 30 min per day, in less than 3 days were coded as 'no exercise'. Participant who drank more than 2 drinks per day for men and more than 1 drink per day for women were considered as regular users of alcohol.

Adherence to antihypertensive medication was measured with the Morisky self-reported scale. A 'yes' answer attracted a score of Zero (0) and a 'no' answer a score of one. Patients who scored 8 were considered highly adherent, a score of 6- < 8 was classified as medium adherence and a score below 6 was classified as low adherence. The paired sample T test was used to compare means of end of study outcomes (SBP, DBP, adherence and BMI) within the IG and the CG. McNemar test was run to determine if there was any difference in the proportion of subjects who ate salty food, consumed alcohol and exercised pre and post intervention. The general linear model (repeated measures) analysis was run to compare the difference (SBP, DBP, adherence and BMI) between the two groups at baseline and after 6 months. Then the Wilks Lambda test was used to determine if there was any differences between the two groups. The Fishers exact test of association was employed to determine any association between the intervention offered and achievement of blood pressure goal. Cramer's V test was used to determine the strength of the association; values of 0–0.30 were considered weak, 0.31–0.70 moderate, and 0.71–1.0 strong. In the analysis of data, all p values less than 0.05 were deemed significant.

Results

One hundred and eighty hypertensive patients were recruited. Eight patients in the intervention group dropped out of the study because they moved out of the region while 6 patients were not reachable for subsequent follow-ups. Nineteen patients in the control group were unreachable for follow up after the 6th month. Participants who finally completed the study were thus 75 and 71 for the intervention and control groups respectively.

Demographics characteristics of subjects at baseline

The mean age for the intervention group was 56.56 ± 9.197 whiles that for the control group was 53.45 ± 8.299. There was no significant difference in demographic characteristics of the two groups at baseline (Table 2).

Drug therapy problems identified among the intervention group and solutions provided

Pharmaceutical care issues identified were related to effectiveness of therapy, side effects and adherence to therapy. Tables 3, 4 and 5, illustrate the various categories of pharmaceutical problems and actions taken to resolve them. The mean time spent in offering the pharmaceutical care to hypertensive patients was 14.88 mins ±3.78818 (Range10–32 min).

Table 1 Outcome Measures

	Outcome	Measure
1	Blood pressure (systolic and diastolic BP)	A validated automated blood pressure monitor (Omron M6) was used in measuring the blood pressure. Blood pressure was measured after the subject had rested for 5 min. Each blood pressure measurement recorded was based on an average of two blood pressure readings.
2	Body Mass Index (BMI)	BMI was determined with an equipment (Height And Weight Scale TZ 120) that measured the client's weight and height. Then the formulae "weight in kg /Height in m ^{2}"was used in computing the BMI.
3	Level of adherence to antihypertensive	Patient's self-report using the 8 item Morisky scale
4	Alcoholic Status and frequency	Subject's answer (Yes/No) to drinking alcohol The amount of alcohol consumed in a day was self-reported
5	Consumption of salty food	Yes/No to question "Do you eat salty food?
6	Frequency of exercise	Whether the subject exercised or not (Yes/No) Amount of aerobic physical activity (e.g., brisk walking, Skipping) undertaken within a week
7	Modifications in life style modifications	The number of hypertensive patients who reported adopting healthy life style practices at the end of the study
8	Pharmaceutical care issues	The number of pharmaceutical care issues identified and the action taken to resolve it.
9	Patient Satisfaction	Survey

Table 2 Baseline characteristics of Subjects

Demographic Characteristics		Intervention Group	Control Group	*p*-value
Sex n (%)	Male	33(44)	29 (40.8)	0.700
	Female	42(56)	42 (59.2)	
Age n (%)	36–45	12 (16.0)	15 (21.1)	0.166
	46–55	22 (29.3)	26 (36.6)	
	56–65	28 (37.3)	23 (32.4)	
	Above 65	13 (17.3)	7 (9.9)	
Educational Background n (%)	No education	10 (13.3)	8 (11.3)	0.497
	Basic	14 (18.7)	10 (14)	
	Middle School	17 (22.6)	19 (26.7)	
	Secondary	18 (24)	20 (28.2)	
	Tertiary	16 (21.3)	14 (19.7)	

Outcome measures after 6 months follow up

There was an association between the intervention and the mean SBP: both groups showed a decrease in SBP at the end of the study. However the mean SBP difference between the two groups for the time period was not statistically significant. ($F = 101.569$, $p = 0.697$ partial $\eta 2 = 0.001$). There was an association between the intervention and the mean DBP during the time period: the intervention group showed a decrease in DBP and the control group showed an increase in DBP at the end of the study (Table 6). The mean DBP difference comparing the two groups was significant. ($F = 20.250$, $p = .000$ partial $\eta 2 = .123$) There was also a statistically significant association between the intervention offered and attainment of BP goal [OR, 2.509 95% CI, 1.683–3.739, $p = 0.21$] however the association was weak (=ϕ .177). There was an association between the intervention and adherence, the intervention group showing an increase in mean adherence score and the control group showing a decrease in adherence scores at the end of the study. The difference in the mean adherence scores between the two groups was statistically significant. [$F = 218.851$, $p = .000$ partial $\eta 2 = 0.228$].

Patient satisfaction with intervention

Patients were satisfied with the medicines use review and health education conducted by the pharmacists. As some patients put it. Seventy three percent of patients within the intervention group were most of the time satisfied with the service provided by the pharmacist (Table 7).

The pharmacist explains the possible side effects that my medication may cause and also the service has helped me in taking my medicines. P1

The pharmacist makes sure that I understand how to take my medication and if I have a question about my medicines the pharmacist is always available to help me. P2

I am very satisfied with the service offered by the pharmacist, the advice given by the pharmacist has helped me change some unhealthy life style practices. P3

However there was some mixed opinions on whether the pharmacists should be paid for offering the service.

Table 3 Pharmaceutical issues related to effectiveness of therapy and action taken to resolve them

Pharmaceutical care issues	n (%)	Recommendations to clinician and action taken by clinician to resolve it (italicized)
Effectiveness of therapy (B)		
Patients whose blood pressure levels were above or equal to 160/100	15(20)	Dosage adjustments and/or add on therapy. [a]*Changed dosage of antihypertensive (n = 9)* [a]*Added an additional antihypertensive (n = 5)*
Aspirin prescribed when BP was not controlled.	5(6.67)	Aspirin be discontinued. [a]*Aspirin discontinued(n = 3)*
Atenolol and carvedilol prescribed as monotherapy for the management of hypertension.	2(2.60)	Beta blocker be changed to calcium channel blocker or a diuretic [a]*Beta blocker changed to a diuretic (n = 2)*
Furosemide prescribed for the management of hypertension	1(1.33)	Furosemide to be changed to bendrofluazide [a]*Furosemide substituted with bendrofluazide*

[a]Action taken by the physician on referral

Table 4 Pharmaceutical problem Related to side effects of medicine and Action Taken to resolve them

Safety (C)	n (%)	Recommendations and action taken to resolve it
Side effects of medicines		
Drowsiness and dizziness on taking methyldopa, nifedipine, lisinopril bendrofluazide	1 (1.33)	Advised patient to take lisinopril and nifedipine at night if sleep disruptions are minimal or to take medication with meals.
Blurred vision with hydrochlorothiazide	1(1.33)	Recommended to clinician that hydrochlorothiazide changed to calcium channel blocker. *Hydrochlorothiazide changed to Nifedipine*
Headache due to Nifedipine	8(10.67)	Advised patients: To take paracetamol for headache To take nifedipine at night Referred two patients with persistent headache to clinician. *Paracetamol prescribed for one and nifedipine substituted with amlodipine for other one.*
Sexual weakness with methyldopa	1(1.33)	Recommended patient to clinician for change of antihypertensive [a]*Methyldopa not changed*
Cough due to lisinopril	3 (4.00)	Recommended that Lisinopril should be changed to losartan. *Lisinopril changed to Bendrofluazide* *Lisinopril changed to amlodipine* *Lisinopril changed to losartan*
Frequent urination due to bendrofluazide	5(6.67)	Advised patients to always take bendrofluazide in the morning
Constipation with furosemide	1(1.33)	Advised patient to take in lots of fluids and referred to clinician for change in therapy. *Furosemide substituted with bendrofluazide*

[a]**Action taken by the physician italicized**

Table 5 Pharmaceutical problem Related to nonadherence of therapy and Action Taken to resolve them

Adherence (D)		
Nonadherence	n (%)	Recommendations and action taken to resolve it
Patient has not taken medication for the past two weeks because she feels blood pressure is low. She was given lisinopril 20 mg instead of 10 mg daily on her last visit to the hospital	1 (1.33).	Agreed with the patients on measures that would aid adherence to therapy, such as; • To always check blood pressure in a health facility and seek assistance when she feels her BP is low • Education on the need for continuous medication use.
Patient decided to double the dosage of Nifecard to 30 mg twice daily as she was not well	1(1.33)	Recommended that patient seeks advice from a health practitioner before adjustment on dosages is done.
Patient only takes medicines when symptoms such as headache or dizziness are felt.	11(14.6)	Agreed with patients on regular medication use and offered education on the advantage of continuous medicines administration.
Stopped taking antihypertensive and currently on herbal medicines.	5 (6.67)	Advised to see herbal medicine practitioner at the Kumasi South Hospital.
Noncompliance to doctor's appointment	10(13.3)	Agreed with patient on measures that would ensure adherence to the doctor's appointment These measures were; • The pharmacist/family member reminding patients of the appointment • Seeking financial help for transportation to the hospital • Prompt renewal of national health insurance Offering education on the importance of adhering to the doctor's appointment.
Using antihypertensive with herbal medicine for fever	3 (4.0)	Advised patient not to take medicines together.
Patient has not taken medication because antihypertensive is finished and has not visited the hospital for a refill.	9(12.0)	Agreed with patient on measures that would ensure continuous administration of medication and ways to acquire a refill when medicines were finished. Such measures were: • Keeping the medicines pack and consulting a community pharmacist for few days refill • Visiting the hospital for a refill before medicines get finished. • Pharmacist/family member reminding patients of refill appointments • Education by pharmacist on the importance of continuous medicines administration.
Sub Total	40	

[a]**Action taken by the physician on referral**

Table 6 Clinical Characteristics of Subjects at baseline and end of Study

		Intervention group (IG)				Control Group (CG)			
Variables		Baseline	After 6 Months	Mean difference (95% CI)	*p*-Value	Baseline	After 6 months	Mean difference (95% CI)	*p*-Value
Blood Pressure	SBP Mean	152.3	143.4	9.28 (12.79 to 5.79)	0.000	147.2	145.8	1.34 (4.95 to −2.28)	0.463
	DBP Mean	87.6	78.5	9.040 (12.77 to 5.30)	0.000	90.7	91.2	−0.535 (1.77 to −2.84)	0.644
BMI	Mean	27.5	26.0	1.463 (2.33 to −0.59)	0.001	27.1	27.6	−0.098 (0.66 to −0.86)	0.798
Adherence	Mean	5.5	6.2	−0.693 (−0.08 to −1.30)	0.027	4.3	3.9	0.408 (0.765–0.052)	0.026
Smoking	n (%)	2 (2.7)	2 (2.7)		1.000	0 (0)	0(0)		1.102
Consumption of Salty foods	n (%)	28 (37.3)	15 (20.0)		0.011	19 (26.8)	16 (22.5)		0.508
Alcohol n (%)	Regular n (%)	8 (10.6)	2 (2.7)		0.000	9 (12.7)	3 (4.2)		.005
Exercise n (%)	n(%)	24 (32.0)	58 (77.3)		0.000	32 (45.1)	22 (31.0)		0.031

The pharmacist should be paid for offering such a service and this service should be provided to all hypertensive patient P4

Although the service provided by the pharmacist has helped me in taking my medicines, I cannot regularly pay for such a service. P5

Discussion

Pharmaceutical care issues identified among the pharmacist intervention group and solutions provided

The common care issues identified was nonadherence to antihypertensive therapy. These were missed doses, lack of medicines and missed doctor's appointments. Some studies among hypertensive patients have also reported nonadherence as a major care issue commonly encountered [15]. Another category of pharmaceutical problems reported was experiencing side effects of the antihypertensive; an issue often associated with chronic diseases [16]. Solutions provided were mostly changes in therapy because if patients continued experiencing side effects it was likely they would not take their medicines.

Low dose aspirin is an antiplatelet and its long term use is associated with major gastrointestinal and extracranial bleeding [17]. Patients whose blood pressure are not optimised are at risk of complications such as stroke and this could be haemorrhagic if patients are on low dose aspirin. Therefore low dose aspirin is recommended for the primary prevention of cardiovascular events in hypertensive patients aged over 50 years with a baseline CVD risk level > 20% and whose blood pressure has been controlled to an audit standard of 150/90 [18]. However some subjects were still on dispersible aspirin although their blood pressure was not controlled.

Another drug therapy problem encountered was the use of beta blockers as monotherapy in the management of hypertension. Beta blockers are often recommended as add on therapy when drugs such as diuretics and calcium channel blockers have not worked [19, 20]. Compared with placebo beta blockers are effective in reducing the blood pressure, however the blood pressure lowering efficacy of beta blockers are suboptimal compared to other antihypertensive. Furthermore there is evidence suggesting that beta blockers do not reduce mortality [21].

Outcome measures after 6 months

The intervention studied led to a statistically significant mean DBP difference between the IG and the CG and there was an association between the intervention offered and achievement of BP Goal. Thus, subjects who were offered the intervention were more likely to achieve BP Goal than those who were not. A similar intervention

Table 7 Patient Satisfaction Survey

Variables	Most of the time	Sometimes	Very rarely	Never
I have to wait for a long time before my blood pressure is measured	4 (5.3)	7 (9.3)	50 (57.6)	14 (18.7)
I have to wait for a long time before my weight and height is taken	5 (6.7)	21 (28.0)	39 (52.0)	10 (13.3)
The pharmacist spends as much time with me as necessary	24 (32.0)	42 (56.0)	7 (9.3)	2 (2.7)
I have trouble understanding the education given to me	3 (4)	12 (16.0)	33 (44.0)	27 (36.0)
The pharmacy staff are friendly	45 (60)	25 (33.3)	5 (6.7)	0 (0.0)
Follow up appointments are helpful	32 (42.7)	34 (45.3)	6 (8.0)	3 (4.0)
The advice given by the pharmacist helped me in taking my medicines	48 (64.0)	23 (30.7)	3 (4.0)	1 (1.3)
I am very satisfied with the pharmacy service received	55 (73.3)	18 (24.0)	2 (2.7)	0 (0.0)

(medicines review, adherence and counselling) for 118 hypertensive patients in a randomized study in Canada caused a significant reduction in SBP in the intervention group compared to placebo. The difference in the number of subjects who had their blood pressure controlled was also statistically significant. The average age of participants, 58 years, was similar to that in our study [22]. Achievement of BP control is essential as there is evidence that suggests that patients whose blood pressure is controlled to less than 140/90 often have a low incidence of cardiovascular complications such as stroke, myocardial infarction and death [19].

The mean adherence difference between the IG and the CG was also statistically significant and there was a moderate association between the intervention offered and adherence. Thus subjects who were offered the intervention were more likely to adhere to treatment than those who were not. Some studies on pharmacist intervention on adherence have shown similar or conflicting results. There was a significant difference in adherence level in the intervention and control groups in randomised studies in Thailand and United Kingdom [8, 10]. However another randomized controlled study showed no significant difference in adherence between the intervention and control groups [9].

Implications of findings on practice

At baseline adherence levels of subjects in both groups was quite low. It is therefore essential that measures and polices are established to achieve high adherence levels among hypertensive patients. In most clinical settings in Ghana hospital folders lack documentation of adherence to therapy for patients with chronic diseases. Ideally adherence to medication should be assessed in the consultation room during each review visit before decisions on medicines are taken. In addition, adherence could also be assessed by the pharmacist before medicines are dispensed. This practice could enable these health care personnel to identify and address any adherence concerns of the patient.

The Ghanaian community pharmacist should be encouraged to monitor and offer similar interventions to patients with hypertension who come to refill their medications; as this can improve blood pressure control and adherence and enhance the public image of the pharmacy profession in the country. For such pharmaceutical services to be effectively rolled out in Ghanaian community pharmacies it is very important for some laws and policies to be updated. For instance the Ghana Pharmacy Act 489, (1994) which has been repealed and subsumed by the Health Professions Regulatory Bodies Act 867, is silent on the extended responsibilities of the community pharmacists for patients with chronic diseases [5]. The Pharmacy Council, Ghana in conjunction with the Community Pharmacy Pharmacist Association (CPPA) of Pharmaceutical Society of Ghana (PSGH) could determine policy guidelines on care services the community pharmacist can provide. However there is the need to explore measure to reduce the number of patients lost to follow up because pharmacy owners might not want to invest their time in offering such a service if clients are going to disappear.

Offering the intervention described in this study, is time consuming. The mean time spent with subjects was fourteen minutes and several phone calls and SMS were made in an attempt to remind them of follow up dates. It is therefore essential that the pharmacist is offered some remuneration as was done in the study and also there is the need to explore the cost effectiveness of the service. Over half of hypertensive patients agreed that the pharmacist should be paid for rendering such services and should offer it to all hypertensive patients. In the United Kingdom the community pharmacist is mandated to offer so many pharmaceutical services apart from their primary role and are paid a commission by the National Health Service (NHS) for each care service they offer [23].

Limitations of the study

Some patients in the Control Group (CG) were mostly lost to follow up, probably because the first follow up occurred six months after the first encounter. Another reason why follow up appointments were missed was that in some instances the telecommunication coverage was poor, hence some clients were unreachable. The study also assumed that all patients who liked salty food consumed salty food. Furthermore a quasi-experiment design was chosen for the evaluation of the pharmaceutical care of hypertensive patients instead of a randomised controlled study which is the gold standard due to the lack of documentation of clients medical and medication history in the community pharmacy.

Conclusions

It is feasible for Ghanaian community pharmacists to extend their services and continually offer pharmaceutical care (conducting medication reviews, assessing adherence and counselling) to patients with hypertension. This could lead to the identification and resolution of drug related problems and improvement in blood pressure control and adherence. However, for community pharmacies to effectively and continually offer these services, national policies would have to be enacted to provide some remuneration for the service. Community pharmacists in low income countries with increasing low levels of blood pressure control could adopt such an intervention. However, it is important that they consider their pharmacist staffing level and pharmacy setting. This is because this service

requires the continuous presence of a pharmacist and space for offering pharmaceutical care to ensure privacy.

Abbreviations

BMI: Body Mass Index; BP: Blood Pressure; CG: Control Group; CPPA: Community Pharmacists Association; CVD: Cardiovascular Diseases; DBP: Diastolic Blood Pressure; IG: Intervention Group; OR: Odd Ratio; P1-P5: Patients; PSGH: Pharmaceutical Society of Ghana; SBP: Systolic Blood Pressure; SOAPO: Subjective, Objective, Analysis, Plan and Outcome; SPSS: Statistical Package for social sciences

Acknowledgements

All community pharmacies, pharmacists and hypertensive patients who agreed to be part of the study.

Funding

The work was partially funded by the Commonwealth Pharmacists Association. (CPA).

Authors' contributions

Conception, design, acquisition and analysis of data - AFAM and FTOD. Drafting of manuscript and revising it - AFAM and FTOD. Revising and approval of final manuscript to be published: FTOD and AFAM.

Competing interests

The authors declare that they have no competing interests.

References

1. Guwatudde D, Nankya-Mutyoba J. Kalyesubula. BMC Public Health. 2015;15:1211. https://doi.org/10.1186/s12889-015-2546-z
2. Bosu WK. Epidemic of hypertension in Ghana: a systematic review. BMC Public Health. 2010;10:418.
3. Awuah RB, Anarfi JK, Agyemang C, Ogedegbe G, Aikins AD. Prevalence, awareness, treatment and control of hypertension in urban poor communities in Accra, Ghana. J Hypertens. 2014;32(suppl 6):1203–10.
4. Addo J, Agyemang C, Smeeth LA, De-Graft Aikins A, Edusei AK, Ogedegbee O. Review of population-based studies on hypertension in Ghana. Ghana Medical Journal. 2012;46(suppl 2):4–11.
5. Marfo AFA, Owusu-Daaku FT, Opare Addo MNA, Saana IB. Ghanaian hypertensive patients understanding of their medicines and life style modification for managing hypertension. Int J Pharm Pharm Sci. 2014;4:165–70.
6. Parliament of Ghana Health Professions Regulatory Bodies Act 857 Part four Establishment of the Pharmacy Council [Available at URL: http://www.pcghana.org/wp-content/uploads/2017/02/Health-Professions-Regulatory-Bodies-Act.pdf Accessed: 17 July 2014.
7. Smith F. The quality of private pharmacy services in low and middle-income countries: a systematic review. Pharm World Sci 2009;31Suppl 3:351–361.
8. Sookaneknun P, Richards RME, Sanguansermsri J. Pharmacist involvement in primary care improves hypertensive patient clinical outcomes. Ann Pharmacother. 2004;38:2023–8.
9. Zillich AJ, Sutherland JM, Kumbera PA. Hypertension outcomes through blood pressure monitoring and evaluation by pharmacists. (HOME study). J Gen Intern Med. 2005;20:1091–6.
10. Blenkinsopp A, Phelan M, Bourne J, Dakhil N. Extended adherence support by community pharmacists for patients with hypertension: a randomised controlled trial. Int J Pharm Pract. 2000;8:165–75.
11. Chabot I, Moisan J, Grégoire JP, Milot A. Pharmacist intervention program for control of hypertension. Ann Pharmacother. 2003;37:1186–93.
12. American College of Clinical Pharmacist. Clinical Pharmacy Practice Model Available at https://www.accp.com/docs/report/0612_table1.pdf Accessed 12 February 2012.
13. Charan J, Biswas T. How to calculate sample size for different study designs in medical research. Indian Journal of Psychological Medicine. 2013;35(2):121.
14. Kasiulevicius V, Sapoka V, Filipaviciute R. Sample size calculation in epidemiological studies. Gerontology. 2006;7:225–31.
15. Chua SS, Kok LC, Yusof FAM, Tang GH, Lee SWH, Efendie B, Paraidathathu T. Pharmaceutical care issues identified by pharmacists in patients with diabetes, hypertension or Hyperlipidaemia in primary care settings. BMC Health Serv Res 2012; 12Suppl 1: 388.
16. Oparah AC, Adje DU, Enato FEO. Evalution of pharmaceutical care intervention to hypertensive patients in a Nigerian community pharmacy international journal. Pharm Pract. 2006;14:115–22.
17. NICE Hypertension: Clinical Management of Primary Hypertension in Adults Available at https://workspace.imperial.ac.uk/ref/Public/UoA%2002%20-%20Public%20Health,%20Health%20Services%20and%20Primary%20Care/NICE%20hypertension%20guidelines.pdf. Accessed on 12 July 2013.
18. BHS. The Use of Aspirin in Primary Prevention of Cardiovascular Disease [Available at http://www.bhsoc.org/pdfs/Statement%20on%20Aspirin%20Jan10.pdf Accessed 14 September 2014].
19. Chobdanian AV, Barkis GL, Black HR. The seventh report of the joint National Committee on prevention, detection evaluation and treatment of high blood pressure. Journal of American Medical Association. 2003;289:2560–72.
20. Messerli FH, Grossman E, Goldbourt U. Are Beta-blockers efficacious as first-line therapy for hypertension in the elderly a systematic review. Journal of American Medical Association. 1998;279:1903–7.
21. Dahlof B, Sever PS, Poulter NR, Wedel H, Beevers DG, Caulfield M. Prevention of cardiovascular events with an antihypertensive regimen of amlodipine adding perindopril as required versus atenolol adding Bendroflumethiazide as required, in the Anglo-Scandinavian cardiac outcomes trial-blood pressure lowering arm (ASCOT-BPLA): a multicentre randomized Control Trail. Lancet. 2005;366:895–906.
22. Ontario Pharmacists Association and Green Shield Canada. Impact of Community Pharmacist Interventions in Hypertension Management on Patient Outcomes: A Randomized Controlled Trial Available at https://www.opatoday.com/Media/Default/Reports/Hypertension%20Study%20-%20Final%20Report%20(January%208%202014).pdf. Accessed 10 January 2015.
23. NHS Community Pharmacy services a Summary Available at http://psnc.org.uk/wp-content/uploads/2013/08/CPCF-summary-July-2013.pdf. Accessed 10 October 2014.

17

A bibliometric analysis of the global research on biosimilars

Akram Hernández-Vásquez[1*], Christoper A. Alarcon-Ruiz[2], Guido Bendezu-Quispe[3], Daniel Comandé[4] and Diego Rosselli[5]

Abstract

Background: Biosimilars could be a promising option to help decrease healthcare costs and expand access to treatment. There is no previous evidence of a global bibliometric analysis on biosimilars. Therefore, we aimed to assess the quantity and quality of worldwide biosimilars research.

Methods: We performed a bibliometric analysis using documents about biosimilars published until December 2016 in journals indexed in Scopus. We extracted the annual research, languages, countries, journals, authors, institutions, citation frequency, and the metrics of journals. The data were quantitatively and qualitatively analyzed using Microsoft Excel 2013. Additional information about authors' participation was obtained using the R-package Bibliometrix. Publication activity was adjusted for the countries by population size. Also, author co-citation analysis and a term co-occurrence analysis with the terms included in the title and abstract of publications was presented as network visualization maps using VOSviewer.

Results: A total of 2330 biosimilar-related documents identified in the Scopus database, most of them were articles (1452; 62.32%). The number of documents published had an exponential increased between 2004 and 2016 ($p < 0.001$). The United States was the country with the highest production with 685 (29.40%) documents followed by Germany and UK with 293 (12.58%) and 248 (10.64%), respectively. Switzerland (11.05), Netherlands (5.85) and UK (3.83) showed the highest per capita ratio. The highest citation/article ratio were for the Netherlands (28.06), Spain (24.23), and France (20.11). *Gabi Journal* published 73 (3.13%) documents; both *Biopharm International* and *Pharmaceutical Technology* and *Mabs,* 41 (1.76%). Three out of top ten journals were Trade publications. Amgen Incorporated from the USA was the most prolific institution with 51 documents followed by Pfizer Inc. with 48. Terms about specific diseases and drugs were found in recent years, compared with terms such as legislation, structure, protein, dose and generic in the early years.

Conclusions: Research production and publication of documents on biosimilars are increasing. The majority of publications came from high-income countries. The trends in terminology use are according to state of the art in the topic, and reflects the interest in the utilization of biosimilars in diseases who are expected to obtain benefits of its use.

Keywords: Biosimilar pharmaceuticals, Bibliometrics, Biomedical research (source: MeSH NLM)

Background

A biosimilar, or "similar biological product", is a highly similar product to an already approved biological product regarding structure, function, potency, quality, clinical efficacy and safety [1]. Currently, there are already 5 and 39 biosimilars products approved in the United States [2] and Europe [3], respectively. The number of approved biosimilars might increase in the next year due to manifest interest from different healthcare systems and international organizations [4].

The development of biological products represented a significant advance in the therapy of many diseases that did not have effective treatments. Nonetheless, these products require a vast expenditure of money and resources to develop, leading to an increase in the cost of these therapies for both patients and the health sector [5, 6]. The field of biosimilars could be a promising option to help decrease healthcare costs and expand access to treatment [7] particularly when many patents have already expired or will do so soon [8].

* Correspondence: akram.hernandez.v@upch.pe
[1]Universidad Privada del Norte, Lima, Peru
Full list of author information is available at the end of the article

Few studies had evaluated the clinical evidence in support of different biosimilars: there are only three cancer related-biosimilars products whose safety/efficacy have been published [9], while five biosimilars for chronic inflammatory diseases have six clinical trials comparing them with their reference drug [10]. This situation of scarce evidence may lead physicians [11], pharmacists [12] and patients to have low confidence their safety and efficacy [13].

Bibliometric analysis is a useful method to objectively measure current research of a certain subject and its international scientific influence as an aspect of scientific quality [14]. However, to our knowledge, there is no previous evidence of a global bibliometric analysis on biosimilars. Our study aimed to assess the quantity and quality of worldwide biosimilars research.

Methods

Study design

We performed a bibliometric analysis using documents published until December 2016 in journals indexed in Scopus (https://www.scopus.com/). While there are a variety of document types, only articles, reviews, editorials and letters were included.

Source of information

Scopus (Elsevier BV Company, USA) is the largest abstract and citation database of scientific peer-review literature including more than 22,000 titles from international publishers. We decided to use this database because it includes all MEDLINE documents and includes further characteristics such as country of all the authors and citations per document, information that is relevant for this study [15–17].

Search strategy

A literature search was conducted by a research librarian in Scopus for publications on a single day, October 18, 2017, and used the following MeSH and free terms in the title and abstract field: biosimilar pharmaceutical OR biosimilar*. The validity of the search strategy was tested by manually reviewing retrieved articles.

Data analysis

All data were collected by two authors and downloaded in csv format (Additional file 1: Dataset). The data were imported to Microsoft Excel 2013 and quantitatively and qualitatively analyzed. The Scopus database presents some disadvantages for bibliometric applications [17]. For this reason, it was necessary to standardize the data. We detected documents mistakenly attributed to the domain of author name and affiliation. Therefore, a standardization was carried out manually by the authors.

Bibliometric indicators were extracted from the data and with the option "Analyze Results" in Scopus, including annual research, languages, countries, journals, authors, institutions, and citation frequency. Scopus Journal Metrics was used to extract the metrics of journals. The contributions of countries were evaluated based on paper and citation numbers, and the research output of each country was adjusted according to population size (https://www.cia.gov/library/publications/the-world-factbook/geos/ag.html). To describe more information about author participation in research production about biosimilars, we use the open-source Bibliometrix R-package (http://www.bibliometrix.org/) to obtain the mean of articles per author, the mean of authors per article, the mean of articles' citation and the number of articles with only one or more than one author.

Author co-citation analysis (ACA) to analyze the relations among highly cited references and productive authors, and a term co-occurrence analysis with the terms included in the title and abstract of publications was presented as network visualization maps using VOSviewer version 1.6.6 (Leiden University, Leiden, Netherlands) techniques [18].

Research ethics

The data were downloaded from Scopus and as secondary data, did not involve any interactions with human subjects. There were no ethical questions about the data. Approval of an ethics committee was not necessary.

Results

A total number of 2330 documents indexed on Scopus were retrieved from 2004 to 2016. The majority of papers were articles (1452; 62.32%) followed by reviews (642; 27.55%), editorials (138; 5.92%), and letters (98; 4.21%). In 2004, three publications were identified compared to 521 in 2016 (Fig. 1); this increase in the amount of papers was statistically significant ($p < 0.001$). In general, 83 countries contributed to research articles about biosimilars. Table 1 listed the top ten countries, which represented 84.12% of the total. Seven of the top ten publishing countries are European. United States was the country with the highest production with 685 (29.40%) documents followed by Germany and UK with 293 (12.58%) and 248 (10.64%), respectively. European countries such as Switzerland (11.05), Netherlands (5.85) and UK (3.83) showed the highest per capita ratio. The highest citation/article ratio were for the Netherlands (28.06), Spain (24.23), and France (20.11).

The analysis of the subject area, Table 2 shows that most documents were included in the broad category "Medicine" with 1453, followed by "Pharmacology, toxicology and pharmaceutics" with 946 and "Biochemistry, Genetics and Molecular biology" with 607.

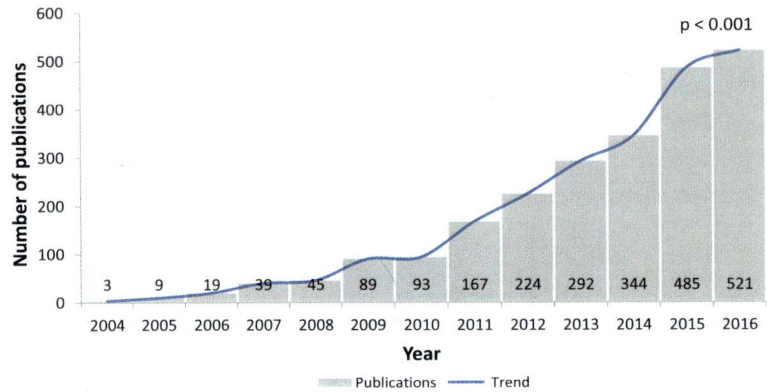

Fig. 1 Annual scientific documents of biosimilar research, Scopus 2004–2016

The total of documents retrieved were published in 803 journals, but top ten journals account for 18.82% of the total (Table 3). The top journals included in first place *Gabi Journal* with 73 (3.13%) documents, followed by *Biopharm International* and *Pharmaceutical Technology* and *Mabs* both with 41 (1.76%). Three out of ten titles were Trade publications. *Mabs* journal had the greatest SJR 2016 (1.62).

Table 4 presents a ranking of the Top ten institutions that published in biosimilars. Amgen Incorporated from the USA was the most prolific institution with 51 documents followed by Pfizer Inc. with 48. Seven of this top 10 list are European institutions, the others from USA. Four institutions were pharmaceutical companies. Based on the citations, academic institutions obtained higher positions compared to pharmaceutical companies being Medizinische Universitat Wien the institution with the highest number of citations and citations per articles ratio.

There were 6344 authors in the documents on biosimilars. The mean of articles per author was 0.4 and there were 420 documents with only one author. A co-authorship analysis that included authors with at least five publications is shown in Fig. 2. There were 143 authors; each circle represents one author, the closer the circles the closer the collaboration.

We show the top 10 cited articles in biosimilars in Table 5. The article "EULAR recommendations for the management of rheumatoid arthritis with synthetic and biological disease-modifying antirheumatic drugs: 2013 update" published in 2014 received the highest citation (962) within the retrieved documents. The top 10 include five articles and five reviews. All of the top ten cited articles were published in scientific journals. In general, the mean of citations per article was 9.6.

In the analysis of terms co-occurrence (Fig. 3), we used words in the titles and abstracts related to specific diseases and drugs. Rheumatoid arthritis, ulcerative colitis, rheumatism, infliximab, etanercept, and tofacitinib were found in recent years, compared with terms such as legislation, structure, protein, dose and generic in the early years.

Discussion

Biosimilars' cost-saving potential is their best attribute, making them an attractive option in the close future [19]. Also, the mandatory research that they have to do prior of their approval, and their large utility in diverse diseases, such as cancer, hemophilia, autoimmune diseases, and rare genetic conditions, make biosimilars an

Table 1 Top ten countries with more publications on biosimilars, and there average citation rate. Scopus 2004–2016

Rank	Country	Number of documents	% of articles	Number of articles per million inhabitants	Citations (up 2016)	Citations/Article
1	United States	685	29.40	2.10	6768	9.88
2	Germany	293	12.58	3.64	4373	14.92
3	United Kingdom	248	10.64	3.83	3824	15.42
4	Italy	149	6.39	2.40	2097	14.07
5	France	132	5.67	2.10	2654	20.11
6	Netherlands	100	4.29	5.85	2806	28.06
7	Spain	91	3.91	1.86	2205	24.23
8	Switzerland	91	3.91	11.05	1783	19.59
9	India	86	3.69	0.07	338	3.93
10	Canada	85	3.65	2.39	794	9.34

Table 2 Subject areas for documents published on biosimilars, Scopus, 2004–2016

Rank	Subject area	Documents published	% of documents
1	Medicine	1453	37.92
2	Pharmacology, Toxicology and Pharmaceutics	946	24.69
3	Biochemistry, Genetics and Molecular Biology	607	15.84
4	Immunology and Microbiology	219	5.72
5	Health Professions	165	4.31
6	Chemistry	137	3.58
7	Chemical Engineering	136	3.55
8	Business, Management and Accounting	68	1.77
9	Engineering	62	1.62
10	Mathematics	39	1.02

interesting field to make research. This explains the growing interest by many groups, including patients, health insurers, and providers, as well as the pharmaceutical industry. This interest is evidenced in the exponential increased of documents published on biosimilars between 2004 and 2016. High-income countries seem to dominate research in the field of biosimilars where the United States and Western European countries contributed to most of the world's research on biosimilars, and receive the most of the citations.

Authors from the United States published the highest number of scientific publications and received more citation compared to other countries. This result is not surprising, since the US leads the rankings in worldwide research, including medicine [20–22]. Majority of top-ranking countries were European. Although Switzerland, Netherlands, and United Kingdom do not have as many papers but go to the top of the list when we adjust by population. On the other hand, Netherlands, Spain, and France have the greatest citation per article. Those situations are similar in other biomedical fields: Rheumatology [20], arthroscopy [23], foot and ankle [24], and probiotics in pediatrics [25], but it differs from endocrinology and metabolism field [26] and research on tramadol [27]. It would perhaps be better to adjust by the number of researchers, instead of inhabitants, but this information is not easily accessible [26].

"Gabi Journal" and "Mabs" were the most productive peer-review journals in the topic of biosimilars. Besides, "Biopharm International", a trade publication journal, occupied the second most productive journal on biosimilars. It is remarkable that three trade publication journals, perhaps showing the industry's interest in promoting their products, were in the top 10 most productive journals, but they do not receive that many citations. This may reflect the fact that they might be considered less trustful, or that they are not necessarily targeted at researchers [28]. Both "Mabs" and "Expert Opinion on Biological Therapy" are rated much higher in CiteScore 2017, SJR 2016, and SNIP 2016, despite having less publications. These suggest that at least in the field of biosimilars quantity is not necessarily correlated with quality. This situation differs from other biomedical fields like spine surgery [29].

Only three of the top 10 institutions were from America, the other seven were from Europe. This reflects the fact that biosimilars are a subject of interest in many different countries. Additionally, institutions with most citations and mean citation rate were from universities, which might indicate its better quality. Also, there is less risk that universities have conflicts of interest in developing research papers in biosimilars, so their results might be more trustful.

The top five most cited papers were original articles. The top two were guidelines for management of clinical conditions (rheumatoid arthritis and febrile neutropenia). This could be explained because three biosimilars are available to treat rheumatoid arthritis and others are in the way to approval [30], and the recent

Table 3 Top ten journals publishing on biosimilars ($N = 2330$). Scopus 2004–2016

Rank	Source title	Publication type	Documents published	% of articles	CiteScore 2016	SJR 2016	SNIP 2016
1	Gabi Journal	Journal	73	3.13	0.28	0.23	0.08
2	Biopharm International	Trade Publication	41	1.76	0.17	0.16	0.08
3	Mabs	Journal	41	1.76	4.66	1.62	1.25
4	Biodrugs	Journal	40	1.72	2.98	1.01	1.13
5	Bioprocess International	Trade Publication	39	1.67	0.26	0.23	0.25
6	Pharmaceutical Technology	Journal	39	1.67	0.09	0.14	0.16
7	Biologicals	Journal	34	1.46	1.65	0.62	0.74
8	Contract Pharma	Trade Publication	30	1.29	0.02	0.12	0
9	Journal of Generic Medicines	Journal	28	1.20	0.12	0.14	0.39
10	Expert Opinion on Biological Therapy	Journal	27	1.16	3.14	1.14	0.75

Table 4 Top ten institutions publishing on biosimilars, and their citations. Scopus 2004–2016

Rank	Institution Name	Country	Number of papers	Citations	Citations/Article
1	Amgen Incorporated	United States	51	394	7.73
2	Pfizer Inc.	United States	48	201	4.19
3	Utrecht University	Netherlands	44	898	20.41
4	Duke University	United States	37	763	20.62
5	Sandoz International GmbH	Germany	33	460	13.94
6	Medizinische Universitat Wien	Austria	23	1538	66.87
7	KU Leuven	Belgium	22	227	10.32
8	Erasmus University Medical Center	Netherlands	20	929	46.45
9	Universita degli Studi di Milano	Italy	20	152	7.6
10	Novartis International AG	Switzerland	19	174	9.

approval process of granulocyte-colony stimulating factor biosimilars, a useful drug to treat febrile neutropenia [31]. Moreover, clinical practice guidelines from any field generally have a lot of cites. The fourth and fifth most cited articles were randomized controlled clinical trials of the infliximab biosimilar CT-P13. This is the first biosimilar monoclonal antibody approved by the European Medicines Agency [32]. Overall, those two clinical trials help to understand and accept their interchangeability with infliximab as a feasible and safe strategy to be applied in real-life clinical practice [33]. On the other side, there were five reviews in the top 10. Mostly, they try to better explain biosimilars to health professionals, especially clinician [34], that could have some reluctance about the use of biosimilars [35]. These reviews focus on improving the uptake of biosimilars, educating the physicians, and motivating to adopt them in routine clinical practice [36].

Words included in the title and abstracts of biosimilars research papers and their main year when they were published were: Legislation (2011), enzyme (2012), structure, protein, dose, antibody, interchangeability (2013), glycosylation, receptor, phase, adverse event (2014), and rheumatoid arthritis, ulcerative colitis,

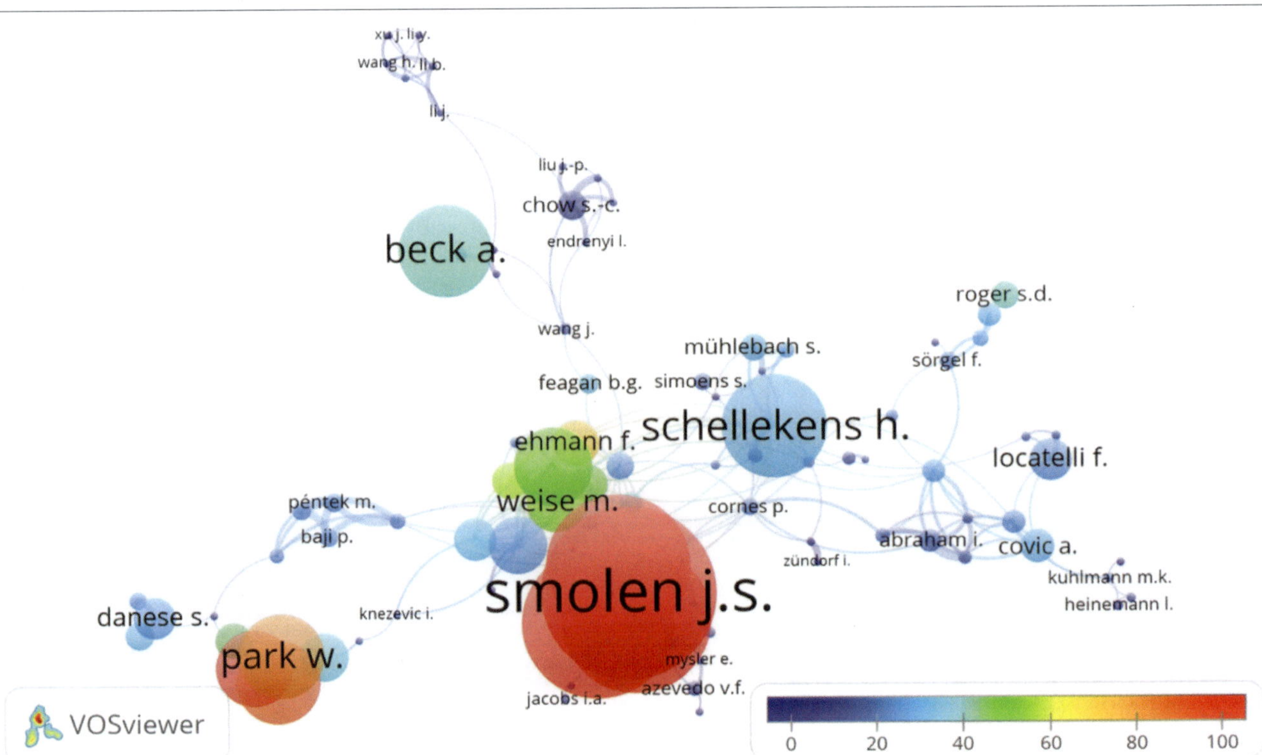

Fig. 2 Author co-authorship analysis with VOSviewer for biosimilars publications. Minimum of five documents per author, 143 authors were included. Weighted by citations and scores by average of citations

Table 5 Top 10 cited documents of biosimilars research. Scopus 2004–2016

Rank	Title	Year	Journal name	Cited by	Type of document
1	EULAR recommendations for the management of rheumatoid arthritis with synthetic and biological disease-modifying antirheumatic drugs: 2013 update	2014	Annals of the Rheumatic Diseases	962	Article
2	2010 update of EORTC guidelines for the use of granulocyte-colony stimulating factor to reduce the incidence of chemotherapy-induced febrile neutropenia in adult patients with lymphoproliferative disorders and solid tumours	2011	European Journal of Cancer	498	Article
3	Biopharmaceutical benchmarks 2014	2014	Nature Biotechnology	275	Article
4	A randomised, double-blind, parallel-group study to demonstrate equivalence in efficacy and safety of CT-P13 compared with innovator infliximab when coadministered with methotrexate in patients with active rheumatoid arthritis: The PLANETRA study	2013	Annals of the Rheumatic Diseases	269	Article
5	A randomised, double-blind, multicentre, parallel-group, prospective study comparing the pharmacokinetics, safety, and efficacy of CT-P13 and innovator infliximab in patients with ankylosing spondylitis: The PLANETAS study	2013	Annals of the Rheumatic Diseases	250	Article
6	Analytical tools for characterizing biopharmaceuticals and the implications for biosimilars	2012	Nature Reviews Drug Discovery	215	Review
7	PEG-modified biopharmaceuticals	2009	Expert Opinion on Drug Delivery	201	Review
8	The challenge of biosimilars	2008	Annals of Oncology	178	Review
9	Sublingual immunotherapy: World Allergy Organization position paper 2013 update	2014	World Allergy Organization Journal	172	Review
10	Biosimilars: What clinicians should know	2012	Blood	158	Review

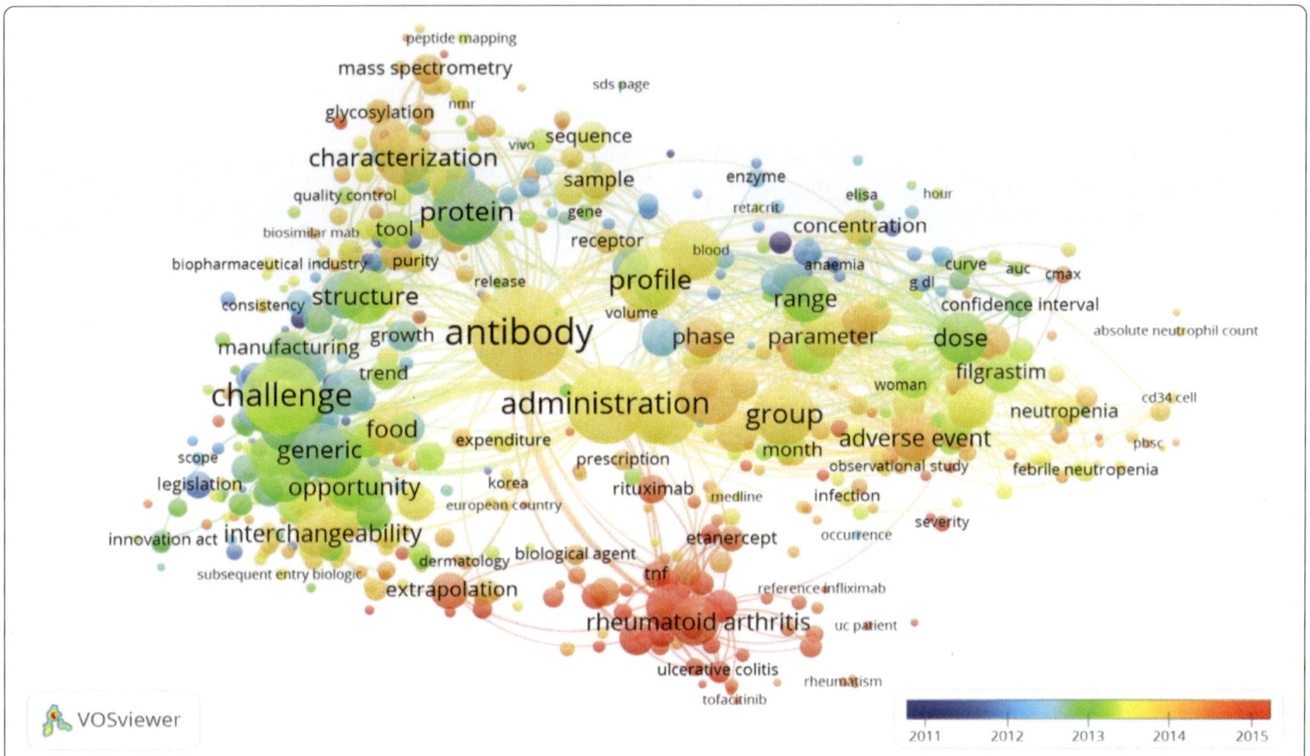

Fig. 3 Terms co-occurrence analysis of tittles and abstracts (overlay visualization) and their temporal evolution with VOSviewer for biosimilars publications. Binary counting method, choose threshold (10 terms). Term "conclusion" was excluded

extrapolation, rituximab, etanercept (2015). This suggests that the emphasis of biosimilars research responds to a subject that is very new to researchers and should follow the law of the development of a new discipline. This find is similar to a report in a previous bibliometric analysis on exomes [37]. In the field of biosimilars, there are requirements for their approval, including to demonstrate similarity, safety, and effectiveness [38]. These terms were more frequently found in the early.

The present research shows an overall view about biosimilars research and their distribution mostly in high-income countries where they have policies to their approval. Although markets like BRICS (Brazil, Russia, India, China, and South Africa), MIST (Mexico, Indonesia, South Korea, and Turkey) [39], and Latin America [40] provides an emerging future to biosimilars, they do not represent an important influence in biosimilars research. Also, the present study like previous bibliometric analyses has some limitations. First, our study did not include articles published in non-Scopus databases. However, Scopus is a reliable and significant source for bibliometric studies in general. Second, it is difficult to distinguish articles that focus on biosimilars from those that only mention the term or tangentially address it. However, using correct keywords and given its original subject, this study still provides a comprehensive picture of biosimilar research productivity, which could be used to track overall trends and identify topics of interest.

Conclusions

In summary, the results of the present study showed that documents published in journals about biosimilars are increasing. The majority of publications came from high-income countries, being the US the most productive country in biosimilars followed by European countries. To the best of our knowledge, this is the first study conducted in the analysis of research production and citations in biosimilars. The trends in terminology use are according to state of the art in the topic that comes from issues of safety and efficacy to the study of new biosimilar products in specific diseases.

Abbreviations

MeSH: Medical subject heading; SNIP: SCImago journal rank; SRJ: Source normalised impact per paper; UK: United Kingdom; USA: United States of America

Funding

This research received no specific grant from any funding agency.

Authors' contributions

AHV conceived the idea for the study; AHV and DC collected the data; AHV and GBQ did the statistical analysis; AHV, GBQ, CAAR and DR drafted the manuscript; all authors contributed in the writing and preparation of the manuscript. All authors read and approved the final manuscript.

Competing interests

The authors declare that they have no competing interests.

Author details

[1]Universidad Privada del Norte, Lima, Peru. [2]Facultad de Medicina, Universidad Ricardo Palma, Lima, Peru. [3]Universidad Peruana Cayetano Heredia, Lima, Peru. [4]Institute for Clinical Effectiveness and Health Policy (IECS), Buenos Aires, Argentina. [5]Departamento de Epidemiología Clínica y Bioestadística, Facultad de Medicina, Pontificia Universidad Javeriana, Bogotá, Colombia.

References

1. Declerck P, Danesi R, Petersel D, Jacobs I. The language of Biosimilars: clarification, definitions, and regulatory aspects. Drugs. 2017;77(6):671–7.
2. US Food and Drug Administration. Purple Book: Lists of Licensed Biological. US Department of Health and Human Services, Food and Drug Administration, Center for Biologics Evaluation and Research (CBER). 2017 [cited 2017 August 13]. Available from: https://www.fda.gov/downloads/Drugs/DevelopmentApprovalProcess/HowDrugsareDevelopedandApproved/ApprovalApplications/TherapeuticBiologicApplications/Biosimilars/UCM560162.pdf.
3. Biosimilars approved in Europe. Generics and Biosimilars Initiative July 7, 2017 [cited 2017 August 13]. Available from: http://www.gabionline.net/Biosimilars/General/Biosimilars-approved-in-Europe.
4. Bennett S. WHO to begin pilot prequalification of biosimilars for cancer treatment. 2017 [cited 2017 November 05]. Gineva: World Health Organization; [Nov 05, 2017]. Available from: http://www.who.int/mediacentre/news/releases/2017/pilot-prequalification-biosimilars/en/.
5. Blackstone E, Fuhr J. Innovation and competition: will biosimilars succeed? Biotechnol Healthcare. 2012;9(1):24–7.
6. Prince FH, van Suijlekom-Smit LW. Cost of biologics in the treatment of juvenile idiopathic arthritis: a factor not to be overlooked. Paediatr Drugs. 2013;15(4):271–80.
7. Boccia R, Jacobs I, Popovian R, de Lima LG, Jr. Can biosimilars help achieve the goals of US health care reform? Cancer Manag Res. 2017;9:197–205.
8. Ventola CL. Biosimilars. Part 1: proposed regulatory criteria for FDA approval. P T. 2013;38(5):270–4. 277, 287
9. Jacobs I, Ewesuedo R, Lula S, Zacharchuk C. Biosimilars for the treatment of Cancer: a systematic review of published evidence. BioDrugs. 2017;31(1):1–36.
10. Olteanu R, Zota A, Constantin M. Biosimilars: an update on clinical trials (review of published and ongoing studies). Acta Dermatovenerol Croat. 2017;25(1):57–66.
11. Cohen H, Beydoun D, Chien D, Lessor T, McCabe D, Muenzberg M, et al. Awareness, knowledge, and perceptions of Biosimilars among specialty physicians. Adv Ther. 2017;33(12):2160–72.
12. Beck M, Michel B, Rybarczyk-Vigouret MC, Leveque D, Sordet C, Sibilia J, et al. Knowledge, behaviors and practices of community and hospital pharmacists towards biosimilar medicines: results of a French web-based survey. MAbs. 2017;9(2):383–90.
13. Jacobs I, Singh E, Sewell KL, Al-Sabbagh A, Shane LG. Patient attitudes and understanding about biosimilars: an international cross-sectional survey. Patient Preference Adherence. 2016;10:937–48.

14. Van Raan T. The use of bibliometric analysis in research performance assessment and monitoring of interdisciplinary scientific developments. Technikfolgenabschautzung - Theorie und Praxis. 2003;1:20–9.
15. Falagas ME, Pitsouni EI, Malietzis GA, Pappas G. Comparison of PubMed, Scopus, web of science, and Google scholar: strengths and weaknesses. FASEB J. 2008;22(2):338–42.
16. Kulkarni AV, Aziz B, Shams I, Busse JW. Comparisons of citations in web of science, Scopus, and Google scholar for articles published in general medical journals. JAMA. 2009;302(10):1092–6.
17. Agarwal A, Durairajanayagam D, Tatagari S, Esteves SC, Harlev A, Henkel R, et al. Bibliometrics: tracking research impact by selecting the appropriate metrics. Asian J Androl. 2016;18(2):296–309.
18. van Eck NJ, Waltman L. Software survey: VOSviewer, a computer program for bibliometric mapping. Scientometrics. 2010;84(2):523–38.
19. Nabhan C, Parsad S, Mato AR, Feinberg BA. Biosimilars in oncology in the United States: a review. JAMA Oncol. 2017;4(2):241–7.
20. Cheng T, Zhang G. Worldwide research productivity in the field of rheumatology from 1996 to 2010: a bibliometric analysis. Rheumatology. 2013;52(9):1630–4.
21. Li Q, Jiang Y, Zhang M. National representation in the emergency medicine literature: a bibliometric analysis of highly cited journals. Am J Emerg Med. 2012;30(8):1530–4.
22. Zhang WJ, Ding W, Jiang H, Zhang YF, Zhang JL. National representation in the plastic and reconstructive surgery literature: a bibliometric analysis of highly cited journals. Ann Plast Surg. 2013;70(2):231–4.
23. Liang Z, Luo X, Gong F, Bao H, Qian H, Jia Z, et al. Worldwide research productivity in the field of arthroscopy: a bibliometric analysis. Arthroscopy. 2015;31(8):1452–7.
24. Luo X, Liang Z, Gong F, Bao H, Huang L, Jia Z. Worldwide productivity in the field of foot and ankle research from 2009-2013: a bibliometric analysis of highly cited journals. J Foot Ankle Res. 2015;8:12.
25. Sweileh WM, Shraim NY, Al-Jabi SW, Sawalha AF, Rahhal B, Khayyat RA, et al. Assessing worldwide research activity on probiotics in pediatrics using Scopus database: 1994-2014. World Allergy Organ J. 2016;9:25.
26. Zhao X, Ye R, Zhao L, Lin Y, Huang W, He X, et al. Worldwide research productivity in the field of endocrinology and metabolism–a bibliometric analysis. Endokrynologia Polska. 2015;66(5):434–42.
27. Sweileh WM, Shraim NY, Zyoud SH, Al-Jabi SW. Worldwide research productivity on tramadol: a bibliometric analysis. SpringerPlus. 2016;5(1):1108.
28. Oklahoma State University. Article Types and indentification: Trade Publications [Internet]. Oklahoma: Oklahoma State University, Library; 2016 [cited 2017 Sep 23]. [Available from: info.library.okstate.edu/c.php?g=151701&p=998800.
29. Wei M, Wang W, Zhuang Y. Worldwide research productivity in the field of spine surgery: a 10-year bibliometric analysis. Eur Spine J. 2016;25(4):976–82.
30. Rein P, Mueller RB. Treatment with biologicals in rheumatoid arthritis: an overview. Rheumatol Ther. 2017;4(2):247–61.
31. Schulz M, Bonig H. Update on biosimilars of granulocyte colony-stimulating factor - when no news is good news. Curr Opin Hematol. 2016;23(1):61–6.
32. McKeage K. A review of CT-P13: an infliximab biosimilar. BioDrugs. 2014; 28(3):313–21.
33. Becciolini A, Raimondo MG, Crotti C, Agape E, Biggioggero M, Favalli EG. A review of the literature analyzing benefits and concerns of infliximab biosimilar CT-P13 for the treatment of rheumatologic diseases: focus on interchangeability. Drug Des, Dev Ther. 2017;11:1969–78.
34. Eleryan MG, Akhiyat S, Rengifo-Pardo M, Ehrlich A. Biosimilars: potential implications for clinicians. Clin Cosmet Investig Dermatol. 2016;9:135–42.
35. van Overbeeke E, De Beleyr B, de Hoon J, Westhovens R, Huys I. Perception of originator biologics and Biosimilars: a survey among Belgian rheumatoid arthritis patients and rheumatologists. BioDrugs. 2017;31(5):447–59.
36. Gyawali B. Biosimilars in oncology: everybody agrees but nobody uses? Recenti Prog Med. 2017;108(4):172–4.
37. Wang Y, Wang Q, Wei X, Shao J, Zhao J, Zhang Z, et al. Global scientific trends on exosome research during 2007-2016: a bibliometric analysis. Oncotarget. 2017;8(29):48460–70.
38. Sullivan PM, DiGrazia LM. Analytic characterization of biosimilars. Am J Health Syst. 2017;74(8):568–79.
39. Farhat F, Torres A, Park W, de Lima LG, Mudad R, Ikpeazu C, et al. The concept of Biosimilars: from characterization to evolution-a narrative review. Oncologist. 2017;22:1–7.
40. Garcia R, Araujo DV. The regulation of Biosimilars in Latin America. Curr Rheumatol Rep. 2016;18(3):16.

Evaluating inter-rater reliability of indicators to assess performance of medicines management in health facilities in Uganda

Belinda Blick[1], Stella Nakabugo[1], Laura F. Garabedian[2], Morries Seru[3] and Birna Trap[1*]

Abstract

Background: To build capacity in medicines management, the Uganda Ministry of Health introduced a nationwide supervision, performance assessment and recognition strategy (SPARS) in 2012. Medicines management supervisors (MMS) assess performance using 25 indicators to identify problems, focus supervision, and monitor improvement in medicines stock and storage management, ordering and reporting, and prescribing and dispensing. Although the indicators are well-recognized and used internationally, little was known about the reliability of these indicators. An initial assessment of inter-rater reliability (IRR), which measures agreement among raters (i.e., MMS), showed poor IRR; subsequently, we implemented efforts to improve IRR. The aim of this study was to assess IRR for SPARS indicators at two subsequent time points to determine whether IRR increased following efforts to improve reproducibility.

Methods: IRR was assessed in 2011 and again after efforts to improve IRR in 2012 and 2013. Efforts included targeted training, providing detailed guidelines and job aids, and refining indicator definitions and response categories. In the assessments, teams of three MMS measured 24 SPARS indicators in 26 facilities. We calculated IRR as a team agreement score (i.e., percent of the MMS teams in which all three MMS had the same score). Two sample tests for proportions were used to compare IRR scores for each indicator, domain, and overall for the initial assessment and the following two assessments. We also compared the IRR scores for indicators classified as simple (binary) versus complex (multi-component). Logistic regression was used to identify supervisor group characteristics associated with domain-specific and overall IRR scores.

Results: Initially only five (21%) indicators had acceptable reproducibility, defined as an IRR score ≥ 75%. At the initial assessment, prescribing quality indicators had the lowest and stock management indicators had the highest IRR. By the third IRR assessment, 12 (50%) indicators had acceptable reproducibility, and the overall IRR score improved from 57% to 72%. The IRR of simple indicators was consistently higher than that of complex indicators in the three assessment periods. We found no correlation between IRR scores and MMS experience or professional background.

Conclusions: Assessments of indicator reproducibility are needed to improve IRR. Using simple indicators is recommended.

Keywords: Data reproducibility, Inter-rater reliability, IRR, Medicines management indicators, Data quality audit, Performance assessment quality, Simple indicators, Complex indicators

* Correspondence: birna.trap@gmail.com
[1]Management Sciences for Health, Plot 15, Princess Anne Drive, Bugolobi, P.O. Box 71419, Kampala, Uganda
Full list of author information is available at the end of the article

Background

Like many other developing countries, Uganda faces serious financial and human resource constraints in the health sector [1]. For every 100,000 citizens, there are only 1.6 pharmacists; only 8% of public sector pharmacist posts and 61% of pharmacy technician posts were filled in 2013/14 [2]. Because of the inadequate number of pharmacy professionals, health workers from different cadres are often called on to perform tasks related to medicines management in their facilities despite their lack of appropriate training [2]. This results in problems that negatively affect service delivery (e.g., drug stock-outs) and waste limited resources through inappropriate management. Surveys in public sector facilities depict a challenging environment; in 2010, less than 10% of facilities had all six vital tracer medicines available, no facilities had correctly filled stock cards, and only 1% of facilities provided the correct treatment for a simple cough and cold [3, 4]. The Ministry of Health's traditional approach of providing short training courses to address the knowledge and skills gap in medicines management has not produced significant or sustainable improvements [3, 5].

Using multi-pronged approaches to build capacity and change behaviors has proven to be more effective compared to single approaches [6, 7], and in 2012, following pilot results, Uganda's Ministry of Health introduced a new national multi-pronged approach to build health worker capacity—the supervision, performance assessment and recognition strategy (SPARS). SPARS combines supervision—in the form of "supportive supervision"—with performance assessment to identify problem areas, guide supervision, and track improvements. A recognition strategy rewards good performance. Selected district health facility staff members trained as medicines management supervisors (MMS) are tasked to build capacity at health facilities by implementing SPARS [8].

The MMS assess medicines management performance in five SPARS domains: 1) stock management, 2) storage management, 3) dispensing, 4) prescribing, and 5) ordering and reporting quality. They use a standardized indicator-based assessment tool that includes 25 indicators. The SPARS indicators in the five domains are listed in Table 1. As part of their training, the MMS receive an orientation on how to use the tool that includes the indicators' background and purpose; data sources and data collection method; and indicator calculation, analysis, and interpretation. MMS gather indicator data during each supervisory visit by interviewing exiting patients, observing health workers' practices, and auditing records; the data gathering method used depends on the indicator. They receive netbooks and internet modems to facilitate data entry, analysis, and reporting [8].

The SPARS facility assessment data are reported upward to district health offices and national program managers through a computerized national pharmaceutical management information system. High-performing health facilities, district health officers, and MMS are recognized with rewards such as mobile phone air and modem time, T-shirts, tea, calendars, soap, branded wall clocks, and mugs. Since SPARS started piloting at the end of 2010, MMS have submitted more than 12,000 SPARS facility reports. Using medicines management performance data, managers can identify problems more quickly and make data-informed decisions. Facilities supervised to date have documented improvements in medicines management [9].

Many indicators have been developed to assess various aspects of medicines management and pharmaceutical sector performance, and country programs use indicators to identify problems and monitor progress [10, 11]. Too often, however, programs apply well-known and well-tested indicators, such as the World Health Organization rational drug use indicators, without assessing the quality of data or indicator reproducibility or investing the time and effort needed to assure that the standards of data collection and interpretation are met [10, 12, 13].

To ensure data quality and reproducibility of indicator-based tools, it is important that the data collector has enough training and practice to develop a sufficient understanding of what the indicators are measuring and how to use them [10, 14, 15]. Data reliability is a critical issue, especially when data are used to make program and policy decisions. Suggested strategies to improve data quality include inter-rater reliability (IRR) assessments that measure agreement among independent raters about their rating of a characteristic or behavior plus efforts to improve IRR, if it is insufficient [16–18].

From the outset, the Ministry of Health's Pharmacy Department prioritized efforts to assure data reliability, because the SPARS data would be used to make programmatic and policy decisions for the sector. The Ministry of Health uses the SPARS facility scores to implement a performance and certification program; therefore, it is critically important that the SPARS scores are reliable and independent of the rater (MMS) assessing the performance.

As part of the development of the SPARS facility assessment tool, we carried out a small exploratory study in July 2011 to assess IRR of the SPARS indicators. The low IRR scores in this initial assessment led to targeted efforts to increase IRR. The research question for the current study was to assess IRR for SPARS indicators and to evaluate if targeted interventions improved inter-rater reliability. The study objectives were to assess IRR for 24 SPARS indicators collected by well-trained MMS at three different time points and to examine whether IRR increased after efforts to improve reproducibility,

Table 1 List of the 25 SPARS indicators by the five domains

Dispensing quality	Description
1. Dispensing time*	Measures active/interactive dispensing time for 6 patients. Excludes any interruptions and time spent on communication unrelated to the patient condition or medication
2. Packaging material	Measures availability of appropriate dispensing materials like envelopes for solid dosage forms and bottles for liquid dosage forms. Paper cones and reused bottles were considered inappropriate
3. Dispensing equipment	Measures availability of dispensing equipment for both liquid and solid dosage forms like spoon, spatula, measuring cylinder, tablet counting tray to ensure that tablets are not counted by bare hands
4. Services available at the dispensing area	Measures access to privacy, chairs and benches, hand washing facilities at the facility and drinking water for patients within the dispensing area
5. Patient care*	Measures discrepancy between dispensed and prescribed medications and adequacy of information provided to patients at dispensing (dose, frequency, duration, why to take and other information required for adherence to medication)
6. Labeling*	Measures adequacy of information on the label (medicines name, strength, quantity, date, dose, name of patient and facility)
7. Rationing of antibiotics	Measures the practice of rationing antibiotics when in short supply. Antibiotic quantities prescribed and dispensed for 5 patients are compared to establish rationing, using amoxicillin and cotrimoxazole as examples
Prescribing quality	Description
8. Correct use of prescription recording system	Measures appropriate recording of 10 prescriptions dispensed (date, OPD/IP number, diagnosis, medicine and prescribers' name, quantity of medicine prescribed and dispensed)
9. Rational prescribing*	This standard World Health Organization indicator measures appropriate prescribing medicines in 20 prescriptions, assessing average number of medicines prescribed per patient, percent of products prescribed as generics, percent of prescriptions containing antibiotics, percent of prescriptions containing injections, and percent of prescriptions with diagnosis recorded
10. Adherence to STG for diarrhoea	Measures adherence to STG for non-bloody diarrhoea treatment. Appropriate treatment is ORS and zinc only
11. Adherence to STG for common cough/cold (simple respiratory tract infection)	Measures adherence to STG for cough/ cold. Appropriate treatment is optional antipyretic/ analgesic without use of antibiotics
12. Adherence to STG for malaria	Measures adherence to STG for treatment of non-complicated malaria. Appropriate treatment with antimalarials only should always follow a positive test
Stock management	Description
13. Availability of stock card	Measures availability of stock cards based on basket of 15 stock items
14. Correct filling of stock card	Measures correct filling of stock cards (medicines name, strength, dosage form, average monthly consumption, special storage conditions)
15. Does physical count agree with recorded stock card balance	Measures whether stock balance according to stock card agrees with counted physical stock
16. Stock book** correctly used	Measures correct use of stock book (all column information is appropriately filled and calculated, including average monthly consumption and quantity to order)
Storage management	Description
17. Cleanliness of the pharmacy	Measures cleanliness of the dispensary and main store (floor, wall, shelves and medicines are checked)
18. Hygiene of the pharmacy	Measures availability, functionality, and hygiene of designated sanitary facilities for dispensary staff (toilet, toilet paper, hand washing and soap).
19. System for storage of medicines and supplies	Measures if medicines in the facility are stored on shelves/cupboards in an appropriate and systematic manner and the shelves are labelled
20. Storage conditions (main store)	Measures appropriate physical storage conditions and steps taken to assure quality and safety of medicines in storage (sign of pest, protection from light, temperature monitoring and regulation, roof condition, storage space, lockable storage, fire safety equipment, cold storage, separate storing of medicines/vaccines appropriately in refrigerator, recording temperature in refrigerator)
21. Storage practices of medicines in pharmacy (stores & dispensary)	Measures adherence to good storage practices (incorrect storage on the floor, expired items recorded and stored separately, FEFO, opened bottles labelled with opening date, and lids on all containers)
Ordering and reporting	Description

Table 1 List of the 25 SPARS indicators by the five domains *(Continued)*

Dispensing quality	Description
22. Reorder level calculation	Measures ability of the facility to correctly calculate reorder quantity
23. Timeliness of order & distribution***	Measures adherence to order and delivery schedules (only applicable for higher level facilities)
24. Accuracy of HMIS reports	Measures if the health facility staff update the HMIS 105 report with accurate information on medicines availability during the previous month from stock management records. Stock card and HMIS 105 information are compared for consistency for a basket of 6 EMHS.
25. Filing	Measures appropriate filing of previous orders, delivery notes and discrepancy reports

Notes: OPD=outpatient department; IP=inpatient; ORS=oral rehydration solution; STG=standard treatment guidelines; FEFO=First expiry first out; HMIS=Health Management Information System; EMHS=essential medicines and health supplies
*World Health Organization indicators or sub indicators; **Stock book summarize in one line the monthly transactions from the stock card ***Excluded from assessment

which included revisions of the tool, development of guidelines, and additional MMS training.

Methods

MMS selection

To assess IRR, we used teams composed of three MMS each. The MMS who participated in the IRR assessments were randomly selected from the pool of all active MMS at the time of the study. In the first assessment, 54 MMS were active, which increased to 151 by the second assessment, and 224 by the third assessment. The active MMS were grouped into "experienced" or "less experienced" based on the number of SPARS facility assessments that the MMS had completed prior to the IRR assessment. At the initial assessment, the threshold for MMS to be considered experienced was seven or more SPARS facility assessments; this threshold increased to ≥12 visits in the following two assessments because MMS had more time to complete additional visits and thereby gain experience. In all three assessments, the MMS were randomly selected from the two different experience groups to make up rater teams with two experienced MMS and one less-experienced MMS. The initial assessment included only two rater teams, which increased to 10 rater teams per assessment in the second and third assessments. A total of 66 MMS participated.

The three IRR assessments

The initial IRR assessment in July 2011 was conducted to determine baseline IRR. The second (March–June 2012) and third (February–April 2013) IRR assessments were specifically designed and carried out to evaluate whether the revision of the tool, new guidelines, and additional MMS training had contributed to improved IRR scores. In the initial assessment, the two MMS teams each assessed three facilities (six facilities total). In the two following assessments, the 10 teams each assessed two facilities, and each facility was assessed by two teams, totaling 26 facilities in all three assessments (Table 2).

We selected the facilities purposefully to consider accessibility from the facilities the MMS had planned to supervise. The initial baseline assessment included two higher level facilities. The next two assessments only included lower level facilities, which are higher in number (93%) and only have one medicine store, making it faster to collect data for stock management indicators.

Data collection

When the MMS team visited a facility, each team member independently collected the data needed and scored the SPARS indicators using the standardized SPARS data collection tool and method (Additional files 1 and 2). One SPARS indicator (#23) was excluded from the assessment because it only applied to higher-level facilities. A study investigator oversaw each assessment to ensure that the MMS did not communicate with each other during the SPARS data collection. The investigator did not influence or interfere in the data collection. We recorded the characteristics of MMS teams to explore possible relationships of IRR scores and rater team composition, including gender, profession, and experience.

The MMS did not receive additional training or orientation on the purpose of the study prior to the IRR assessment. For SPARS indicators that required record sampling (e.g., outpatient register records and dispensing log), the investigator pre-selected the records to be used by all team members. Patient exit interviews were conducted with the same patient; one MMS conducted the interview, but all MMS recorded their assessments independently. MMS assessed dispensing time for the same patients, but individually. In the stores, MMS observed the storage conditions and collected stock management and ordering and reporting information individually as per their basic MMS training.

Once each MMS independently completed the assessment at the health facility using the SPARS tool, the study investigator collected the tools and compiled the scores from each MMS for each indicator in an Excel spreadsheet. For the purpose of the IRR analysis, we classified the 24 SPARS indicators into two groups based on their complexity (Table 3). *Simple* indicators are

Table 2 Summary of efforts to improve reproducibility and IRR assessments

Efforts flow	Timing	Number of MMS rater teams (total # of MMS)	# IRR facility assessments by each team	Total # of IRR assessments	# facilities by level of care (High/Low)
IRR assessment: 1	Jul 2011	2 (6)	3	6	2 High, 4 Low
Effort: 1	Jan 2012	All MMS receive effort 1			
IRR assessment: 2	Mar-Jun 2012	10 (30)	2	20	10 Low
Effort 2	Sep 2012	All MMS receive effort 2			
IRR assessment: 3	Feb-Apr 2013	10 (30)	2	20	10 Low
Total	Jul 2011-Apr 2013	22 (66)	Not applicable	46	2 High, 24 Low

those that require binary yes or no answers, and *complex* indicators are composites with sub-indicators that require sampling and calculations.

Scoring

We looked at the SPARS scores to assess agreement across the three-person team (i.e., team agreement score) to calculate an IRR score for each indicator. We used a slightly different approach to assess team agreement score depending on the type of indicator:

- For yes or no responses, the team agreement score was 100% if all the three MMS agreed; otherwise, it was 0% [18].
- In a continuous scale, a team agreement score of 100% was given if all three MMS had a SPARS score within +/− 10% of the median value for the group. If not, the team agreement score was 0%.
- For the indicator *dispensing time*, a team agreement score of 100% was given if all three MMS assessed the average dispensing time for the patients within +/− 15 s of the median value for the group. If not, the IRR score was 0%.

For indicators that had sub-questions or sub-indicators, the team agreement score was separately assessed for each sub-question and then averaged across the sub-questions for that indicator. We calculated the average percentage agreement across all MMS teams to measure the IRR for an indicator (i.e., the proportion of teams that scored 100%). An illustration of the IRR score calculation for indicators, sub-indicators, and domains is provided (Additional file 3).

Table 3 Classification of SPARS indicators by complexity

Simple indicators (13/24)	Complex indicators (11/24)
2. Packaging material	1. Dispensing time
3. Dispensing equipment	5. Patient care
4. Services available at dispensing areas	6. Labelling
7. Rationing of antibiotics	8. Correct use of prescription recording system
13. Availability of stock card	9. Rational prescribing
14. Correct filling of stock card	10. Adherence to STG for diarrhea
16. Stock book correctly used	11. Adherence to STG for cough/cold
17. Pharmacy cleanliness	12. Adherence to STG for malaria
18. Pharmacy hygiene	15. Physical count agrees with stock card balance
19. Storage system for medicines and supplies	22. Reorder level calculation
20. Storage conditions	24. Accuracy of HMIS reports
21. Storage practices in store and dispensary	
25. Filing	

Inter-rater reliability was deemed “acceptable” if the IRR score was ≥75%, following a rule of thumb for acceptable reliability [19]. IRR scores between 50% and < 75% were considered to be moderately acceptable and those < 50% were considered to be unacceptable in this analysis.

Statistical analysis

For each of the three IRR assessment periods, we calculated the average IRR for each of the 24 indicators, indicator category (simple or complex), the five SPARS domains and overall SPARS score and compared the IRR scores of the three IRR assessment periods using a two-sample test for proportions.

To determine whether there was an association between MMS group characteristics and SPARS reliability, we used logistic regression to estimate the odds ratio and the 95% CI associated with having a score of ≥75% for each SPARS domain by MMS team composition type. The MMS team composition characteristics that we assessed were gender (i.e., number of males on the team), profession, and experience based on the average number of SPARS visits carried out by the team prior to the IRR assessment. All these analyses were conducted using STATA, Version 13 and Excel 2007.

Efforts to improve measurement reliability

Prior to making SPARS a national strategy, we piloted the performance assessment tool with simple instructions over 12 months and made several adjustments during that time. In 2010 the tool was finalized for national rollout and became the basis for the MMS two-week classroom training and five-day practical training.

In July 2011, we carried out the first exploratory IRR assessment, and although the sample was small, the findings led to the development of training programs to increase IRR scores (Table 2). We then applied interventions that are proven to be effective in increasing reliability [20]. To increase IRR by reducing errors in measurement procedures and interpretation, we developed guidelines, refined indicator wording and definitions in the tool to increase clarity, and re-trained MMS in the problematic indicators identified by the IRR assessments (< 75% IRR score).

Starting in January 2012, detailed data collection guidelines were developed to supplement the simple instructions. We now included in the data collection tool descriptive information on each indicator that had been highlighted during training, including information on the background, purpose, and operational definitions of indicators, and guidelines on methods to collect, analyze, and interpret data. Some indicator response categories were simplified to make MMS assessment more straightforward; for example, *cleanliness of dispensary and main store* was revised from the possible response categories—*very clean/tidy (score 1), acceptable clean/tidy (score 0.5),* and *not clean/untidy (score 0),* to only two categories: *clean/tidy (score 1)* and *not clean/untidy (score 0).* For other indicators, MMS were given examples of what they should look for in their assessment, for example for *presence of pests in the store,* we advised them to check for wasp nests, cobwebs on the ceilings, termites along the walls, and small droppings of bats or rats. These efforts were followed by the second IRR assessment in March–June 2012 (Table 2).

In September 2012, we issued a second revision of the tool and guidelines that further clarified challenging indicators. The final SPARS data collection guidelines are provided in Additional file 2. After the introduction of the revised tool, all MMS attended a targeted two-day training course that focused on the problematic indicators and other frequent errors. We focused heavily on the complex indicators that involve several steps, including multiple calculations, to produce the SPARS indicator score and the correct use of zero and "not applicable" and how to address blank fields. To test individual MMS' understanding of the focus indicators, we incorporated practical exercises using multiple choice questions. An example of such an exercise is given in Fig. 1. The group would discuss the answers to achieve a common understanding.

We realized that MMS' calculation skills differed considerably because they come from diverse health-related professional backgrounds, and that we needed to consider this in the training design. Consequently, we added more test examples to give them ample practice. We refined the standard operating procedures for SPARS data management to clarify information on tracking facility visits, data cleaning, data security, and reporting. The September 2012 revision and training were followed by the third and final IRR assessment in February–April 2013 (Table 2). To reduce errors, we also shifted from a manual tool to an electronic tool that automatically calculates the scores for some of the indicators. However, the electronic SPARS data collection was not rolled out until December 2013, after the study period.

Ethical considerations

This study evaluated IRR of medicines management data as part of the national capacity-building strategy SPARS carried out by MMS under the Ministry of Health, Uganda. The study did not involve patients, human or personal health data, human tissue, or animals. Therefore, the study did not require ethical approval or a waiver. All observations and data collection were conducted with the permission of Ministry of Health, the District Health Officers, the facility in-charges, and the MMS.

The study constituted a Ministry of Health initiated data quality evaluation and is approved by the Ministry of Health.

Results

Table 4 presents the average IRR scores for the 24 indicators, the two indicator categories, the five domains, and overall scores from each of the three IRR assessments. The IRR scores for the rational drug use sub-indicators are presented in Additional file 4.

I. Overall IRR score (all 24 indicators)

The overall IRR score across all indicators improved from 57% in 2011 to 72% in 2013. The number of indicators with an acceptable IRR score (≥75%) increased from five indicators (21% of the 24 indicators) in 2011 to 12 indicators (50% of the indicators) in 2013.

Of the 24 indicators, the IRR scores of 17 (71%) improved between the initial and third assessments. The average IRR indicator improvement for the 17 indicators was 24 percentage points (range: 4%–68%). The IRR scores for seven indicators got worse between the first and third assessment with an average reduction of 11% points (range: – 2% to – 25%) (Table 4). The number of indicators with unacceptable IRR scores (i.e., IRR < 50%) fell from seven to only one following the two interventions (Fig. 2). Figure 3 depicts the IRR scores for each indicator presented by domains at the first and third assessments. Between the first and third assessment the IRR score ranges narrowed with more indicators having an IRR score of 75%, indicating improvement in reproducibility and data quality over the study period from 2011 to 2013.

II. IRR scores for indicator and domains

Dispensing quality

Two indicators in this domain, *packaging material* and *labelling,* had an acceptable IRR score of ≥75% at all three assessments. Three additional indicators had an

1. You are assessing if privacy can be observed during dispensing. Which situation(s) would you accept as privacy? More than one situation can be correct.

No	Situation	Correct 1(yes)/0 (no)
1	Distance to other patients is 2 meters and other patients cannot hear the conversation	1
2	Distance to the other patients is 1 meter	0
3	Other patients are behind a clearly marked line on the floor to create a significant gap	1
4	Medicines are dispensed from a separate room	1
5	Dispenser speaks softly and other patients cannot hear conversation	0
6	Dispenser is loud and other patients can hear conversation	0

2. You are assessing if labeling is done correctly and are specifically looking at the medicine name. What would you consider correct? There can be more than one correct answer.
   a. The generic name is written on the medicines
   b. Brand and generic names or generic alone are written on the dispensing envelope
   c. No name is indicated
   d. Medicine generic name appears by abbreviation
   e. Medicine brand name appears by abbreviation

Fig. 1 Example of SPARS indicator exercise from the MMS training

acceptable reproducibility score at the third intervention (not significant improvement): *dispensing equipment, services available at dispensing area,* and *no discrepancy between prescribed and dispensed medicine—cotrimoxazole/amoxicillin.* Two indicators, *dispensing time* and *patient care,* were below the acceptable reproducibility score by more than 10 percentage points at the final assessment. The overall IRR score for the dispensing domain at the third assessment was acceptable (76%).

Prescribing quality

Of the five indicators in this domain, only one, *rational prescribing,* had acceptable reproducibility at only the second assessment, after improving significantly from the first to second assessment ($p = 0.038$). Three indicators, *correct use of recording system, rational prescribing,* and *adherence to treatment guidelines for malaria,* improved considerably between the first and third assessments (not significant), but did not reach the acceptable reproducibility benchmark. Overall, the prescribing quality domain IRR score improved but remained not acceptable at the final assessment (64%).

Stock management

Three of the four indicators, *availability of stock card, agreement between stock card and physical count* and *stock book filled correctly,* had acceptable reproducibility scores at the third assessments, although the IRR for the latter two declined over time (not significant). One indicator, *availability of stock card,* improved significantly from the first to the third assessment ($p = 0.002$). *Correct filling of stock card* continued to be difficult to assess in a unified manner and had a low IRR score despite our efforts to improve IRR. Overall, however, the stock management domain IRR score was acceptable at the final assessment (76%).

Storage management

One indicator in this domain, *storage conditions,* had an acceptable reproducibility score at all three assessments. By the third assessment, two other indicators also achieved an acceptable reproducibility score: *hygiene of the pharmacy* and *systems of storage.* One indicator, *cleanliness of the pharmacy,* had the largest improvement between the first and third assessments (not significant) but with an IRR score far below the acceptable reproducibility threshold of ≥75%. The overall IRR score for the storage domain remained just below the acceptable threshold (73%).

Ordering and reporting

Of the three indicators in this domain, one—*reorder level calculation*—achieved an acceptable IRR score by the third assessment with a significant improvement between the first and third assessment ($p = 0.001$). *Accuracy of the health management information system (HMIS) report* declined from moderately acceptable reproducibility to unacceptable (not significant). The domain IRR score improved following the interventions, but remained just below the acceptable threshold of ≥75% (70%).

III. IRR scores for simple or complex indicator categories

In the initial assessment, neither of the two indicator categories, simple or complex, had an acceptable IRR score. IRR scores improved following two assessments for both categories, with the simple indicators improving by 15 percentage points between the initial and third assessments ($p = 0.475$) and complex indicators improving by 13 percentage points ($p = 0.558$).

Table 4 Average IRR scores (%) for 24 SPARS indicators and tests of change, by domain and indicator category

	Assessment			Assessments		
	1	2	3	1 to 2	2 to 3	1 to 3
Number of teams (facilities assessed by each team)	2 (3)	10 (2)	10 (2)			
Number of assessments	n=6	n=20	n=20	iwo sample test lor proportions		
Dispensing quality domain						
1. Dispensing time	67	55	60	0.602	0.749	0.757
2. Packaging material	83	100	100	0.060	-	0.060
3. Dispensing equipment	71	90	80	0.245	0.376	0.641
4. Services available at dispensing area	67	81	78	0.470	0.814	0.583
5. Patient care	37	72	64	0.117	0.588	0.240
6. Labeling	79	83	75	0.823	0.535	0.841
7. No discrepancy between prescribed and dispensed medicines cotrimoxazole/ amoxicillin- Rational prescribing	50	45	75	0.829	0.053	0.245
Dispensing quality domain	**65**	**75**	**76**	**0.630**	**0.941**	**0.593**
Prescribing quality domain						
8. Correct use of prescription recording system	33	65	70	0.164	0.736	0.102
9. Rational Prescribing	30	76	63	0.038	0.372	0.154
10. Adherence to standard treatment guidelines diarrhea	67	60	60	0.757	1.000	0.310
11. Adherence to standard treatment guidelines cough and cold	67	45	65	0.345	0.204	0.928
12. Adherence to standard treatment guidelines malaria	25	65	63	0.084	0.895	0.101
Prescribing quality domain	**44**	**62**	**64**	**0.434**	**0.896**	**0.382**
Sto ck management do main						
13. Availability of stock card/ledger book	17	55	85	0.102	0.038	0.002
14. Correct filling of stock card	50	50	55	1.000	0.752	0.829
15. Does physical count agree with stock card	100	75	90	0.173	0.212	0.420
16. Stock book correctly filled	100	95	75	0.576	0.077	0.173
Sto ck management do main	**67**	**69**	**76**	**0.926**	**0.62**	**0.66**
Storage management domain						
17. Cleanliness of the pharmacy	33	40	55	0.757	0.342	0.345
18. Hygiene of the pharmacy	57	77	75	0.337	0.882	0.395
19. System of storage of medicines and supplies	63	84	79	0.267	0.684	0.425
20. Storage conditions	79	88	88	0.578	1.000	0.578
21. Storage practices of medicines in pharmacy (stores and dispensary)	64	77	68	0.524	0.524	0.855
Storage management domain	**59**	**73**	**73**	**0.513**	**1.00**	**0.513**
Ordering and reporting domain						
22. Reorder level calculation	33	50	95	0.464	0.001	0.001
24. Accuracy of HMIS report	67	70	45	0.889	0.110	0.345
25. Filing	50	45	70	0.829	0.110	0.366
Ordering and reporting domain	**50**	**55**	**70**	**0.829**	**0.327**	**0.366**
Overall Score	**57**	**67**	**72**	**0.653**	**0.731**	**0.488**
Indicator categories						
Complex	**55**	**65**	**68**	**0.657**	**0.841**	**0.558**
Simple	**60**	**71**	**75**	**0.611**	**0.776**	**0.475**

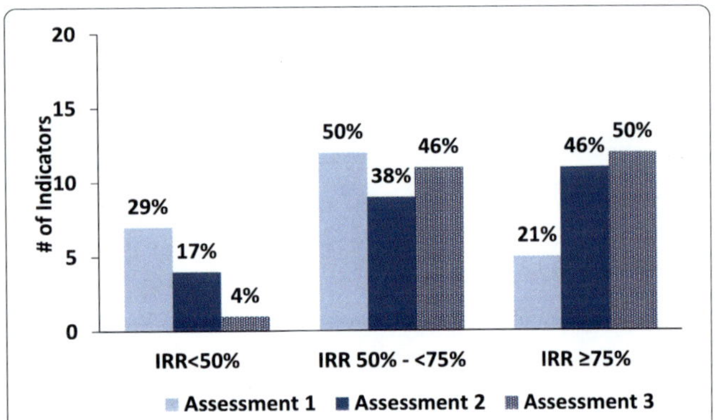

Fig. 2 Distribution of indicators by IRR score, at first, second, and third assessments

The complex category did not reach the ≥75% threshold of acceptable reproducibility by the third assessment, however, the simple indicator category just reached the 75% cut-off (Fig. 3).

IV. IRR scores and rater (MMS) team characteristics

We found no statistically significant relationship between the IRR scores and any of the characteristics of the MMS raters—gender, profession (e.g., clinical officer), or average number of prior SPARS supervisory visits completed (Additional file 5).

Discussion

This study measured IRR for the 24 SPARS medicines management indicators used to assess performance in the Ugandan pharmaceutical sector at three different time points and examined whether IRR increased after efforts to improve reproducibility. The SPARS data collection tool uses well-known indicators, the tool was thoroughly piloted, and the MMS received three weeks of combined classroom and practical training. Despite this preparation, we found that initially the MMS' IRR scores for the medicines management indicators in the SPARS assessment was poor; only five of the 24 indicators achieved an acceptable IRR of ≥75%. Our findings highlight the fact that IRR must be considered when designing indicator-based assessments, even when using well-known and globally recognized indicators and extensively trained data collectors.

Pharmaceutical sector indicators that assess rational drug use and supply chain performance are used to guide policies and system change [10, 11, 14]. These indicators are widely accepted as an objective and standard measure of rational use of medicines and medicines management and have been used in more than 30 mainly developing countries [21]. However, very few programs make the effort to assess the temporal and inter-rater reliability of the indicators they use. Therefore, little is known about the reproducibility of pharmaceutical sector indicators [13]. A systematic literature review of the use of medicine-related indicators in Southeast Asia found little information on validity, reliability, and feasibility of these indicators, especially those not promoted by World Health Organization [13]. The World Health Organization drug use indicators have been developed using appropriate methods, tested in numerous countries, applied in a standardized way in many studies and are widely

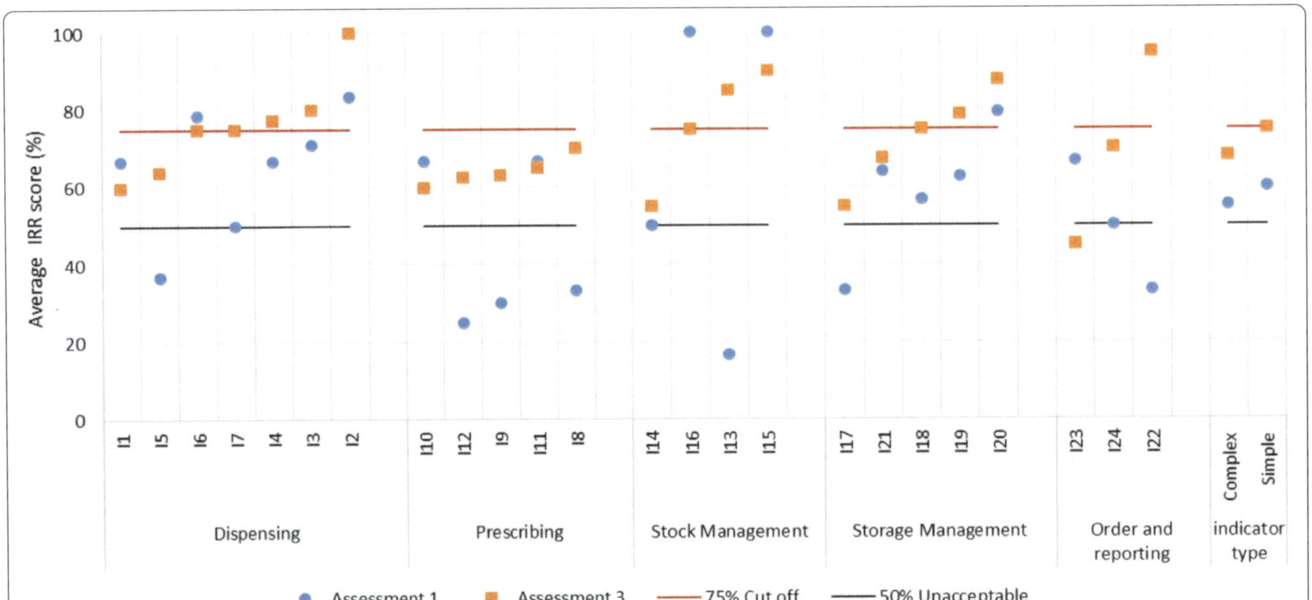

Fig. 3 Inter-rater reliability scores for 24 SPARS indicators and complex & simple indicator types at first and third assessments for 2011–2013. *Optimal IRR score is 100%, acceptable score of ≥75% marked with red line and 50% marked with black line

accepted [10, 13, 22, 23]. Nevertheless, we found that both World Health Organization and non- World Health Organization indicators had poor inter-rater reliability. Our study is one of the first that measures and documents the IRR of pharmaceutical and rational drug use indicators. Moreover, we suggest multi-pronged interventions to increase IRR of problematic pharmaceutical sector indicators.

This study suggests that focused and practical training and tailored instructions may improve IRR scores for pharmaceutical and medicines management indicators; at the final assessment half (12) of the 24 indicators achieved an acceptable ≥75% IRR and only one had an IRR of less than 50%. IRR of indicators in all five domains improved following the interventions, reaching acceptable or almost acceptable scores; only the prescribing quality domain indicators continued to have low IRR. Both the IRR and the effectiveness of our efforts to improve IRR depended greatly on the type of indicator. Not surprisingly, indicators that involve complex calculations, detailed sampling, and a high degree of judgement required the most effort to achieve acceptable reliability. Prescribing domain indicators are all complex indicators and have very specific data collection methods. The MMS were trained in sampling and the complicated calculations; however, correctly assessing these complex indicators remained a challenge for many MMS, even with extra attention. Therefore, although the domain had the highest improvement in IRR score overall, it remained the domain with the lowest reproducibility in scores.

Despite overall improvement, the IRR score did not improve for all SPARS indicators. IRR for two indicators decreased by over 20 percentage points: *stock book is filled in correctly* and *accuracy of the HMIS report*. At the time of the first assessment in 2011, most facilities had not yet received the new stock book, and the indicator could therefore only be scored "not applicable." Later when all the facilities received stock books, the MMS needed to know how to fill in the stock book correctly to assess the indicator, causing reproducibility to decline. Each facility reports data on a monthly basis into a centralized HMIS. The HMIS report includes data on availability of a selected basket of medicines and health supplies and patient attendance figures. A new HMIS form was introduced to the health facilities at the end of 2012. Assessing accuracy of the data reported in the new HMIS form is likely to have declined due to the introduction of the new HMIS form without related training for the MMS.

This study has multiple limitations. Although the overall IRR score increased over the three assessments, we cannot attribute the improvement to the revised tool and training because we did not use a controlled design; other changes, such as MMS gaining more experience over time, changes in the MMS used as raters, or changes in the sample of facilities assessed could have contributed to the improvement in the IRR scores. MMS experience increased across assessments as they made more visits, and the threshold for MMS to be considered experienced increased from ≥7 SPARS facility visits initially to ≥12 SPARS visits in the last two assessments. Though the composition of the assessment team remained consistent with one less experienced and two experienced MMS's, the number of visits that comprised the definition of "experienced" rose after the first assessment; therefore, the teams became more experienced overall. However, because we observed improvements in both the second and third assessment with same threshold for experience (≥12), the revised tool and training likely contributed to reproducibility improvements.

The study is also limited by the small number of observations in the initial assessment, which resulted in insufficient power to detect statistically significant differences between the three assessments. We included the initial findings because they demonstrated the need to improve IRR. We limited the later assessments to lower level facilities because they manage fewer pharmaceutical products than higher level facilities and have only one medicines storage area, which shortens the time MMS need to collect the SPARS data and allows more time for supportive supervision; lower level facilities also constitute 93% of all public sector health facilities.

We chose to measure IRR using percentage agreement instead of Fleiss kappa coefficient, which measures inter-rater agreement among three raters, because we did not have a sufficient number of facilities per MMS team to calculate kappa [18, 24]. Compared to other IRR methods, the percentage agreement approach tends to overestimate IRR due to chance agreement. However, our method was conservative, requiring agreement among three raters instead of the more commonly used agreement between two raters. Finally, we did not assess the validity of the indicators because we did not have a gold standard.

Measuring performance using the SPARS indicators has been proven to be feasible and useful to identify medicines management problems and to track the impact of SPARS in health facilities in Uganda. Uganda now has in place a strong capacity building strategy with indicators, training approaches, and data collection methods that ensure reproducible results for most of the indicators, not only for guiding the supervision and tracking improvements, but also for informing national pharmaceutical policy.

Conclusion

Health program managers must have access to reliable information to identify problems, monitor progress accurately, and make evidence-based decisions. Often such information is obtained through indicator-based tools, but the reliability of these indicators is unknown. By testing the IRR of the SPARS assessment indicators, we identified problems in how supervisors understood and calculated the indicators. Our study suggests that targeted and multi-pronged efforts including training, tool revisions, and repeated instructions can improve reproducibility of the SPARS indicator ratings. We now have a set of indicators with an average IRR score of 72%, just shy of the acceptable level, and three of five domains that achieved an acceptable IRR of ≥75%. We learned that, where possible, it is best to use simple binary indicators when designing an indicator-based assessment tool and that assessing and improving IRR should be an iterative process. Having uniform data reproducibility standards, assessment methods, and guidelines for best practices to evaluate IRR of indicators would make it easier for more programs in resource-limited countries to improve their data quality.

Additional files

Additional file 1: SPARS indicator based data collection and performance assessment tool dated January 2013. (PDF 964 kb)

Additional file 2: The final SPARS data collection guidelines October 2011. (PDF 246 kb)

Additional file 3: Illustrative example of IRR score calculation for SPARS indicators, sub-indicators, and domains across the rater teams. (PDF 99 kb)

Additional file 4: IRR score for the rational drug use sub indicators assessments 1–3. (PDF 502 kb)

Additional file 5: Relationship assessment using logistic regression between MMS group characteristics and domain score measures by IRR scores ≥75% categorized as acceptable. (PDF 321 kb)

Abbreviations

HMIS: Health management information system; IRR: Inter-rater reliability; MMS: Medicines management supervisors; SPARS: Supervision performance assessment and recognition strategy

Acknowledgements

This study was funded by the United States Agency for International Development (USAID). USAID did not have any role in the study design, data analysis, or writing of this paper or in the decision to submit the paper for publication. We thank the medicines management supervisors for their willingness to be part of the study and the district health officers and facility staff for participating in the study. We gratefully acknowledge the input of Dr. Dennis Ross-Degnan and Dr. Anita Katharina Wagner on earlier versions of the manuscript and Richard Musoke who contributed to the analysis of the data.

Funding

This study was funded by the United States Agency for International Development (USAID). USAID did not have any role in the study design, data analysis, or writing of this paper or in the decision to submit the paper for publication.

Authors' contributions

BB and BT conceived of, designed, and oversaw the study. They developed the study methods, oversaw and took part in the implementation, and drafted and edited the manuscript. SN contributed to developing the study methods, implementation, and article writing. MS contributed to the design, writing, and quality assurance. LG contributed to data analysis, interpretation, and writing of the manuscript. All authors read and approved the final version.

Competing interests

The authors declare that they have no competing interests.

Author details

[1]Management Sciences for Health, Plot 15, Princess Anne Drive, Bugolobi, P.O. Box 71419, Kampala, Uganda. [2]Harvard Pilgrim Health Care Institute, 401 Park Drive Suite 401,, Boston, MA 02215, USA. [3]Ministry of Health, Pharmacy, Division, Lourdel Road, Wandegeya, Kampala, Uganda.

References

1. Wane W, Martin GH. Education and health Services in Uganda - data for results and accountability. Serv Deliv Indic - Educ Heal. 2013;18:1–13. Report # 82666. http://hdl.handle.net/10986/16683.
2. Ministry of Health Uganda, "Annual Pharmaceutical Sector Performance Report 2013–2014," 2015. [internet]. 2015. [cited 2017 June 2]. Available from: http://www.health.go.ug/content/report-pharmacy
3. Ministry of Health Uganda, "Uganda Pharmaceutical sector report 2010," 2010. [internet]. 2010. [cited 2017 June 2]. Available from: http://library.health.go.ug/publications/medical-products-technologies/pharmaceuticals-and-drugs/uganda-pharmaceutical-sector
4. Ministry of Health Uganda, "Uganda Pharmaceutical sector report 2011," 2011. [internet]. 2011. [cited 2017 June 2]. Available from: http://health.go.ug/content/uganda-pharmaceutical-sector-report-2011
5. Ssengooba F, Rahman SA, Hongoro C, Rutebemberwa E, Mustafa A, Kielmann T, McPake B. Health sector reforms and human resources for health in Uganda and Bangladesh: mechanisms of effect. Hum Resour Health. 2007;5:3.
6. D. Ross-Degnan, R. Laing, B. Santoso, D. Ofori-Adjei, C. Lamoureux, and H. Hogerzeil, "Improving pharmaceutical use in primary care in developing counties: a critical review of experience and lack of experience.," 1997.
7. Rowe AK, De Savigny D, Lanata CF, Victora CG. How can we achieve and maintain high-quality performance of health workers in low-resource settings? Lancet. 2005;366(9490):1026–35.
8. Trap B, Ladwar DO, Oteba MO, Embrey M, Khalid M, Wagner AK. Article 1: supervision, performance assessment, and recognition strategy (SPARS) - a multipronged intervention strategy for strengthening medicines management in Uganda: method presentation and facility performance at baseline. J Pharm Policy Pract. 2016;9(1):1–15.
9. Ministry of Health Uganda, Pharmacy Department.Performance Report SPARS. 2015. [cited 2017 June 2]. Available from: http://health.go.ug/content/national-performance-report-medicines-management-july-september-2015
10. World Health Organization, "How to investigate drug use in health facilities," 1993. [internet]. 1993. [cited 2017 June 2]. Available from: http://apps.who.int/medicinedocs/en/d/Js2289e/
11. Hogerzeil H, Ross-Degnan D. Field tests for rational drug use in twelve (12) developing countries. Lancet. 1993;342:1408–10.
12. Rahbar MH, Gonzales NR, Ardjomand-Hessabi M, Tahanan A, Sline MR, Peng H, Pandurengan R, Vahidy FS, Tanksley JD, Delano AA, Malazarte RM, Choi EE, Savitz SI, Grotta JC. The University of Texas Houston Stroke Registry (UTHSR): implementation of enhanced data quality assurance procedures improves data quality. BMC Neurol. 2013;13(1):61.
13. Nguyen HT, Wirtz VJ, Haaijer-Ruskamp FM, Taxis K. Indicators of quality use of medicines in south-east Asian countries: a systematic review. Trop Med Int Heal. 2012;17(12):1552–66.

14. Management Sciences for Health, *MDS-3: Managing Access to Medicines and Health Technologies*. 2012. [internet]. 2012. [cited 2017 June 2]. Available from: http://apps.who.int/medicinedocs/documents/s19577en/s19577en.pdf
15. Suh S, Moreira P, Ly M. Improving quality of reproductive health care in Senegal through formative supervision: results from four districts. Hum Resour Health. 2007;5:26.
16. Kimaro H, Twaakyondo H. Analysing the hindrance to the use of information and technology for improving efficiency of health care delivery system in Tanzania. Tanzan Heal Res Bull. 2005;7(3):189–97.
17. Mphatswe W, Mate KS, Bennett B, Ngidi H, Reddy J, Barker PM, Rollins N. Improving public health information: a data quality intervention in KwaZulu-Natal, South Africa. Bull World Health Organ. 2012;90(3):176–82.
18. McHugh ML. Interrater reliability: the kappa statistic. Biochem Med. 2012; 22(3):276–82.
19. Norcini JJJ. Standards and reliability in evaluation: when rules of thumb don't apply. Acad Med. 1999;74(10):1088–90.
20. Forrester L, Collet JC, Pelude L, Henderson E, Vayalumkal J, Leduc S, Ghahreman S, Weir C, Gravel D. How reliable are national surveillance data? Findings from an audit of Canadian methicillin-resistant Staphylococcus aureus surveillance data. Am J Infect Control. 2012;40(2):102–7.
21. Laing R, Hogerzeil H, Ross-Degnan D. Ten recommendations to improve use of medicines in developing countries. Health Policy Plan. 2001;16(1):13–20.
22. P. Brudon, J. Rainhorn, and M. R. Reich, "Indicators for monitoring national drug policies a practical manual," 1999, no. 1.
23. World Health Organization. and DACP, "Using indicators to measure country pharmaceutical situations. Fact book on WHO level 1 and level II monitoring indicators," 2006. [internet]. 2006. [cited 2017 June 2]. Available from: http://www.who.int/medicines/publications/WHOTCM2006.2A.pdf
24. McQuillian S. Inter-rater reliability testing for utilization management staff. Managed Care. 2001;10(6):49–50. 53–59

19

Assessment of primary labeling of medicines manufactured by Nepalese pharmaceutical industries

Ramesh Sharma Poudel[1*], Shakti Shrestha[2], Santosh Thapa[3], Bhupendra Kumar Poudel[4] and Muniraj Chhetri[5]

Abstract

Background: Appropriate labeling of marketed medicines is necessary to fulfill the regulatory provisions and ensure patient medication safety. This study aimed to assess the primary labeling of medicines manufactured and marketed by Nepalese pharmaceutical industries.

Methods: We assessed the primary labeling of all medicines available at the pharmacy of Chitwan Medical College Teaching Hospital (CMCTH), Chitwan, Nepal, between November 2017 to December 2017. Medicines were assessed as required by Drug Standard Regulation, 2043 (1986 AD) of Nepal. Appropriate classification of all the medicines and content of over-the-counter (OTC) medicines (where certain information should be in Nepali language) was also assessed. Descriptive statistics was performed.

Results: Seven hundred fifty-nine medicines manufactured by 37 Nepalese pharmaceutical industries were assessed. While all pharmaceutical products had the name of the drug (brand), only76.8% of them stated drug quantity. Almost all products were found to declare category of the drug, with only a few (4.1%) mentioning the sub-category. The system of medicine was stated in 9.9% of the products. Active ingredients and their quantity, manufacturer's information, serial number for the production of drug and the date of production, storing methods, and information on the quantity used were mentioned in almost all the products. Similarly, all the products had batch number and the date of expiry. But, 11% of the products lacked the name of pharmacopoeia to which the drug belongs and all the products lacked the serial number for establishment of pharmaceutical industry. Similarly, 5.3% of the products did not list their price, and 2.4% of prescription medicines lacked caution labeling. Unfortunately, the majority of the products (84.4%) did not provide the directions of use. Appropriate drug classification was found in 89.6% of products. None of the over-the-counter medicines totally adhered to the requirements for writing certain information in Nepali language.

Conclusions: Majority of the products did not meet the regulatory standards of primary labeling of Nepalese pharmaceutical products. This study highlights the necessities for improvement from all stakeholders.

Keywords: Counterfeit drug, Low-income countries, Labeling, Regulatory standard, Pharmaceutical industry, Nepal, Patient safety

* Correspondence: pharmacistsharma23@gmail.com
[1]Hospital Pharmacy, Chitwan Medical College Teaching Hospital, Bharatpur, Chitwan, Nepal
Full list of author information is available at the end of the article

Background

Labeling of medicines is a legislative requirement for conveying information about medicines to patients. It provides information on brand, type of drug enclosed within the packaging, strength and quantity of product, appropriate users, instructions, indications, contraindications and side-effects [1]. Therefore, appropriate labeling of medicines is crucial for ensuring patient medication safety, while its ambiguity is associated with administration errors due to incorrect interpretations of products [2]. It has been suggested that medication compliance, distinction, and their readability are affected by medicine labeling that includes design features such as signal word, color, format, wording, language etc. [3]. Evidences demonstrate that marketed pharmaceutical products have, at times, failed to meet the standard labeling requirements [4, 5]. Moreover, studies have also claimed that dispensed pharmaceutical medicines lacked the prescribed labeling requirements [6, 7]. As there are inadequacies in identification and reporting of such requirements in Nepal, Department of Drug Administration (DDA), which is the national medicine regulatory authority, should be more vigilant on such issues [8–10]. In Nepal, allopathic drugs are classified as "a", "b", or "c", with respective subcategories. Category "a" consists narcotic and poisonous drugs; category "b" consists antibiotics, hormones etc. that require a prescription for dispensing from pharmacies; and category "c" usually consists over-the-counter (OTC) drugs. It has been made obligatory by DDA for pharmaceutical companies to properly label their pharmaceutical products according to the provisions mentioned in Drug Standard Regulation, 2043 (1986 AD) of Nepal [11]. At times, inabilities to follow foreign-language labeling of OTC drugs have resulted in adverse outcomes [12]. To overcome this, DDA has mandated to mention at least name of the drug, directions of use, category/caution, price of the drug, date of production, batch number and expiry date of twenty category "c" medicines in Nepali language [13]. Still then, Nepalese pharmaceutical industries are striving harder to meet the regulatory requirements [14]. It has also been reported that the same generic medicine is placed in two different categories by different pharmaceutical industries [14]. However, the data on this issue is rare in literatures. Therefore, we aimed to assess the primary labeling of medicines manufactured and marketed by Nepalese pharmaceutical industries.

Methods

Primary labeling of medicines manufactured by Nepalese pharmaceutical industries was assessed between November to December 2017. Only the medicines available at CMCTH, a tertiary hospital located in Chitwan district, Nepal, was assessed. CMCTH was purposefully selected because its pharmacy dispenses most products manufactured by Nepalese Pharmaceutical industries. This hospital only practices allopathic medicines; hence this study only included such medicines. The primary labeling of marketed medicines was assessed as required by Drug Standard Regulation, 2043 (1986 AD) of Nepal [11]. The regulation states that the marketed medicines for human use should contain 16-points information in primary labeling that includes Drug name and quantity; Category and sub category of the drug; System of medicine; Name of active ingredient, quantity and the pharmacopoeia; Name of the drug production company, address and the country; Serial number for the establishment of drug industry; Serial number for the production of the drug; Batch number; Date of production; Date of expiry; Price; Storing methods (techniques) and management of the drug; Caution in Group "a" and "b" (may not be sold without the prescription of a registered medical practitioner); Quantity; Method of use; and additional information on External preparation (only for external use). The primary labeling should contain at least the name of the drug, method of use, category/caution, price, date of production, batch number, and date of expiry of 20 category "c" drugs in Nepali language [13]. A checklist was developed to assess these aforementioned requirements of primary labeling of all kinds of dosage forms. A market basket method (total collection of all available branded generic medicines) was used for sample collection. The appropriateness of classification was also assessed according to Drug Standard Regulation, 2043 (1986 AD) [11]. Descriptive statistics was performed using IBM SPSS version 20 (IBM Corporation, Armonk, NY, USA). The collected generic medicines were categoried according to therapeutic categories and expressed as frequency and percentage.

Results

This study assessed primary labeling of 759 medicines manufactured by 37 Nepalese pharmaceutical industries. The types of dosage forms assessed are depicted in Table 1.

Table 1 Type of dosage form assessed ($n = 759$)

*Dosage form	n(%)
Tablet and Capsule	617(81.3)
Oral Solution, Syrup, Suspension and Drop	65(8.6)
Ointment, Cream and Gel	40(5.3)
Injection	21(2.8)
Nasal Drop	5(0.7)
Eye and Ear Drop	4(0.5)
Mouth Gargle	3(0.4)
External solution and lotion	3(0.4)
Powder	1(0.1)

*Percentage do not add up to 100 due to single decimal place

Of 759 medicines, majority belongs to antimicrobial drugs (20.2%), followed by antihypertensive drugs (13. 6%) and vitamins and minerals (8.5%). Details about the therapeutic categories of drugs assessed during study were illustrated in Table 2.

Primary labeling of all pharmaceutical products had the name of the drug (brand); however, only over three-quarters of products had stated the quantity of the drug. Similarly, almost all the products declared the category of the drug while only a few products (4.1%) mentioned the sub-category. The system of medicines was stated in around one out of 10 products. Active ingredients and their quantity were mentioned in almost all products. But, 11% products lacked the name of pharmacopoeia belonging to the drug. None of the products mentioned serial number for establishment of pharmaceutical industry. Almost all products stated drug production company, address and country, serial number for production of drug, date of production, storing methods [but keep out of reach of children was not mentioned in 46(6%) products] and information on quantity used. Similarly, all products had the batch number and the date of expiry. However, five out of 100 products did not list their selling price. Few Group "a" and Group "b" products (2.4%) lacked caution labeling (not to be sold without the prescription of a registered medical practitioner). More importantly, approximately seven percentage of products were found to provide misleading information with respect to caution [example: stating 'not to be sold without the prescription of a registered medical practitioner' in case of OTC drugs (Group "c")]. Unfortunately, majority of products (84.4%) did not provide information on directions of use. The appropriate drug classification was found in 89.6% of products (Table 3).

Out of 88 OTC products studied, almost all mentioned the drug name and category of drug in Nepali language as provisioned in the DDA's requirements. As shown in Table 4, some information were not assessed because they were lacking. While a total of 18.2% OTC products stated directions of use, only 14.8% of products mentioned it in Nepali language. Most of the OTC products (84.1%) mentioned only necessary precautions in Nepali

Table 2 Classification of drugs based on therapeutic categories ($n = 759$)

Therapeutic Categories of Drugs	n(%)
Antidepressants	35(4.6)
Antidiabetics	58(7.6)
Antihypertensives	103(13.6)
Antimicrobials	153(20.2)
Lipid- lowering Drugs	23(3.0)
Hypnotics and sedatives	18(2.4)
Antipsychotics	15(2.0)
Corticosteroids	16(2.1)
Vitamins and minerals	65(8.5)
Anti-cold and Cough preparations	13(1.7)
Anticoagulants	5(0.7)
Analgesic, Anti-inflammatory Drugs and Antipyretics	55(7.2)
Antiepileptics	12(1.6)
H_1-antihistamines	32(4.2)
Proton-pump inhibitors	27(3.6)
Antiemetics	9(1.2)
Antispasmodics	15(2.0)
Bronchodilators and Anti-asthma Drugs	14(1.8)
Muscle relaxants	14(1.8)
Antigout Drugs	7(0.9)
Tropical Nasal Decongestants	5(0.7)
Miscellaneous	65(8.6)

Table 3 Information mentioned in primary labeling of medicines ($n = 759$)

Information	Categories	n(%)
Drug name (Brand)	Yes	759(100)
Drug quantity	Yes	583(76.8)
Category of drug	Yes	757(99.7)
Sub-category of drug	Yes	31(4.1)
System of medicine	Yes	75(9.9)
Active ingredient and quantity	Yes	758(99.9)
Pharmacopoeia	Yes	676(89.1)
Drug production company, address and country	Yes	758(99.9)
Serial number for establishment	Yes	0(0)
Serial number for production	Yes	757(99.7)
Batch number	Yes	759(100)
Date of production	Yes	752(99.1)
Date of expiry	Yes	759(100)
Price	Yes	719(94.7)
Storage	Yes	759(99.9)
*Caution in Group "a" and "b" (not to be sold without the prescription of a register medical practitioner)	Yes	588(77.5)
	No	18(2.4)
	Misleading information	52(6.9)
	Not applicable (Category c)	101(13.3)
Quantity to be used	Yes	743(97.9)
Method of use	Yes	116(15.3)
External preparation (only for external use) ($n = 55$)	Yes	54(98.2)
Appropriateness of drug category	Appropriate	680(89.6)
	Inappropriate	77(10.1)
	Unable to assess	2(0.3)

*Percentage do not add up to 100 due to single decimal

Table 4 Assessments of labeling of OTC (DDA listed) medicines where certain information required to write in Nepali language ($n = 88$)

Information	Categories	n(%)
Drug name (brand) in Nepali language	Yes	87 (98.9)
Method of use in Nepali language	Yes	13(14.8)
	No	3(3.4)
	Unable to assess	69(78.4)
Category of drug in Nepali language	Yes	85(96.6)
Precaution taken in Nepali language	Yes	74(84.1)
	No	13(14.8)
	Unable to assess	1(1.1)
*Price Nepali language	Yes	15(17.0)
	No	67(76.1)
	Unable to assess	6(6.8)
Date of production in Nepali language	Yes	14(15.9)
	No	73(83)
	Unable to assess	1(1.1)
Date of expiry in Nepali language	Yes	14(15.9)
Batch number in Nepali language	Yes	14(15.9)

*Percentage do not add up to 100 due to single decimal

language, but majority of them were found without batch number (84.1%), date of production (83%), date of expiry (84.1%) and price (76.1%) in Nepali language (Table 4).

Other labeling errors were also encountered during the assessment of primary labeling. This included duplication of same information in two products (0.3%), while sticker with new price by erasing original price, inappropriate dosage information, incorrect method of use, no printed information (except batch number, date of production, date of expiry and price), erasing of drug category with permanent marker, each of which were observed in different single product (0.1%).

Discussion

The pharmaceutical sector of Nepal continues to grow, with over 15,000 registered products, over 300 registered manufacturing facilities and over 16,000 pharmacy outlets. This growth demands additional human resources for the regulatory authority (DDA) to improve regulation and smooth functioning of the authority body [15]. As a consequence, the gap between regulatory provision and actual practice has been documented. [8–10]. To keep this in check, primary labeling of medicines should be assessed on a regular basis.

Studies have demonstrated that labeling and packaging are causal factors for medication errors [2, 16–18]. Therefore, appropriate labeling of marketed medicines is necessary for fulfilling the regulatory provision and ensuring patient medication safety [3]. As observed in this study, nearly a quarter of products were lacking information on quantity or strength of the drug. This might be due to difficulty in stating strength along with their brand name in those products containing multiple active ingredients. However, it was observed that almost all products had information on active ingredient(s) and respective quantity to communicate the composition of products. Majority of products had not mentioned subcategory of drugs on their labeling but mandatory presence of this information from the perspective of consumers still remains controversial. Similarly, most of the products were found to lack information on system of medicine they belong to. Practice of categorizing drugs as "a", "b" or "c" was observed. Pharmacopoeial standard of product, which essentially reflects standard of the product, [19] was missing in some of the labels. Perhaps, this issue should be of serious concern for stakeholders because this is considered important for drug safety and is of special concern for consumers. Drug Standard Regulation, 2043 (1986 AD) mentions that products need to have serial number for establishment of pharmaceutical industries [11]. This provision was found ignored on labelling of all medicines of all drug companies that were assessed. This might be because it is considered less relevant to patients and healthcare professionals. In this study, all products were observed to include storage information, except for 6% of them that did not have information regarding "keep out of reach of children". Study in Nigeria reported 89.6% pharmaceutical products had adequate storage instructions [5]. However, this study also included products other than requiring prescription (OTC, antiseptics, disinfectants, detergents, household items, insecticides and consumables). Similarly, majority of medicines stated caution (not be sold without the prescription of a registered medical practitioner) (77.5%) and quantity to be used (97.9%) in this study. Printed words were not always in red or orange, and some products were found to lack 'signal words' (e.g. caution, warning) in this study. Printing of such words in colors other than red or orange have been known to lower the perceived hazard and higher proportion of compliant behavior, with red conveying it the strongest [20]. Similarly, it has been demonstrated that the presence of a 'signal word' increases perceived product hazard compared to its absence [21]. During this study, we also observed caution mentioned in group 'c' drugs, which might be misleading. In Nigeria, a lower proportion of pharmaceutical products adequately mentioned warning and dosage instruction on the labeling of pharmaceutical products [5] but we argue that in Nepal products such as household items, insecticides, detergents and consumables do not come under Drug Act, which was included by this study. However, this study has performed a detail investigation on warning including exploration of first aid instructions as well as sign and symptoms of product toxicity and their treatment. Most of the products in this study had no directions of use, which is important to avoid medication errors [22], especially for modified-release products. For instance, labeling "swallow tablet as a whole without breaking or cursing" on controlled released tablets and "tablets should be chewed before swallowing" on chewable tablets are needed to ensure that patients use it in the intended manner. Studies in SriLanka [6] and Malaysia [7] have also reported insufficient labeling of dispensed medicines as required by the regulatory authorities. The study done in SriLanka used WHO manual for household survey, and included both Western and traditional medicine but did not evaluate repackaging by family members and their understanding of medication administration instruction [6]. Similarly, study in Malaysia used simulated client method to explore labeling requirement of dispensed medicine using a case of common cold but limits itself to single simulated case, observer bias and being a pilot study [7]. Therefore, improved assessment and monitoring of primary labeling of marketed medicines is a dire need.

Medication labeling is rarely available in languages other than English, placing patients with limited English proficiency at greater risk of misunderstanding medication instructions and warnings [23–26]. To overcome this, DDA has necessitated to write at least name of the drug, method of use, category/caution, price, date of production, batch number and date of expiry of 20 category "c" drugs in Nepali language. However, this study demonstrated that none of the products under study totally adhered to this requirement. Besides this, the print size of label was also very small to read. Studies have shown an association between the print sizes and medication errors [27, 28]. This might contribute to increased medication errors particularly by the elderly people. Therefore, pharmaceutical industries should consider the use of medium and large print to increase readability [28], at least for OTC medicines. Other alternative may be to include comprehensive, clear drug leaflets in individual packs of OTC medicines as they are frequently self-administered without consultation with healthcare professionals. Moreover, confusion between look-alike products can be reduced by using Tall man (capital) letters to write drug names [29]. In this study, labeling errors such as the use of sticker with new price to cover the original price, duplication of same information, and so on were also observed. Different countries have their own regulatory provisions for labeling of pharmaceuticals products, because of which, it was not completely compatible with labeling requirement of other countries [4]. Therefore, foreign manufacturers should also comply with labeling requirements before registration of their product in the country of their interest.

Issues on such labeling errors should be removed through strict assessment of medicine labeling by the DDA and also by stakeholders (Manufacturers, Importers and pharmacy outlets). To overcome this, DDA has implemented Drug administration and management system (DAMS) software and warranted all manufacturers to put detailed information of the products in the software before registration/renewal of their products. Additionally, some sort of hologram, for example, as issued by regulatory authority itself, can also be conceptualized to remove counterfeits related to labels.

This study is the first of its kind in Nepal that assessed the scenario of primary labeling inadequacy and suggests stakeholders to rectify them. This is also useful to identify counterfeit and falsified medicines from true ones, which is an overwhelming problem in Nepal. However, this study has certain limitations that should be taken into account while approaching its findings. Limited number of products from only one system of medicine and from single pharmacy outlet were assessed. Also, this study does not cover factors influencing primary labeling of medicine manufactured by Nepalese pharmaceutical industries.

The results of this study highlight the need for stringency in assessment and evaluation of labels of medicines prior to their approval. Further, the regulatory authority need to closely inspect those approved labels for compliance to the provisions during periodic inspections. The Nepalese pharmaceutical industries should also improve their labeling standards/requirements as a part of GMP compliance. Therefore, all stakeholders should take into consideration that improving labeling requirements will eventually improve patients' safety, products' quality and provides thorough information like usage and storage requirements.

Conclusions

The present study demonstrates a gap between regulatory provisions for primary labeling of Nepalese pharmaceutical products and their actual labeling in medicines. It highlights the need for continued monitoring, reassessment and improvement of labeling of pharmaceutical products manufactured by Nepalese pharmaceutical industries.

Abbreviations

CMCTH: Chitwan Medical College Teaching Hospital; DAMS: Drug administration and management system; DDA: Department of Drug Administration; OTC: Over-the-counter; SPSS: Statistical Package for social sciences

Acknowledgements

We are grateful to Mr. Bijaya Basyal, Pharmacist, hospital pharmacy, Chitwan Medical College for his help during data collection and Mr. Praves Lamichhane, Faculty of Science, The University of Sydney, Sydney, Australia, for English editing.

Authors' contributions
RSP is the principal investigator and conceived the study. All authors collaboratively designed the study. Data acquisition, analysis and interpretation were performed by RSP and SS. All authors contributed in manuscript writing. All authors read and approved the final manuscript.

Competing interests
The authors declare that they have no competing interests.

Author details
[1]Hospital Pharmacy, Chitwan Medical College Teaching Hospital, Bharatpur, Chitwan, Nepal. [2]Department of Pharmacy, Shree Medical and Technical College, Bharatpur, Chitwan, Nepal. [3]Hospital Pharmacy, Ashwins Medical College and Hospitals Pvt. Ltd, Lalitpur, Nepal. [4]Department of Drug Administration, Ministry of Health, Kathmandu, Nepal. [5]School of Public Health, Chitwan Medical College Teaching Hospital, Bharatpur, Chitwan, Nepal.

References

1. Moore S. Labelling and its role in pharmaceutical packaging. International Pharmaceutical Industry. 2012;4(3):114–8.
2. Guchelaar HJ, Kalmeijer MD, Jansen ME. Medication error due to ambiguous labelling of a commercial product. Pharm World Sci. 2004;26(1):10.
3. Hellier E, Edworthy J, Derbyshire N, Costello A. Considering the impact of medicine label design characteristics on patient safety. Ergonomics. 2006; 49(5–6):617–30.
4. Veronin M. Packaging and labeling of pharmaceutical products obtained from the internet. J Med Internet Res. 2011;13(1):e22.
5. Nonyelum SC, Nkem N, Ifeyinwa CN, Orisakwe OE. Safety warnings and first aid instructions on consumer and pharmaceutical products in Nigeria: has there been an improvement? J Pak Med Assoc. 2010;60(10):801–4.
6. Athuraliya N, Walkom EJ, Dharmaratne S, Robertson J. Assessing medication packaging and labelling appropriateness in Sri Lanka. J Pharmaceutical Policy Pract. 2016;9:38.
7. Neoh CF, Hassali MA, Shafie AA, Awaisu A, Tambyappa J. Compliance towards dispensed medication labelling standards: a sross-sectional study in the state of Penang, Malaysia. Curr Drug Saf. 2009;4(3):199–203.
8. Poudel A, Mohamed Ibrahim MI, Mishra P, Palaian S. Assessment of the availability and rationality of unregistered fixed dose drug combinations in Nepal: a multicenter cross sectional study. Glob Health Res Policy. 2017;2:14.
9. Poudel BK, Ishii I, Khakurel B. Assessment of regulatory compliance in selected pharmacy outlets of Nepal. J Pharm Health Serv Res. 2016;7(1):31–6.
10. Gyanwali P, Humagain BR, Aryal KK, Pandit A, Acharya T, Bista B, et al. Surveillance of quality of medicines available in the Nepalese market: A study from Kathmandu Valley. J Nepal Health Res Counc. 2015;13 (31):233–40.
11. Department of Drug Administration. Drugs Standard regulation, 2043(1986). http://www.dda.gov.np/content/drug-standard-regulation-2043. Assessed 12 Nov 2017.
12. Maciejewski CS. The dilemma over foreign-language labeling of over-the-counter drugs. J Leg Med. 1994;15(1):129–54.
13. Department of Drug Administration. Notice (151/073/74) (Nepali). Department of Drug Administration, Kathmandu, Nepal.
14. Khadka DB. News related to misclassification of drug by Nepalese Pharmaceutical industries (Nepali). http://swasthyakhabar.com/news-details/1321/2016-10-27. Assessed 12 Nov 2017.
15. World Health Organization, Regional Office for South East Asia. Medicines in health care delivery Nepal: Situational analysis 2014. http://www.searo.who.int/entity/medicines/nepal2014.pdf. Assessed 10 Dec 2017.
16. Orser B. Reducing medication errors. CMAJ. 2000;162(2):1150–1.
17. Brass EP, Weintraub M. Label development and the label comprehension study for over the counter drugs. Clin Pharmacol Ther. 2003;74(5):406–12.
18. Peterson GM, Wu MS, Beggin JK. Pharmacists' attitudes towards dispensing errors, their causes and prevention. J Clin Pharm Ther. 1999;24(1):57–71.
19. Wieniawski W. Role and functions of the international pharmacopoeia. Ann Ist Super Sanita. 1975;11(3–4):204–10.
20. Braun CC. Silver NC. Interaction of signal words and color on warning labels: differences in perceived hazard and behavioral compliance. Ergonomics 1995;38. 11:2207–20.
21. Wogalter MS, Jarrard SW, Simpson SN. Influence of warning label signal words on perceived hazard level. Hum Factors. 1994;36(3):547–56.
22. Aronson JK. Medication errors: what they are, how they happen, and how to avoid them. QJM. 2009;102(8):513–21.
23. Leyva M, Sharif I, Ozuah PO. Health literacy among Spanish-speaking Latino parents with limited English proficiency. Ambul Pediatr. 2005;5(1):56–9.
24. Bradshaw M, Tomany-Korman S, Flores G. Language barriers to prescriptions for patients with limited English proficiency: a survey of pharmacies. Pediatrics. 2007;120(2):e225–35.
25. Weiss L, Gany F, Rosenfeld P, Carrasquillo O, Sharif I, Behar E, et al. Access to multilingual medication instructions at new York City pharmacies. J Urban Health. 2007;84(6):742–54.
26. Sharif I, Lo S, Ozuah PO. Availability of Spanish prescription labels. J Health Care Poor Underserved. 2006;17(1):65–9.
27. Watanabe RK, Gilbreath K, Sakamoto CC. The ability of the geriatric population to read labels on over-the-counter medication containers. J Am Optom Assoc. 1994;65(1):32–7.
28. Wogalter MS, Vigilante WJ Jr. Effects of label format on knowledge acquisition and perceived readability by younger and older adults. Ergonomics. 2003;46(4):327–44.
29. Filik R, Purdy K, Gale A, Gerrett D. Drug name confusion: evaluating the effectiveness of capital (tall man) letters using eye movement data. Soc Sci Med. 2004;59:2597–601.

20

Regulatory requirements for the registration of generic medicines and format of drug dossiers: procedures in Sri Lanka in comparison with selected regulatory authorities

D. Thambavita*, P. Galappatthy and R. L. Jayakody

Abstract

Background: The regulatory requirements for approval of generic medicines and the format of compiling drug dossiers vary among regulatory authorities. The variation is particularly wide between High-income countries (HIC) and lower and middle-income countries (LMIC) with different regulatory frameworks. In this study, document requirements for approval of generic products, approval timelines, and consideration of bioequivalence and/or biowaiver data by Regulatory Authorities (RAs) of 10 selected jurisdictions was studied.

Methods: The guidelines and procedures from 5 purposively chosen RA of HIC and4 regional RAs relevant for Sri Lanka were compared with the Sri Lankan National Medicines Regulatory Authority (NMRA). Information available in the official websites of the selected RAs, published journal articles and via personal communication was collected in2016. Drug approval timelines achieved in Sri Lanka was obtained from data available from another study.

Results: Common technical dossier (CTD) format of the International Council on Harmonization (ICH) for registration of pharmaceuticals (ICH:CTD) or the Association of South East Asian Nations (ASEAN) CTD format (ACTD) was used by all RAs studied except Sri Lanka which use its own dossier format. Nine out of ten RAs studied request BE data or justification for not submitting BE data for generic medicines. Sri Lanka requested BE studies only for antimicrobials, antiepileptic drugs and narrow therapeutic index drugs. Biowaivers are allowed for Biopharmaceutics Classification System (BCS)-based Class 1drugs in Singapore and India. USA, EMA, Canada and South Korea allowed biowaiver for BCS Class1and Class 3drugs but Sri Lanka does not accept BW at present. Nine NMRAs out of the ten studied reported legislated timelines for approval of generic pharmaceuticals except Sri Lanka.

Conclusions: Streamlining the drug regulatory systems in LMIC such as Sri Lanka with that of HIC would facilitate an effective drug regulatory system based on reliance on decisions made by stringent regulatory authorities. Findings of this study encourage Sri Lanka to adopt a CTD format for regulatory submission of drug dossiers. Expanding the BE requirement drug list and accepting BCS-based biowaivers for BSC class 1 and 3 drugs during registration of generic drugs when it is scientifically justified is also recommended for Sri Lanka.

Keywords: Dossier, Generic drugs, Bioequivalence, Biowaiver, DRA process

* Correspondence: tmdhanusha@pharm.cmb.ac.lk; tmdhanusha@yahoo.com
Department of Pharmacology and Pharmacy, Faculty of Medicine, University of Colombo, Kynsey Road, Colombo 08, Sri Lanka

Background

The primary goal of a national medicine Regulatory Authority (RA) of a country is to approve efficacious, safe and quality drugs to the people of the country. The RAs meet two types of drugs, viz., new drugs (NDs) and generic or multisource medicines. With increasing use of generic medicines, a considerable amount of time of a RA would be spent on evaluating and approving generic medicines. Evaluation of the quality of the generic products becomes crucial for RAs of the lower and middle-income countries (LMIC). The situation becomes more complicated with biologics and bio-similar products, as they are not identical to innovator products. During the regulatory review process, the interchangeability of the generic product with the originator product was evaluated. Most RAs use bioequivalence (BE) data when evaluating their interchangeability [1–4]. BE is determined by administering the generic and a comparator medicine to a group of healthy volunteers and measurement of serial blood concentrations over a 24-h period. Most RAs recommend either the innovator product or an already approved brand-named product to use as the comparator product. As BE studies involve human volunteers and measurement of very low concentrations of the drug in blood they are very expensive to carry out. Moreover, the RAs will need to have experienced evaluators to evaluate BE data and to check their authenticity. To overcome some of these difficulties, the concept of biowaiver (BW) was introduced based on the Biopharmaceutics Classification System (BCS) of Active Pharmaceutical Ingredients (APIs) which can be applied for Immediate Release (IR) solid oral generic drug products. In BW studies, comparative dissolution testing is carried out between a comparator and generic product in 3 different pH media representing gastric, duodenal and intestinal pH. These in vitro BW studies are much cheaper to carry out when compared to the in vivo BE studies particularly for LMIC [5]. Therefore, most countries including the High Income Countries (HIC) are now resorting to accept BW data in place of BE data for selected drugs [4, 6–8]. Granting BW is based on the solubility and permeability of the API, and in vitro dissolution of the finished product. However, one of the challenges faced by RAs of LMIC is lack of properly trained, experienced technical staff to evaluate the BE/BW data, interpret and advice on the data. Thus, some RAs in LMIC have regulatory systems that rely on the review process already done by ICH member countries or ICH observer countries. This process would be easier if a common dossier format is used during regulatory submission. Another factor that is important to the industry is to know how quickly they can get the registration of their products. Thus, most RAs have published drug approval timelines in order to establish an efficient and transparent drug regulatory process in their countries. They revise these timelines based on past performance [9].

Sri Lanka is a LMIC in South Asian region and vast majority of the medicines used in the country are generic medicines. The medicines regulation in Sri Lanka underwent a major revision recently with the implementation of a new National Medicines Regulatory Authority Act of 2015 passed in parliament and the establishment of a new National Medicines Regulatory Authority (NMRA) in 2015 [10]. The NMRA replaced the Cosmetics Devices and Drugs Authority (CDDA) and the CDDA Act of 1982. Although the establishment of the NMRA is considered a significant improvement in medicines regulation in Sri Lanka, we believe that the medicines regulatory system in Sri Lanka could be further improved. In this background, this study was planned to study the generic medicines approval process in Sri Lanka, compared to the regulatory process used in purposively selected 9 other countries. The generic medicine approval process was compared on the use of a common technical dossier (CTD) and the acceptance of BE and BW data. In addition, the legislated timelines for registration, the target time lines and achieved time taken for both generic and new drug product approvals was studied across the selected RAs. We also planned to make recommendations to the Sri Lankan NMRA to improve its generic drug approval process based on our findings.

Methods

The purposively selected RAs for the study included those generally considered as 'stringent' regulatory authorities (SRAs) and the regional authorities that are relevant to Sri Lanka, from which it was possible to obtain data required from the official websites. The definition of 'stringent' used by the Global Fund was used in this study [11]. Accordingly, SRA means a regulatory authority which is (a) a member of the ICH or (b) an ICH Observer, being the European Free Trade Association (EFTA) as represented by Swiss Medic, Health Canada and World Health Organization (WHO) or (c) a regulatory authority associated with an ICH member through a legally binding mutual recognition agreement including Australia, Norway, and Iceland. Using this definition of SRAs, as all ICH member countries have similar or comparable generic medicine approval systems, three jurisdictions from ICH-member countries, one from ICH-observers and one from ICH-associate countries were selected as the five SRAs for the study. The international SRAs included were three ICH- members i.e. European Medicines Agency (EMA), United States Food and Drug Administration (US FDA) and Pharmaceuticals and Medical Devices Agency (PMDA) of Japan, one ICH-observer i.e. Health Canada (HC), and one ICH-associate i.e. the Therapeutics Goods Administration (TGA) of Australia. The four regional agencies selected were Central Drugs Standard Control Organization (CDSCO) of India, National Pharmaceutical Control Bureau (NPCB) of Malaysia, Health Sciences Authority (HSA) of Singapore and Food and Drug Administration of South Korea (KFDA). Requirements of these RAs were compared with the processes adopted by the NMRA of Sri Lanka.

Data were collected from July–December 2016 for the comparison study from the selected RAs. Data for the achieved drug approval time in Sri Lanka was obtained from data available from another study conducted by the authors from January to May 2014 [12]. The generic medicine approval process comparison was conducted through the information available on the official websites of the selected NMRAs and published articles in books and journals. Journal articles were searched using Google Scholar and PubMed. Recommended drug dossier format for regulatory submission of generic medicines, use of BE and BW data were compared in the websites of selected RAs and data available from published literature. Information about the NMRA, Sri Lanka was obtained through documents available with the officials of the NMRA. Legislated drug approval times and targeted drug approval times of these jurisdictions were obtained for both generic medicines and New Drug Application (NDA). Data on these drug approval times were obtained from the official websites and achieved drug approval times were obtained from published literature. As there were no mandated or targeted timelines available for Sri Lanka, achieved median drug approval time for Sri Lanka was calculated using unpublished primary data collected for another study conducted by the authors [13]. In that study on quality of registered amoxicillin products', data on 8 imported generic amoxicillin dossiers were audited based on 'clock- stop' method excluding client's time [14]. The approval time considered was from the date of submission of the dossier until the date of approval of the medicinal product. The Median time for generic medicine registration was calculated using the time taken for registering these generic dossiers of imported products of amoxicillin. For other RAs, the drug approval times reported in the official websites and literature were obtained and reported. Guidelines and regulations pertaining to drug approval were also obtained from the official websites of the selected jurisdictions.

Results

Definition of generic drugs used by RAs

Definition and subsequent explanations provided for 'generic medicine' by the selected RAs in their guidelines contained common criteria [7, 8, 10, 14–19] of active drug substance being qualitatively and quantitatively same with an already approved product, having the same or comparable dosage form, having the same route of administration, and demonstrating bioequivalence with a reference product.However, there were differences in consideration of salts or esters as the same active (or drug) substance, in the reference product. With regards to active pharmaceutical ingredient, USA, EU, Australia and Singapore accept different salts as the same active (or drug) substance, if it is the same active moiety in the reference product. However, Japan does not consider different salts as the same active substance.

Generic drug dossier format

Nine out of the ten RAs studied were using one of two common technical dossier (CTD) formats. Australia [20], Canada [21, 22], EU [23], India [24, 25], Japan [26], US [27] and South Korea [28] were using the ICH:CTD format. Association of Southeast Asian Nations (ASEAN) CTD format (ACTD) was used by Malaysia [29]. Singapore accepted dossiers in either formats [30]. Sri Lanka was using a format which it had developed based on the WHO recommendations for drug registration but not claimed to be either ICH:CTD or ACTD [31]. This drug dossier format used in Sri Lanka consisted of 79 criteria out of 126 recommended by the WHO [32]. ICH:CTD and ACTD formats are similar in many aspects as the ACTD format has been derived from ICH:CTD format. In the ICH: CTD format, information should be organized into 5 modules. The ACTD format consists of four parts which corresponds to modules 1, 3, 4 and 5 of the ICH: CTD format. ACTD format does not have a part corresponding to Module 2 of the ICH: CTD, which contains summaries of Modules 4 and 5. Data on animal and clinical studies and bioavailability studies are included in Modules 4 and 5 of ICH: CTD and in Parts III and IV of the ACTD format for innovator medicines. These are replaced by the bioequivalence data in generic drug dossiers. Of the 10 NMRAs studied, except Sri Lanka all other nine DRAs accept drug dossiers through either electronic version of the CTD format (eCTD), or data via e-Drug Service in South Korea (ezfiling) or electronic filing of the data submitted through hard copies in India.

Requirement of bioequivalence data

All the RAs except Sri Lanka used their own or adopted guidelines in establishing interchangeability of generic drugs but in Sri Lanka, there is no written BE guideline. Australia, EU, India and Canada required BE data at the time of registration for all solid oral dosage forms of generic drugs (Table 1). Therefore, for a drug to be qualified as a 'generic', it needed to demonstrate either in vivo or in vitro BE (for drugs for which BCS-based BW is accepted) with the originator product. Singapore requires BE for all prescription only medicines (PoMs) and Japan requires in vivo BE for first approval of all generic drugs. Australia requests BE or justification for not

Table 1 Bioequivalence data requirements and biowaiver data acceptance by the selected RAs

Jurisdiction	Bioequivalence data requirement	Biowaiver data acceptance
Australia	POM and for an identified list of OTC medicines.	BCS Class1drugs
Canada	Required for all solid oral generic drugs	BCS Class1 and Class 3 drugs [7]
EU	solid oral generic drugs	BCS Class1and Class 3 drugs [46]
India	solid oral generic drugs	BCS Class 1 drugs and Schedule Y drugs[a] and drug already approved for new claims, new indication, new dosage form/ new route of administration, modified release dosage form [25]
Japan	solid oral generic drugs. (In vivo BE is required for first approval of all generics).	Does not accept BCS-based biowaiver for first approval of generic drugs. Accepts dissolution studies[b] for minor changes in the formulation and the dose strength
Malaysia	solid oral generic drugs	BCS Class 1drugs. A list for which biowaiver can be considered is provided [16, 29]
Singapore	POM and for over the counter medicines not included in the list of medicines exempted from BE	BCS Class 1drugs and for additional strengths of the drug if doses are proportional [8]
South Korea	solid oral generic drugs	BCS Class 1 and Class 3drugs
Sri Lanka	antiepileptic, narrow therapeutic index drugs, sustained release products and antimicrobials (from 2014)	Does not accept BW data
USA	solid oral generic drugs	[c]BCSClass1and3drugs [6, 47, 48]

[a] New drugs which require human clinical pharmacology data for registration under the rules for Schedule Y of Drugs and Cosmetics rules of Central Drugs Standard Control Organization (CDSCO), India
[b] Multimedia dissolution tests
[c] For first time registration

submitting BE for all PoMs. For over the counter (OTC) medicines they have given a list of medicines not requiring BE. Since 2014 Sri Lanka requires BE data for antimicrobials, antiepileptic drugs and narrow therapeutic index drugs as per a circular issued by the NMRA. However, NMRA, has not given a definition that it uses for narrow therapeutic index drugs but the drugs that are generally considered to have a narrow therapeutic index as given in standard text books are considered under this category during their regulatory decisions on "case by case basis".

Requirement of biowaiver data

USA, Canada, EMA and South Korea accept BCS-based biowaiver for both BCS Class1and Class 3drugs. Australia, India, Malaysia, and Singapore accept BCS-based BW for BCS Class 1drugs (Table 1). Japan does not accept BCS-based BW when registering generic drugs for the first time. It accepts dissolution test results for minor changes in the formulation and the dose strength, which is allowed for all drugs. Sri Lanka does not have a policy on accepting BW.

Time taken for generic drug registration

Generic drug approval timelines identified and reported from the selected RAs are given in Table 2. Accordingly, 9 out of the 10 RAs studied had mandated drug approval timelines. Achieved times from studies were available only for Sri Lanka and Japan. According to the Melchior [33], in the USA, the target given for standard drug approval for 2010 was 10 months. The performance goal for both USA and Canada for the fiscal year 2010 was to act on 90% of the submission within 10 months [33, 34]. Australia has legislated timelines for drug approval within 40 working days (WD) commitment for informing acceptance or rejection for processing. The, legislated TGA commitment was 255 WD and it was being streamlined to have no more than 300 CD (10 months), including the sponsor time [33]. The 12 months drug approval time in Japan includes 1.5 months applicant response time and 2 months for Good Manufacturing Practices (GMP) inspection time [35]. In practice, the reported regulatory review time was 9 months excluding applicant time in the year 2013 in Japan [33]. Singapore and Malaysia conduct abridged drug dossier evaluation. In Singapore, the approval time for verification dossiers, which are already evaluated and approved by EMA, US FDA, Health Canada, TGA, and UK MHRA is only 60 WD for new drug applications or 120 WD for generic drug applications. According to the reported data, EU has a centralized drug evaluation process with EMA which has legislated timeline of 210 WD. (this is subjected to certain specific National Authority timelines within EU) [33] Malaysia takes 12 months for evaluation of hard copy submissions and 6 months for online submissions [33]. Sri Lanka did not have published legislated or targeted timelines for drug approval. Thus, the study conducted based on an audit of 8 generic dossiers

Table 2 Drug approval timelines of the selected NMRAs

Jurisdiction	Legislated drug approval time		Targeted drug approval time		Achieved drug approval time	Reference
	NDA [g] or NCE [h]	ANDA [i] or generic medicines	NDA or NCE [h]	ANDA [i] or generic medicines	ANDA [i] or generic medicines	
USA	6 months under priority review 10 months under standard review	180 WD	To act on 90% of the submissions within given time	To act on 90% of the submissions within given time		[33]
Australia	255 WD [c d]	175 WD [c d]				[49]
Canada	300 CD [a]	180 CD [a]	To act on 90% of the submissions within given time	To act on 90% of the submissions within given time		[50]
EU	210 WD [c] 150 WD [c] (accelerated assessment)					[51]
Japan	15.3 months	12 months [d]			9 months in the year 2013	[52]
India	180 days	120 days				[53]
Malaysia	245 WD [c d] (Full evaluation)	210 WD [c d] (Full evaluation) 116 WD [c d] (Abridge Single active ingredient) 136 WD [c d](Abridge two or more active ingredients)				[2]
Singapore	180 WD [c] (abridged evaluation) 270 WD [c] (full evaluation) 60 WD [c] (for verification dossiers)	240 WD [c] (abridge evaluation) 120 WD [c] (for verification dossiers)				[30]
Republic of Korea	30 days for INDs [e] 90 days when DMF [f] review is not included 120 days when DMF [f] review is included					[28]
Sri Lanka					90 days (generic medicine)	

[a] CD Calendar dates
[b] The performance goal for the year 2010 was to act 90% of this given timeline
[c] Working days
[d] including client time
[e] Investigational New Drug
[f] DMF: Drug Master File
[g] NDA- New Drug Application
[h] NCE- New Chemical Entity
[i] ANDA – Abbreviated New Drug Application

showed median time of 90 WD with the range of 7 to 379 WD for Sri Lanka.

Discussion

All selected RAs referred to pharmaceutical equivalents to describe term 'generic medicine' in their guidelines. Thus, pharmaceutical equivalents contain identical active drug ingredients which may also can be presented either in same salts or ester forms of the same therapeutic moiety. This definition was similar across the RAs studies except in Japan.

A CTD format was used by all RAs studied except Sri Lanka, when submitting generic drug dossiers for registration. Even though ICH countries initially worked on evaluation and registration of products containing NDAs and new biotechnological products in ICH countries, their guidelines now address quality of generic products [36]. Thus, later versions of ICH guidelines have influenced the generic drug manufacturers in other countries. Notwithstanding the difficulties of implementing highly technical scientific requirements which require considerable cost, there are other countries that have adopted the ICH guidelines [37]. This adoption has given wider acceptability to the ICH standards [37]. According to our study results, three out of four regional RAs selected for the study, i.e. India, South Korea and Singapore, use the ICH: CTD format. Two out of the ten RAs studied used the ACTD format for regulatory submission. ASEAN works on developing reference substances, guidelines and trade agreements with regards to pharmaceuticals in the ASEAN region [38, 39]. The ACTD format aims at establishing a common technical document to harmonize pharmaceutical product dossiers with the ICH [39]. As most of the LMIC in Asia get at least some of their drug products already registered in an ICH jurisdiction, a detailed review of efficacy and safety data is often not required. Further, a country like Sri Lanka can benefit from converting to a CTD format as this facilitates approval based on reliance of judgment made by a SRA.

The local dossier format currently used by the NMRA, Sri Lanka had been developed based on WHO technical guidance at its start in the 1970s [40]. No official updated guidance has been issued since then on the dossier format or other requirements such as BE. Hence the details of BE requirements have so far not been incorporated into it. However, the new NMRA Act of 2015 states that regulations may be made in respect of BE and BW data related to generic medicines submitted for evaluation [10]. Our findings encourage Sri Lanka to have regulations to be made on a CTD format for regulatory submission of drug dossiers. Results also indicate leading well-resourced agencies internationally and regionally facilitating electronic submission of drug dossiers.

Nine out of the ten RAs studied except Sri Lanka had guidelines on BE data requirements. Accordingly, BE data is a mandatory requirement particularly for all prescription only medicines during solid oral generic medicine registration. In vivo BE studies of generic medicines provide greater assurance of BA/BE and consistent therapeutic outcomes. However, BE requirement affects the product cost and timely availability of generic products. The BCS-based biowaiver for solid oral generic products exempts generic drugs belonging to certain BCS classes, from expensive and cumbersome in vivo BE studies. According to Davit et al., presently USA and EU waive in vivo BE for a different strength of BCSClass1 and Class 3drugs which are already approved by those jurisdictions [41]. It further highlights better harmonized BCS-based BW guidance among US FDA, EU and the WHO [41]. EU also considers BW for modified release dosage forms for which acceptable in vitro-in vivo correlation (*IVIVC*) is established [42]. Four RAs studied allow BW for both BCS Class 1 and Class 3 drugs, while five RAs studied allow BW only for BCS Class 1drugs. All RAs in their guidelines documents on application of BW have clearly stated that BW should not be allowed for narrow therapeutic range drugs. The study revealed that the NMRA of Sri Lanka presently does not have any guidelines on application and acceptance of BW. Although the definition of 'generic drug' indicates already proven bioequivalence with a reference product, in Sri Lanka according to the circulars issued only antibiotics, antiepileptic drugs and narrow therapeutic index drugs need to show evidence of bioequivalence. Careful control of the interchangeability of generic medicines is mandatory to have safe generic substitution. As Sri Lanka depends heavily on generic medicines, regulatory decisions are needed for the application of BCS-based biowaiver in establishing interchangeability and waiver of in vivo BE studies for generic medicines. Thus, if Sri Lanka can explicitly apply BCS-based BW it will particularly support the local pharmaceutical manufacturing industry in registering their generic pharmaceuticals by allowing demonstration of interchangeability using low cost BW studies. Furthermore, having guidelines for the industry will facilitate more transparent and effective regulatory system.

Generally, the approval process of a generic drug is considerably simpler and less time consuming compared to a NDA. The drug approval process could be a standard review or expedited review (may be differently named by different RAs). According to Kashyap et al., in the EU, generic drugs are mainly approved through a mutual recognition procedure which has a timeline of 390 days [43]. According to the results of our study nine out of the ten jurisdictions had mandated drug approval timelines. A comparison study on the regulatory review process across five regulatory agencies in the USA, Europe, Canada, Switzerland, and Australia reported overall approval time range across these jurisdictions, which ranged from 368 to 595 days including client times [44]. However, this comparison was conducted in 2007 and now the actual timelines of these jurisdictions may be different. NMRA Sri Lanka did not provide approval timelines. The median drug approval time reported as 3 months from Sri Lanka, was based on the results of an audit conducted on 8 generic drug dossiers. The NMRA of Sri Lanka has registered a considerable number of pharmaceutical products in the recent past [45]. The, the shorter drug approval times indicate expedited review coupled with non-requirement of BE data for most drugs during the generic drug approval in Sri Lanka. Having legislated or targeted drug approval timelines show the transparency in the regulatory process and it is a measure of regulatory efficiency. On the other hand, imposition of hard, legislated time targets could lead to decision errors due to hurried evaluation with adverse consequences. Therefore, instead of unrealistic timelines, it would be better to have performance based time targets for drug approval which would pave the way towards an efficient and timely drug approval process.

Although initial harmonization work was more with NDAs [9] more recent literature by Davit et al. discussed good convergence of US FDA, EU and WHO on BCS biowaiver criteria as applied to generic medicines [41]. Harmonization of the procedures and documentation improved the reliance on stringent regulatory systems. Having an effective drug regulatory system will pave the way towards mutual recognition of regulatory activities among RAs, which would ultimately help to ease the regulatory burden of jurisdictions with limited resource. Although this study highlighted the areas for improvement in generic drug registration process in Sri Lanka, the registration process of biologics, biosimilars, and NCE were not studied. Regulatory timeline was also obtained only for a limited number of generic products registered Sri Lanka. Therefore, further studies are needed to identify registration process for the other categories of medicines and the actual drug approval timelines for a larger number of dossiers submitted for registration in Sri Lanka.

Conclusion

This study evaluated the drug registration process and requirements for registration of generic medicines in Sri Lanka, a LMIC in South Asia, to provide recommendations to NMRA. Adopting a CTD format for regulatory submission and enabling electronic submission would facilitate regulatory review process by speedy review, easy communication with the applicant, reducing regulatory burden and also improving industry compliance. The list of medicines that require BE data needs expansion in Sri Lanka to ensure the quality of generic drugs registered. NMRA should also apply the concept of BCS-based BW for BCS Class 1 and Class 3 drugs when it is scientifically justified. Therefore, we recommend the NMRA Sri Lanka to adopt a CTD format for regulatory submission of drug dossiers, facilitate electronic submission, expand the list of drugs requiring BE and accept BCS based BW for BCS class 1 and 3 drugs when scientifically justified.

Abbreviations

ACTD: Association of Southeast Asian Nations' common technical dossier; API: Active pharmaceutical ingredient; ASEAN: Association of South East Asian Nations; BCS: Biopharmaceutics Classification System; BE: Bioequivalence; BW: Biowaiver; CD: Calendar days; CDDA: Cosmetics Devices and Drugs Authority; CDSCO: Central Drugs Standard Control Organization; CTD: Common technical dossier; eCTD: Electronic common technical dossier format; e-filing: Electronic filling; EMA: European Medicines Agency; EU: European Union; GMP: Good Manufacturing Practices; HC: Health Canada; HSA: Health Sciences Authority; ICH:CTD: International Council on Harmonisation of Technical Requirements for Registration of Pharmaceuticals for Human Use Common Technical Dossier format; IR: Immediate release; IVIVC: In vitro-in vivo correlation; KFDA: Korean Food and Drug Administration; NCE: New chemical entity; NDA: New Drug Application; NMRA: National Medicines Regulatory Authority; NMRAs: National Medicine Regulatory Authorities; NPCB: National Pharmaceutical Control Bureau; OTC: Over the counter; PMDA: Pharmaceuticals and Medical Devices Agency; POM: Prescription only medicines; RA: Regulatory Authority; SRAs: Stringent regulatory authorities; TGA: Therapeutics Goods Administration; USA: United States of America; USFDA: United States Food and Drug Administration; WD: Working days; WHO: World Health Organization

Acknowledgments

Authors wish to thank Research Writing Support Program (RWSP), Faculty of Medicine, University of Colombo, Sri Lanka, and Author AID at INASP for writing assistance.

Authors' contributions

PG and DT conceptualized the study. PG and RLJ contributed to the study design. DT carried out data collection and analysis. All authors contributed to interpretation of results. DT drafted the original manuscript. All the authors read, revised and approved the final manuscript.

Competing interests

The authors declare that they have no competing interests.

References

1. United States Food and Drug Administration. Guidance for industry ANDA submissions — content and format of abbreviated new drug applications, ed. Rockville, USA; 2014. p. 3.
2. National Pharmaceutical Control Bureau Malaysia, Drug registration guidance document. First ed. Selangor Darul Ehsan, Malaysia National Pharmaceutical Control Bureau Ministry of Health, Malaysia. 2014.https://www.pmda.go.jp/files/000204339.pdf. Accessed 15 Dec 2016.
3. World Health Organization. Guidelines on submission of documentation for a multisource (generic) finished product: general format: preparation of product dossiers in common technical document format. In: WHO expert committee on specifications for pharmaceutical preparations. Annex 5 (WHO technical report series, No. 961); 2011.
4. European Medicines Agency. Guideline on the investigation of bioequivalence secondary guideline on the investigation of bioequivalence. 2010. http://www.ema.europa.eu/docs/en_GB/document_library/Scientific_guideline/2010/01/WC500070039.pdf. Accessed 15 June 2015.
5. Polli JE. In vitro studies are sometimes better than conventional human pharmacokinetic in vivo studies in assessing bioequivalence of immediate-release solid oral dosage forms. AAPS J. 2008;10(2):289–99.
6. United States Food and Drug Administration. Guidance for industry: waiver of in vivo bioavailability and bioequivalence studies for immediate-release solid oral dosage forms based on a biopharmaceutics classification system. Rockville, USA; 2015.
7. Health Canada. Guidance document: biopharmaceutics classification system based biowaiver. Ottawa: Health Products and Food Branch, Health Canada; 2014. p. 12.
8. Health Sciences Authority Singapore. Guidance on medicinal product registration in Singapore. 2011. http://www.hsa.gov.sg/content/hsa/en.html. Accessed 1 June 2015.
9. Hill S, Johnson K. Emerging challenges and opportunities in drug registration and regulation in developing countries. Access to medicines. London: Fretwells Ltd; 2004. p. 47.
10. Cosmetics Devices and Drug Regulatory Authority. Legislation: National Medicines Regulatory Authority Act, no. 5 of 2015 Colombo, Sri Lanka; 2016. p. 98.
11. Fund TG. Quality assurance policy for pharmaceutical products. 2018. https://www.theglobalfund.org/media/5894/psm_qapharm_policy_en.pdf. Accessed 15 Feb 2018.
12. Thambawita D, Mannapperuma U, Galappatthy P, Dissanayeke S, Benaragama BVSH, Jayakody RL. Compliance of selected drug dossiers submitted for registration, as per drug regulatory authority requirements and WHO recommendations. Proceedings of international medical congress, Sri Lanka medical association 2015.
13. Wharf C. EMA procedural advice for users of the centralised procedure for generic/hybrid applications. 2016. http://www.ema.europa.eu/docs/en_GB/

document_library/Regulatory_and_procedural_guideline/2009/10/WC500004018.pdf. Accessed 2 Dec 2016.
14. United States Food and Drug Administration. What are generic drugs?. 2015. https://www.fda.gov/Drugs/ResourcesForYou/Consumers/BuyingUsingMedicineSafely/GenericDrugs/default.htm. Accesssed 01 July 2016.
15. European Medicines Agency. Generic medicines. 2012. http://www.ema.europa.eu/ema/index.jsp?curl=pages/special_topics/document_listing/document_listing_000335.jsp&mid=WC0b01ac0580514d5c. Accessed 15 July 2016.
16. Ministry of Health Malaysia. Guidance on Biopharmaceutics Classification System (BCS) based biowaiver. Malaysia: Ministry of Health Malaysia; 2013.
17. Pharmaceuticals and Medical Devices Agency Japan. Approval review of generic drugs in Japan. Second international generic drug regulators meeting. 2012. College Park, MD.
18. Ministry of Food and Drug Safety Republic of Korea. Approval process. 2016. https://www.mfds.go.kr/eng/index.do?nMenuCode=126. Accessed 10 July 2016.
19. Therapeutic Goods Administartion, Australia. Australian regulatory guideline for over-the-counter medicines. 2012.https://www.tga.gov.au/publication/australian-regulatory-guidelines-otc-medicines-argom. Accessed 2 Oct 2016.
20. Therapeutic Goods Administration. Common Technical Document (CTD). 2014. https://www.tga.gov.au/publication/common-technical-document-ctd. Accessed 2 Oct 2016.
21. Health Canada. Draft guidance for industry:preparation of comparative bioavailability information for drug submissions in the CTD format. 2011. http://www.hc-sc.gc.ca/dhp-mps/prodpharma/applic-demande/guide-ld/ctd/draft_ebauche_ctdbe-eng.php. Accessed 11 June 2016.
22. Health Canada. Release of Health Canada's revisions to "1.6 electronic review documents" in draft guidance for industry: preparation of new drug submissions in the CTD format. 2008. http://www.hc-sc.gc.ca/dhp-mps/prodpharma/applic-demande/guide-ld/ctd/notice_avis_ctd-eng.php. Accessed 15 June 2016.
23. European Medicines Agency. ICH topic M 4, common technical document for the registration of pharmaceuticals for human use –organisation CTD secondary ICH topic M 4, common technical document for the registration of pharmaceuticals for human use –organisation CTD. 2004. http://www.ema.europa.eu/docs/en_GB/document_library/Scientific_guideline/2009/09/WC500002721.pdf. Accessed 15 June 2016.
24. Central Drugs Standards Control Organization, India. Guidance for industry on submission of clinical trial application for evaluating safety and efficacy. In: Ministry of Health; 2005. p. 180.
25. Central Drugs Standard Control Organization India. Guidance for industry on preparation of common technical document for import/manufacture and marketing approval. New Delhi: Ministry of Health & Family Welfare Govt. of India; 2010. p. 110.
26. Pharmaceutical Medical Devices Agency Japan. CH-M4 CTD (common technical document). 2015. https://www.pmda.go.jp/int-activities/int-harmony/ich/0035.html. Accessed 10 Oct 2016.
27. United States Food and Drug Administration. Guidance for industry: M4: organization of the CTD.2015. http://www.fda.gov/downloads/drugs/guidancecomplianceregulatoryinformation/guidances/ucm073257.pdf. Accessed 10 Oct 2016.
28. Ministry of Food and Drug Safety Republic of Korea. Guide to drug approval system in Korea. 2017.http://www.masung.co.kr/bbs/board.php?bo_table=s03_01_eng&wr_id=1. Accessed 10 June 2017.
29. National Pharmaceutical Bureau Ministry of Health Malaysia. Generic products containing drug substances/active pharmaceutical ingredients (api) that may be considered for biowaiver. 2014. http://npra.moh.gov.my/images/Guidelines_Central/Guidelines_on_Bioequivalence_BE/Guidance-on-BCS-Based-Biowaiver.pdf. Accessed 7 June 2016.
30. Health Sciences Authority in Singapore. Guidance on medicinal product registration in Singapore. 2011. http://www.hsa.gov.sg/content/dam/HSA/HPRG/Western_Medicine/Overview_Framework_Policies/Guidelines_on_Drug_Registration/Updates%20for%20Guidance%20on%20Medicinal%20Product%20Regist. Accessed 15 June 2016.
31. Cosmetics Devices and Drugs Regulatory Authorty. Application Forms. Secondary Application Forms. http://nmra.gov.lk/index.php?option=com_content&view=article&id=86&Itemid=84&lang=en. Accessed 5 May 2014.
32. Thambavita D, Galappatthy P, Jayakody R. Requirement for bioequivalence and biowaiver data for regulatory decision making: a comparative study of regulatory authorities. Proceeding of the annual scientific session of the Sri Lanka Association of Clinical Pharmacology and Therapeutics Colombo, Sri Lanka: Sri Lanka Association of Clinical Pharmacology and Therapeutics. 2016. p. 24.
33. Melchior R. How transparent are regulatory agencies with regard to review timelines? A global review. Chicago: Thomson Reuters France; 2011.
34. United States Food and Drug Administration. FDA/GPhA quarterly meeting on GDUFA. 2015. http://www.fda.gov/downloads/drugs/developmentapprovalprocess/howdrugsaredevelopedandapproved/approvalapplications/abbreviatednewdrugapplicationandagenerics/ucm442070.pdf. Accessed 7 June 2016.
35. Kuribayashi R, Matsuhama M, Mikami K. Regulation of generic drugs in Japan: the current situation and future prospects. AAPS J. 2015;17(5):1312–6.
36. The International Council on Harmonisation of Technical Requirements for Registration of Pharmaceuticals for Human Use. Quality guidelines. 2015. http://www.ich.org/products/guidelines/quality/article/quality-guidelines.html. Accessed 10 Nov 2016.
37. World Health Organization. The impact of implementation of ICH guidelines in non-ICH countries. 2001. apps.who.int/medicinedocs/pdf/h2993e/h2993e.pdf. Accessed 2 Oct 2016.
38. Ratanawijitrasin S, Wondemagegnehu E. Effective drug regulation a multicountry study. Geneva: World Health Organization; 2002. p. 187.
39. Martin H. Harmonization and standardization of the ASEAN medical industry. Council, US-ASEAN business; 2010. p. 75.
40. World Health Organization. Marketing authorization of pharmaceutical products with special reference to multisource (generic) products: a manual for drug regulatory authorities. 2 ed. Geneva Switzerland; 2011. p. 148.
41. Davit BM, Kanfer I, Tsang YC, et al. BCS biowaivers: similarities and differences among EMA, FDA, and WHO requirements. AAPS J. 2016;18(3):612–8.
42. European Medicines Agency. Guideline on quality of oral modified release products. 2016. http://www.ema.europa.eu/docs/en_GB/document_library/Scientific_guideline/2014/07/WC500170465.pdf. Accessed 10 Oct 2016.
43. Kashyap UN, Gupta V, Raghunandan H. Comparison of drug approval process in United States & Europe. J Pharm Sci Res. 2013;5(6):131–6.
44. Hirako M, McAuslane N, Salek S, et al. A comparison of the drug review process at five international regulatory agencies. Drug Inf J. 2007;41(3):291–308.
45. Galappatthy P, Mythily S, Wickramarathna TN, et al. Availability, prices and registration status of the most commonly prescribed medicines in private pharmacies in Sri Lanka: an island wide survey. Proceedings of the Sri Lanka Association of Clinical Pharmacology and Therapeutics, vol. 31. Colombo: Sri Lanka Association of Clinical Pharmacology and Therapeutics; 2016.
46. The European Agency for the Evaluation of Medicinal Products Evaluation of Medicines for Human Use. Note for guidance on the investigation of bioavailability and bioequivalence. 2001. http://www.ema.europa.eu/docs/en_GB/document_library/Scientific_guideline/2009/09/WC500003008.pdf. Accessed 10 Oct 2016.
47. United States Food and Drug Administration. Guidance for industry- waiver of in vivo bioavailability and bioequivalence studies for immediate-release solid oral dosage forms based on a biopharmaceutics classification system. 2000. https://www.fda.gov/downloads/Drugs/Guidances/ucm070246.pdf. Accessed 20 Sept 2016.
48. United States Food and Drug Administration. CFR-code of Federal Regulations-Bioavailability and bioequivalence requirements. 2013. http://www.accessdata.fda.gov/scripts/cdrh/cfdocs/cfcfr/CFRSearch.cfm?CFRPart=320&showFR=1&subpartNode=21:5.0.1.1.7.2. Accesed 20 Sept 2016.
49. Anand K, Mallu UR, Kuraku M, et al. Pharmaceutical drug products approval procedure in Australia. Exp. 2013;11(3):690–705.
50. Health Canada. Guidance for industry-Management of Drug Submissions. In: Therapeutic products directorate. Ontario: Minister of Public Works and Government Services Canada; 2013. p. 46.
51. Agency EM. The centralised procedure at the EMA. Secondary the centralised procedure at the EMA. 2016. http://www.ema.europa.eu/docs/en_GB/document_library/Presentation/2016/02/WC500201043.pdf.
52. Pacific Bridge Medical. Pharmaceutical and API product registration in the other Asian countries. 2016. http://www.pacificbridgemedical.com/regulatory-services/pharmaceutical/product-registration/others/. Accessed 5 Dec 2016.
53. Central Drugs Standards Control Organization, India. CDSCO Timelines. 2014. http://www.cdsco.nic.in//writereaddata/upTimeline%20CDSCO.pdf.

A qualitative exploration of knowledge, attitudes and practices of hospital pharmacists towards adverse drug reaction reporting system in Lahore, Pakistan

Rabia Hussain[1*], Mohamed Azmi Hassali[1], Furqan Hashmi[2] and Maryam Farooqui[3]

Abstract

Background: Medication safety is a major public health concern and there are well established pharmacovigilance programmes in developed countries. However, there is scarcity of literature on the issue in low and middle income countries. In this context, the current study was aimed to evaluate the knowledge, attitudes and practices of hospital pharmacists towards medication safety and ADR reporting in Lahore, Pakistan.

Methods: A qualitative approach was used to conduct this study. A semi-structured interview guide was developed, 10 hospital pharmacists were recruited and interviewed through convenience sampling technique. All interviews were audio-taped, transcribed verbatim, and were then analyzed for thematic contents analysis.

Results: Thematic content analysis of the interviews resulted in 6 major themes, including (1) Familiarity with medication safety & adverse drug reaction concept (2) Current system of practice and reporting of adverse drug reaction in hospital setting, (3) Willingness to accept the practice change (4) Barriers to adverse drug reaction reporting, (5) Policy change needs and (6) The recognition of the role. Majority of the hospital pharmacists were familiar with the concept of medication safety and ADR reactions reporting however they were unaware of the existence of national ADR reporting system in Pakistan. Several barriers hindering ADR reporting were identified including lack of awareness and training, communication gap between the hospitals and regulatory authorities.

Conclusion: The study revealed that that hospital pharmacists were good in understanding of medication safety and ADR reporting; however they don't practice this in real sense. The readiness of the hospital pharmacist towards the practice change has indicated that they are all set to be actively involved in the provision of medication safety in hospital setting. Involvement of key stake holders from ministry of health, academia, pharmaceutical industry and healthcare professionals is warranted to promote safe and effective use of medicines.

Keywords: Adverse drug reaction, ADR reporting system, Pharmacovigilance, DRAP, Barriers, Hospital pharmacist, Medication safety

* Correspondence: rabia.hussain2010@gmail.com
[1]School of Pharmaceutical Sciences, Universiti Sains Malaysia, Penang, Malaysia
Full list of author information is available at the end of the article

Background

Adverse drug reactions (ADR) represent a significant patient safety concern after being recognized as major cause of morbidity and mortality in hospital admissions [1]. World Health Organization (WHO) defines an ADR as, "a response which is noxious and unintended, and which occurs at doses normally used in humans for the prophylaxis, diagnosis, or therapy of disease, or for the modification of physiological function" [2].

As real-life use of drug is enormously different from the controlled clinical trial due to various reasons. It does not cover the associated effects of drugs for a longer duration of time, a its not a representative of some other populations such as children, elderly and people with different sets of morbidities in those trials [3]. To overcome these problems, the post marketing surveillance is considered as the best tool to recognize the possible effects of a drug [3]. Post marketing surveillance comes under pharmacovigilance (PV) which according to WHO is "the science and activities relating to the detection, assessment, understanding and prevention of adverse effects or any other possible drug-related problems" [4].

WHO established its first pharmacovigilance center in Uppsala, Sweden after the Thalidomide tragedy in 1961 [5]. Now it has collaborating centers all around the world. A pharmacovigilance (PV) center collects reports on possible ADR to detect the ADRs in the post marketing phase [6]. This spontaneous reporting is considered as the most important feature of the system whereby the reports are submitted to the national reporting agency through the healthcare professionals and pharmaceutical manufacturers. These reports are then communicated to WHO pharmacovigilance center [7]. Suspected ADRs reports from member countries of the WHO Programme for International Drug Monitoring are sent to the WHO international database 'VigiBase', which is managed by the WHO Uppsala Monitoring Centre UMC. The reports are reviewed and analysed and the evidence based recommendations are forwarded to the member countries [8].

In UK, according to Yellow Card scheme [9], every year almost 17,000 ADR reports are reported and hospital pharmacists in UK are officially responsible to report ADRs [10]. In US, several major national programs are working on pharmacovigilance including MedWatch, Sentinel Events Reporting Program and Medication Error Reporting Program, whereby the reporting involve both healthcare professionals and public [10–13]. In Canada, Canadian Adverse Drug Reaction Monitoring Program regulates the pharmacovigilance activities and pharmacist are part of this program since its inception [10, 14]. The Centre for Adverse Drug Reactions Monitoring (CARM) monitors adverse drug reactions in New Zealand, and pharmacists are also a part of this programme [15]. In Netherlands, a spontaneous ADR reporting scheme was launched in the 1963, and since then pharmacists have been involved in reporting. ADR reports are submitted by doctors and pharmacists to the Netherlands Pharmacovigilance Centre, and out of these reports about 40% reporting is done by the pharmacists [16]. Contrary to this, ADR reporting is scant in many low and middle come countries and it has impact on use of medicines, patient safety and on policy and practice [17].

Adverse drug reaction monitoring in Pakistan

Pakistan is a lower middle-income country with a population of 207.8 million and ranked as the sixth most populous country in the world [18, 19]. In Pakistan, the healthcare system is comprised of three-tier structure, including primary, secondary and tertiary care [20]. Primary and secondary care centers cater the basic health needs of the population while tertiary care centers involve hospitals based modern facilities [20]. Most of the budget in Pakistan goes to tertiary health care centers [21] and the Ministry of National Health Services Regulation and Coordination (NHSRC) regulates the health system of the country [18].

There was no established pharmacovigilance system in the country until 2011, when a locally manufactured cardiac drug (Isotab 20 mg (Isosorbide mononitrate, batch number J093) caused death of more than 200 patients and hospitalization of 1000 patients in Lahore, Punjab [19, 22]. It turned out that the drug was adulterated and a serious error in quality assurance contributed to this incident [22]. As a result of this incident, Supreme court of Pakistan ordered the federal government to establish an independent drug regulatory authority [23]. To fulfill the order, in 2012, Drug Regulatory Authority of Pakistan (DRAP) was established under DRAP act 2012 [23]. Drug Regulatory Authority of Pakistan (DRAP) is one of the six divisions of Ministry of National Health Services, and Regulation (NHSRC) [23], which regulates the availability, quality, and safety of therapeutic goods including medical devices and medicines in the country [24]. After the establishment of DRAP things have started to get better, few hospitals in the country have pharmacovigilance in place, however overall the pharmacovigilance needs further improvement [25]. Drug Regulatory Authority of Pakistan (DRAP) in collaboration with international bodies including United States Pharmacopoeia and Promoting Quality Medicines (USP-PQM) has developed a framework to carry out post-marketing surveillance of drugs in Pakistan. Drug Regulatory Authority of Pakistan is also planning to obtain the membership of WHO Uppsala centre to access 'Vigiflow', Which is the global database system for pharmacovigilance reporting [26]. This access will help the medical professionals and drug regulators to stay updated with latest safety information about the drugs [27].

Punjab is the most populous province of the country comprising of half of the country's population of 110 million [28]. Lahore is the provincial capital (of the Punjab province) and has a population of over 10 million people [29]. The Punjab Government is the first provincial government to establish provincial office of the pharmacovigilance Centre at the Directorate General Health Services, Punjab [30, 31]. The provincial drug control unit Punjab (PDCUP) is setting up policies and procedures regarding the aspects related to the drug control, it is also publishing medicine safety alerts on regular basis, and since its operation to date total 91 medicine safety alerts have been published [32]. Irrespective of the fact that the data is being updated on regular basis, still the communication gap lies between drug regulatory authorities and the healthcare professionals.

Pharmacists world over are playing an important role to promote the safe use of medicines, however in Pakistan studies on medicines use and pharmacovigilance are scarce. In this context, the present study is being planned to investigate the knowledge, attitudes and practices of hospital pharmacists on Adverse Drug Reaction reporting in Lahore. The study will use qualitative methods to explore attitude, practices and will help to fill the gaps in the literature. The information obtained from this article would be helpful to plan interventions to improve medicines safety.

Methods

Study design

We adopted a qualitative approach (social sciences research methods technique) to collect the data [33]. We opted this design due to certain reasons as the design is flexible and it allows an in-depth understanding that further help in better understanding of participants' experiences and attitudes [34, 35]. Besides, the approach is helpful to generate a number of ideas that how individuals perceive the problem. In addition, qualitative research methods help to identify the gaps that cannot be otherwise identified by the survey based research methods [35, 36].

Study setting

The study setting was Lahore. As it is a metropolitan city of the province of the Punjab (Pakistan) [29]. It has a population of over 10 million and is also a hub for culture, business and healthcare facilities [29, 37].

Development of interview guide

Based on in depth review of literature [38–54] and current practices of hospital pharmacist in Pakistan, a semi structured interview guide was developed. The guide was designed in a way to explore the knowledge about medication safety and ADR reporting and its system. Perceptions and confidence about practice change and future interventions towards improvement in practices were also documented. Prior to data collection, the guide was tested for validity and reliability. The questionnaire was validated by two experienced academicians and researchers at the Universiti Sains Malaysia, Penang, Malaysia. Reliability of the study was assured by face to face interviews with the participants. The guide was piloted on 2 hospital pharmacists (who were excluded from the actual study). The guide was modified accordingly on the basis of pilot results. After obtaining the consent from the experts and interviewees, the interview guide was made available for the study (Appendix).

Respondents and inclusion criteria

Hospital pharmacists working in tertiary care public hospitals as a full time, regular employees were selected for interviews. Contract based hospital pharmacists or pharmacists working in primary or secondary care public or private hospitals were excluded from the study. The study was given the approval by Humans Ethics Committee (HEC), University College of Pharmacy, University of the Punjab, Lahore, Pakistan with reference no. HEC/PUCP/1943.

Sampling and data collection

Pharmacists in our study were purposively selected by using convenience sampling technique [55]. Prior to the participation in the interview, an explanatory statement detailing the objectives of the study was given to each hospital pharmacists and a written consent was obtained from them. Participant's personal information was collected by the self-administered questionnaire attached with the consent form. The interview was conducted by the principal author of this study. The principal author had training in conducting qualitative interviews. The interviews were conducted at a time and place convenient for the participating pharmacist, mostly at the work place of the participants.

The interviews were conducted in English as pharmacy graduates can speak the language and this is the medium of education in the country. Each interview session lasted for 30–40 min. To seek required information where necessary, appropriate probing questions were asked from the respondents and additional field notes were taken. The interviews were audio recorded and transcribed verbatim by the researcher (RH). Data saturation was achieved after 8th interview, however 2 additional interviews were conducted to see if new themes were emerging. The researcher manually analyzed the transcripts line by line for relevant themes and content. The transcripts were independently coded by two researchers (RH and AH). Coding was compared, and consensus was obtained by the co-authors in the study.

Results

Demographics of the participants

A total of 10 hospital pharmacists aged between 25 and 38 years were interviewed. There were 8 female participants and 2 male participants (in Pakistan, female hospitals pharmacists are in majority, they prefer to work in hospital-based setting). Majority of the participants ($n = 7$) were from the age group of 31–40. Six participants had an experience of 1–5 years, while four pharmacists had an experience of 10 or more years of service. Eight of the participants had specialization in their field as Masters or PhD, while two participants were graduates. The demographic distribution of the participants is described as below (Table 1):

Table 1 Demographics of the respondents

Characteristics	Frequency
Gender	
Male	2
Female	8
Age (Years)	
20–30	3
31–40	7
> 40	0
Education	
Graduation	2
Specialization	8
Experience (years)	
1–5	6
6–10	2
> 10	2
ADR reporting	
Yes	2
No	8

Thematic analysis

Thematic content analysis of the interview resulted in 6 major themes. These themes are listed as (1) Familiarity with medication safety & ADR concept (2) Current system of practice and reporting of ADR in the hospital setting (3) Willingness to accept the practice change, (4) Barriers to ADR reporting (5) Policy change needs and (6) Recognition of the role of pharmacists in the reporting.

Theme 1: Familiarity with medication safety and ADR concept

During the interviews, the respondents were asked about their knowledge on medication safety and ADR concept.

> *"Medication safety means that the medicine which you are giving to the patient, should be appropriate, right route of administration, right dose, and drug should be chosen in such a way that there will not be any harm to the patient." (HP-4)*

> *"To protect the patients from harm, from the adversities of the drug related products." (HP-7)*

When asked about the concept of ADR, most participants came up with the standard definition by WHO [1]. This showed that the participants had good knowledge about the ADR.

> *"Adverse drug reactions are the reactions that are abnormal, noxious and can cause life-threatening problems." (HP-1)*

> *"Effects come out which are not coming in a normal dose., allergic reaction due to some idiosyncrasy or something like that for the dose, that was not supposed to produce those effects, which might be due to individualized differences in metabolism...they just occur." (HP-5)*

> *"Any noxious, unintended drug reactions, which even occur at normal dose." (HP-6)*

The hospital pharmacists were also asked about the type of ADRs they will prefer to report and there was mixed response related to this question. Some participants emphasized that only *major* and *severe* ADRs can be reported because they thought that minor ADRs can be handled and they do not require reporting. While some described that even a minor ADR should be reported.

> *"Obviously major or moderate must be reported, minor can be tackled within the hospital." (HP-2)*

> *"Any suspected reactions should be reported, it can be a headache for one person, but for other person, it can be a severe thing." (HP-3)*

Theme 2: Current system of practice and reporting of ADR in hospital setting

The participants discussed about the current system of reporting of ADR in their work settings. The views by participants focused on the lack of interest of hospital administration in the hospital regarding practice of ADR reporting.

> *"Mainly, it's in my mind, because I never reported any ADR report on any form anywhere, its mainly in the conversation, technical discussions, have in meetings all the time instead of reporting. Because again it's not a requirement by the hospital." (HP 9)*

"If patient came with an ADR, then our special team for emergency cases deals with them, we are not involved as such. After the stabilization of patient, we get a report from the ward, then we look if it's a medication error or an adverse drug reaction, but no reporting as such on official basis." (HP 10)

Theme 3: Willingness to accept the practice change

All hospital pharmacists were positive towards improvement in medication safety related practices. They related the practice change with their job satisfaction and quality of life of the patients.

"I feel very positive and I think we should improve the practice and I am satisfied with my job as I am helping my patients." (HP 1)

"It must be patient oriented, we need a positive change regarding strict monitoring of patient related parameters. I think system will benefit the patient, our main goal is to achieve wellness of patients." (HP 2)

"Yes the quality of life of patients will be improved because on the basis of experience you can be more careful choosing the medicines, you have the information based on past experiences." (HP 4)

Theme 4: Training needed to improve ADR reporting

Majority of the hospital pharmacists had no formal training on ADR reporting, although they had basic knowledge during their undergraduate degree program, however there was no implementation in hospital setting. For the better delivery of healthcare services, the hospital pharmacists pointed out that there is a need of necessary training.

"We don't have proper knowledge, training, proper system, don't have access to published data. So, we need more training and awareness to understand what an adverse drug reaction can be.... there is a dire need to change the system." (HP 8)

"They must train a lot of people on their agendas and get the patient safety work done, new protocols must be designed based on international guidelines. A system that can be very vigilant and very aggressive one, I must say." (HP 9)

Theme 5: Barriers related to ADRs reporting

There were many barriers to under reporting of ADRs. Majority respondents stated that they did not report ADRs due to a number of issues including lack of knowledge and training, lack of time, lack of support from colleagues, lack of communication between healthcare professionals and the absence of a reporting mechanism.

"It is difficult actually, I cannot give much time and cannot see the patients individually....and hindrance comes from the attitudes of staff nurses, as they really do not inform pharmacist about any ADR plus there is no ADR reporting system and nobody is serious about that...so, it's difficult for me to report any ADR." (HP-1)

"The key barrier is actually the burden which is on every appointee pharmacist, since there are only a few people appointed by government sector. So, you know by the administration we are actually not prioritizing clinical pharmacy as a priority. This is the problem....it makes reporting difficult because of the burden, lack of training and lack of prioritization." (HP-9)

The participants further identified lack of encouragement, overly burdened staff, legal liability as a barrier to ADR reporting.

"Barriers are the lack of encouragement, unavailability of ADR reporting form, although individual efforts are there. Lack of time and training is there, legal matter can be involved in reporting an ADR." (HP-4)

A systematically functioning reporting system is absent, though the respondents had an idea that what and when to report but they had no idea where to report.

"I don't think so that there is some particular ADR reporting system. As we do not have any knowledge and also maybe there is a lack of interest by government that we are not aware about the existence of the ADR reporting system in Pakistan." (HP-1)

"In files there is a body, yes...DRAP... but in working, it's not functional as such. They have launched the ADR forms, but they have no mechanism to receive the reports and after receiving we don't know what they are doing with those reports." (HP-3)

"Being regulatory authority of Pakistan, they must have approached us, they must have trained us. We never received any email, training or even a circular." (HP 9)

It was interesting to note that the senior pharmacists and peers do not encourage reporting. This was reported as another barrier when pharmacists were interviewed.

"Honestly, pharmacist will never report ADR, because whenever I discuss with any senior about any ADR, they all replied to me the same, that...don't do this, this will blame your position, you will be blamed by hospital authority, and company leaders, so better to stay within your limits." (HP 7)

Theme 6: Recognition of the role as custodian of medicine safety

Majority of the hospital pharmacists were of the view that the healthcare system can be improved, if the role of pharmacist is recognized by the organization, thus medicine safety will be improved.

Participants also expressed their willingness to accept this role as in leadership capacity.

"So, in my opinion if role of pharmacist is implemented well then, no medicine related issue will be there because pharmacist can really take care of safety of medicines." (HP-1)

"I feel, it's now a need of healthcare team, that role of pharmacist should be considered as important. Because, once you are involved in healthcare team, you are at a good position and because you have a good knowledge of medicines right from the selection till the administration, so can advise healthcare team very well. So, I think now role is much more important and the responsibility level is also increased." (HP-4)

"I think pharmacist has a key role in enhancing medicine safety. So, pharmacist have to be visible, be with the medicines." (HP 7)

Discussion

The present study has revealed gaps in the ADR reporting in Pakistan. Though our respondents had a fair knowledge about medication safety and ADR reporting, however the majority were unaware about the existence of any such reporting mechanism in the country. This shows that the pharmacy curriculum is catering the needs of the undergraduate pharmacists to understand the issues. However, the necessary practical training to understand the ADR reporting was found deficient when it came to a practice. This lacking can be attributed by the traditional class room methodology, which is typically followed in Pakistani education system [56]. There is a need to train the pharmacy graduate in real setting by providing the opportunities like internships, trainings and seminars at undergraduate level. Moreover, WHO Uppsala Monitoring Centre (UMC) provides a number of web-based lectures, as well as it also offers distance learning course on signal detection and causality assessment on adverse drug reaction reporting for students as well as for healthcare professionals [17].

In our study we found that the hospitals have basic policies to report and monitor ADR reaction in the setting, but the practice varies from hospital to hospital. Looking at the Pakistani scenario, each provincial government is responsible for the regulation of healthcare facilities in their own province [57]. For example, hospitals in Punjab are regulated by health department, Government of Punjab and it is assumed that all of these hospitals are providing the uniform health care services to the population, however the situation in other provinces may be different [20]. In our study it was observed that the policy implementation related to ADR was not consistent, even within a single hospital, it was observed that different departments were implementing policies differently. As many of the hospitals even do not report a single case, others do report to the provincial health commission or even so to the national pharmacovigilance centre. It was also observed that many public hospitals are still unaware about this online portal and activities by DRAP. Although, The Drug Regulatory Authority of Pakistan has provided a web portal for reporting [24], still the under-reporting of ADR cases is a huge concern. The government officials and policy makers need to form and implement a uniform system regarding the reporting of adverse drug reactions nationwide.

The findings from our study also showed that the hospital pharmacists had a positive attitude towards practice change. This behavior pattern can be explained by employing Trans Theoratical Model (TTM) of change [58]. This model explains the behavior change of an individual and his readiness to accept a new healthier behavior. The model is comprised of six stages of behavior change which develops over a span of time [58]. As the present study focusses on the practices of pharmacist and their readiness to accept if any change comes to the way, therefore the model is believed to be a better explanation of the participants' behavior. The hospital pharmacists working in Lahore had a mixed behavior towards the practice change. The study has revealed that that the pharmacist who were aged between 31 and 40 and had an experience of more than 10 years were at their pre-contemplation stage, while those who were aged between 21 and 30 with an experience of 5 years were in their contemplation stage. So, the newly graduated pharmacist should be trained properly and government bodies need to take interest in the continuous education and training of pharmacists to make them ready for the preparation phase of behavior change.

During the interviews, several barriers were identified which can impact on the reporting of an ADR. Among them workload is a key barrier to the ADR reporting. In Pakistani public hospitals, on every 1200 beds, a pharmacist is appointed, this differs to the world standard of one pharmacist for 50 beds [59]. The government is still unable to meet the minimum health delivery standards [59]. This can be related to 6000 vacant positions of hospital pharmacists in Punjab which are awaiting approval from government. Only 279 hospital pharmacists posts have been sanctioned by the government of the Punjab in last 10 years [60, 61]. This number is so few to cater the needs of a big population. Moreover, many of the public hospitals do not have a clearly defined job structure for the hospital pharmacists. The results from our study showed that most hospitals are not engaging pharmacists to provide clinical services, rather the appointed pharmacists are usually involved with the procurement and supply of drugs at ward level. These findings urge to revise the job structure of pharmacist including pharmacovigilance activities as the responsibility of the pharmacist.

It was noteworthy to state that pharmacist had a basic idea about pharmacovigilance, but majority of the interviewee pharmacist had no idea about the national pharmacovigilance centre by DRAP. Though, already there are few hospital pharmacists in public hospitals, however even they are not aware of the existence of national pharmacovigilance center. This raises questions regarding the communication between healthcare professionals, DRAP and its pharmacovigilance unit. In developed countries, authorities have created effective ways of communication which are both agile and engaging at the same time. Without dynamic and effective communications with key stakeholders of pharmacovigilance it is impossible to achieve the safe use of medicines which requires constant awareness and vigilance [62].

Another identified barrier was a lack of information technology and computertised record system in the public hospitals. The participants shared their concerns that due to the lack of computerized system in hospital, patient records cannot be updated, there is no tracking for the prescription orders and hence no ADR records are available. This strengthens the need for the establishment of an information technology based system in the country where the hospital computers could be linked. If there is a central database then reports from these hospitals can be sent to the national reporting center (DRAP) without any delay. Besides, mobile phones application could be developed and use of social media could also help with the time management issues related to under reporting [63].

During the interviews, hospital pharmacist emphasized on their role as medication safety expert, this is in line with the literature [64] . Another interesting finding came out from participants was the recognition of their roles as the focal person in case of ADR reporting [41, 65]. Majority of the pharmacists were of the view that the medicine safety will improve, if the role of pharmacist is recognized by the organization in which they work [66]. These finding are further strengthened by a Spanish study which pointed out the importance of pharmacist's role in ADR reporting [67].

The respondents in our study also gave suggestions regarding the role of Drug Regulatory Authority of Pakistan to improve the ADR reporting in the country. This includes training and continuing education to health care professionals, providing time for reporting, acknowledging the effort in the form of certificates, incentives and publications. These suggestions were found to be similar with the other incentives reported in the literature [44, 68]. Though the government has already taken many major initiatives to improve ADR reporting including establishment of national pharmacovigilance centre, development of web portal and collaboration with USP-PQM, however the ADR reporting in real time is still not in place. The implementation of drug monitoring is needed both at individual and institutional level to make this programme a success [69]. A strong political will is also important to ensure the multidisciplinary collaboration involving ministry of health, academia, pharmaceutical industry and healthcare professionals regarding safe and effective use of medicines.

Limitations of the study

The study was conducted in Lahore. Though it's the second largest city in the country with a population of about 10 million, however results cannot be generalized to the whole country. There were only 10 hospital pharmacists who were interviewed in the study. Though the number is small however the study is qualitative in nature resulting in useful themes on the issue.

Conclusion

The study showed that the hospital pharmacists were aware regarding medication safety and ADR reporting, however they don't practice this in real sense. Pharmacists showed willingness to change practice provided barriers to ADR reporting could be removed. Identification of barriers by pharmacists are useful to design intervention towards better pharmacovigilance and adverse drug reporting mechanisms. Overall, these findings can serve as primer for policy makers and government to build future work in this area.

Appendix

Hospital Pharmacist's interview guide

Objective: Exploring the knowledge, attitude & perceptions of hospital pharmacists towards medication safety & ADR reporting

Part I

Focus: Knowledge and perceptions about Medication safety

1. What comes to your mind when you hear the word "Medication Safety"?
2. Do you counsel patients on medication safety? If yes which particular aspect of it,under what conditions do you counsel them and why? (condition mean disease state)
3. How long the average counselling/ conversation takes when giving information about medication safety? Do you have enough time and how has this impacted on your workload/practice?

Part II

Focus: Knowledge and attitudes about Adverse Drug Reaction (ADR) reporting

1. What is your understanding of Adverse Drug Reaction?
2. What would you do if you were approached by a patient with a severe ADR (any recent incidence, what was your strategy to deal with the patient)?
3. What type of adverse drug reactions you consider should be reported?
4. In your current practice, how many ADR cases you have seen? (Did you report/ record them by yourself or heard it from some other colleagues)
5. Do you have any guidance on reporting or how to and when to report any ADR? And report to whom and Where?
6. Have you ever sent an adverse drug reaction report to your national reporting agency, when that happened and why did you send it?
7. Have you ever sent an adverse drug reaction report to the responsible pharmaceutical company, when that happened and why did you send it?'
8. Do you think that ADR reporting will influence the quality of life of the patients under your care?
9. In your opinion do you think that ADR reporting contributes to drug safety? If yes, (How)?
10. What are the factors that you think can impact and may encourage pharmacists to report ADRs (why a pharmacist should report an ADR)?
11. In your opinion, what are the possible factors that contribute as the barriers to ADR reporting?
12. Do you think your job in any way makes it easy/ difficult to report ADR.
13. What type of medicine information resources (journal, news, formulary{BNF}) you prefer while reporting ADR?
14. Do you receive and routinely review publications to become aware of medications with error potential?

Part III

Focus: Knowledge about Adverse Drug Reaction reporting system

1. Are you aware about the existence of the regulatory body that regulates ADR reporting in Pakistan? Reasons (if not aware)
2. Do you have any idea about the difference of medication safety and ADR reporting systems between Pakistan and other developed countries?
3. In your opinion, do you think that there is a need to change the system about medicine safety and ADR reporting? What benefit would it have?

Part IV.

Focus: Future perspective

1. What do you think that with the advancements in pharmacy practice, your role has changed and how it can contribute towards medication safety?
2. What could be the possible suggestions to improve ADR reporting (in hospital) in future? Any suggestions?
3. **Conclusion/suggestions**

Would you like to provide any additional comments about medication safety and ADR reporting system in Pakistan?

Abbreviations

ADR: Adverse drug reaction; DRAP: Drug Regulatory Authority of Pakistan; HP: Hospital pharmacist; NHSRC: National Health Services Regulation and Coordination; PV: Pharmacovigilance; UMC: Uppsala Monitoring Centre; WHO: World Health Organization

Acknowledgments

The authors would like to thank all the hospital pharmacists who participated in the study.

Funding

The study received no grant from any funding agency.

Authors' contributions

Conceptualized the study: RH and AH. Collected the data, performed the analysis and drafted the first manuscript: RH and AH. Critically reviewed, revised and approved the manuscript: RH, AH, FH and MF.

Competing interests

The authors declare that they have no competing interests.

Author details

[1]School of Pharmaceutical Sciences, Universiti Sains Malaysia, Penang, Malaysia. [2]University College of Pharmacy, University of the Punjab, Lahore, Pakistan. [3]Unaizah College of Pharmacy, Qassim University, Buraydah, Saudi Arabia.

References

1. Patidar D, Rajput MS, Nirmal NP, Savitri W. Implementation and evaluation of adverse drug reaction monitoring system in a tertiary care teaching hospital in Mumbai, India. Interdiscip Toxicol. 2013;6(1):41–6.
2. WHO. International drug monitoring: the role of the hospital, report of a WHO meeting1969 18–23 1968.
3. Editorial. Improving ADR reporting. Lancet 2002;360(1435.
4. WHO. Safer use of medicines: the basics. World Health Organisation Collaborating Centre for International Drug Monitoring, Uppsala. 2018. https://www.who-umc.org/safer-use-of-medicines/safer-use-of-medicines-the-basics/.
5. WHO. Fast facts on pharmacovigilance. In: Essential medicines and health products. 2015. http://www.who.int/medicines/areas/quality_safety/safety_efficacy/PV_fast_facts/en/.
6. Rolfes L, Wilkes S, Hunsel F, Puijenbroek E, Grootheest K. Important information regarding reporting of adverse drug reactions: a qualitative study. Int J Pharm Pract. 2014;22(3):231–3.
7. Centre UM. WHO Collaborating Centres. Uppsala Monitoring Centre. 2018. https://www.who-umc.org/global-pharmacovigilance/specialist-centres/who-collaborating-centres/. Accessed April 15 2018.
8. UMC. What happens to reports of problems with medicines? Uppsala Monitoring Centre. 2018. https://www.who-umc.org/safer-use-of-medicines/safer-use-of-medicines-the-basics/what-happens-to-reports/. Accessed April 15 2018.
9. MHRA. Yellowcard. Helping to make medicines safer. Medicines and Healthcare products Regulatory Agency. 2018. https://yellowcard.mhra.gov.uk/. Accessed April 19 2018.
10. Rabbur RS, Emmerton L. An introduction to adverse drug reaction reporting systems in different countries. Int J Pharm Pract. 2005;13(1):91–100.
11. FDA. MedWatch: The FDA Safety Information and Adverse Event Reporting Program. U.S. Food and Drug Administration. 2018. https://www.fda.gov/Safety/MedWatch/default.htm. Accessed April 19 2018.
12. AHRQ.gov. Sentinel Event Program. U.S. Department of Health and Human Services. 2013. https://psnet.ahrq.gov/resources/resource/26617/sentinel-event-program.
13. NCCMERP. Medication Errors. United States Pharmacopeial Convention. 2018. http://www.nccmerp.org/. Accessed April 19 2018.
14. Cox A. Broad Spectrum: Embracing ADR reporting could improve pharmacists' standing. Pharm J 2002;269 14.
15. Centre NZP. CARM. 2018. https://nzphvc.otago.ac.nz/carm/. Accessed April 20 2018.
16. Mes K, Berg L, Grootheest AV. Attitudes of community pharmacists in the Netherlands towards adverse drug reaction reporting. Int J Pharm Pract. 2002;10(4):267–72.
17. Palaian. S. Pharmacovigilance Practices and Activities: Issues, Challenges, and Future Direction. In: Ibrahim. M, Wertheimer. A, Babar. Z, editors. Social and Administrative Aspects of Pharmacy in Low- and Middle-Income Countries. Elsevier; 2018. p. 145–162.
18. NHSRC. Achievements. Ministry of National Health Services, Regulations and Coordination, Government of Pakistan. 2018. http://www.nhsrc.gov.pk/index.html. Accessed April 2 2018.
19. Tribunal JI. Batch J093. The Pathology of Negligence (Report of the Judicial Inquiry Tribunal to Determine the Causes of Deaths of Patients of the Punjab Institute of Cardiology, Lahore in 2011–2012)2012.
20. Department H. http://health.punjab.gov.pk/Services_Package. Governemnt of Punjab. 2018. http://health.punjab.gov.pk/Services_Package.
21. Observatory-EMRO RHS. Health Systems Profile-Pakistan. World Health Organization. 2007. http://apps.who.int/medicinedocs/documents/s17305e/s17305e.pdf.
22. WHO. Deadly medicines contamination in Pakistan. World health Organization. 2013. http://www.who.int/features/2013/pakistan_medicine_safety/en/. Accessed April 15 2018.
23. Atif. M, Ahmad. M, Saleem. Q, Curley. L, Zaman. M, Babar. Z. Pharmaceutical Policy in Pakistan. In: Babar. Z, editor. Pharmaceutical Policy in Countries with Developing Healthcare Systems. Springer International 2017. p. 25–44.
24. DRAP. Pharmacy Services Division. 2017. http://dra.gov.pk/Home/PharmacyServicesDivision.
25. Shamim S, Sharib SM, Malhi SM, Muntaha S-u, Raza H, Ata S, et al. Adverse drug reactions (ADRS) reporting: awareness and reasons of under-reporting among health care professionals, a challenge for pharmacists. SpringerPlus. 2016;5(1):1778.
26. Centre UM. VigiFlow. Uppsala Monitoring Centre. 2018. https://www.who-umc.org/global-pharmacovigilance/vigiflow/. Accessed April 15 2018.
27. Wazir HK. DRAP to introduce regulations for post-marketing surveillance of drugs. Pakistan Today. 2017.
28. Department W. Population Profile Punjab. Government of The Punjab. 2017. http://www.pwd.punjab.gov.pk/population_profile. Accessed April 15 2018.
29. Review WP. Lahore Population 2017. 2017. http://worldpopulationreview.com/world-cities/lahore-population/.
30. Punjab PDCU. Pharmacy Pharmacovigilance Division. Provincial Drug Control Unit Punjab. 2017. https://mss.punjab.gov.pk/PublicHome/PharmacyPharmacovigilanceDivision. Accessed April 15 2018.
31. Chaudary A. Punjab reacts to adverse drugs. The Dawn. 2012;
32. Drug Safety Alerts [database on the Internet]. Provincial Drug Control Unit Punjab. 2018. Available from: https://sites.google.com/prod/view/pdcup/divisions/drug-safety-alerts. Accessed: April 10 2018.
33. Smith F. Research methods in pharmacy practice: Pharmaceutical Press; 2002.
34. Kitzinger J. Qualitative research. Introducing focus groups. BMJ Br Med J. 1995;311(7000):299.
35. Berg B. Qualitative research methods for the social sciences, MA: Pearsons education. Inc: Inc. 2009.
36. Dolan Mullen P, Reynolds R. The potential of grounded theory for health education research: linking theory and practice. Health Educ Monogr. 1978;6(3):280–94.
37. Sajjad M, Akhtar S, Ullah MI. Impact of social media marketing on health awareness in Lahore. Pak J Soc Sci (PJSS). 2015;35(1):335–45.
38. Ghulam M, Saeed R, Tahir M. Adverse drug reaction reporting system at different hospitals of Lahore, Pakistan-an evaluation and patient out come analysis. J App Pharm. 2013;4(01):713–9.
39. Iffat W, Shakeel S, Rahim N, Anjum F, Nesar S, Ghayas S. Pakistani physicians knowledge and attitude towards reporting adverse drug reactions. Afr J Pharm Pharmacol. 2014;8(14):379–85.
40. Paveliu MS, Bengea-Luculescu S, Mihai T, Paveliu SF. Perception on adverse drug reaction reporting by physicians working in southern Romania. Maedica. 2013;8(1):17.
41. Vessal G, Mardani Z, Mollai M. Knowledge, attitudes, and perceptions of pharmacists to adverse drug reaction reporting in Iran. Pharm World Sci. 2009;31(2):183–7.
42. Belton K, Group EPR. Attitude survey of adverse drug-reaction reporting by health care professionals across the European Union. Eur J Clin Pharmacol. 1997;52(6):423–7.
43. Belton KJ, Lewis SC, Payne S, Rawlins M, Wood S. Attitudinal survey of adverse drug reaction reporting by medical practitioners in the United Kingdom [see comments]. Br J Clin Pharmacol. 1995;39(3):223–226.
44. Elkalmi RM, Hassali MA, Ibrahim MIM, Liau SY, Awaisu AA. Qualitative study exploring barriers and facilitators for reporting of adverse drug reactions (ADRs) among community pharmacists in Malaysia. J Pharm Health Serv Res. 2011;2(2):71–8.
45. Cheema E, Haseeb A, Khan TM, Sutcliffe P, Singer DR. Barriers to reporting of adverse drugs reactions: a cross sectional study among community pharmacists in United Kingdom. Pharm Pract. 2017;15(3)

46. Jose J, Jimmy B, Al-Ghailani ASH, Al Majali MA. A cross sectional pilot study on assessing the knowledge, attitude and behavior of community pharmacists to adverse drug reaction related aspects in the Sultanate of Oman. Saudi Pharm J. 2014;22(2):163–9.
47. Hadi MA, Neoh CF, Zin RM, Elrggal ME, Cheema E. Pharmacovigilance: pharmacists' perspective on spontaneous adverse drug reaction reporting. Integrated Pharmacy Res Pract. 2017;6:91.
48. Green CF, Mottram DR, Rowe PH, Pirmohamed M. Attitudes and knowledge of hospital pharmacists to adverse drug reaction reporting. Br J Clin Pharmacol. 2001;51(1):81–6.
49. Hadi MA, Helwani R, Long CM. Facilitators and barriers towards adverse drug reaction reporting: perspective of Malaysian hospital pharmacists. J Pharm Health Serv Res. 2013;4(3):155–8.
50. Suyagh M, Farah D, Farha RA. Pharmacist's knowledge, practice and attitudes toward pharmacovigilance and adverse drug reactions reporting process. Saudi Pharm J. 2015;23(2):147–53.
51. Obara T, Yamaguchi H, Satoh M, Iida Y, Sakai T. Prevalence, determinants, and reasons for the non-reporting of adverse drug reactions by pharmacists in the Miyagi and Hokkaido regions of Japan. Adv Pharmacoepidemiol Drug Saf. 2015;4(191):2167–1052.
52. Liu J, Zhou Z, Yang S, Feng B, Zhao J, Liu H, et al. Factors that affect adverse drug reaction reporting among hospital pharmacists in western China. Int J Clin Pharm. 2015;37(3):457–64.
53. Abdel-Latif MM, Abdel-Wahab BA. Knowledge and awareness of adverse drug reactions and pharmacovigilance practices among healthcare professionals in Al-Madinah Al-Munawwarah, Kingdom of Saudi Arabia. Saudi Pharm J. 2015;23(2):154–61.
54. Fadare JO, Enwere OO, Afolabi A, Chedi B, Musa A. Knowledge, attitude and practice of adverse drug reaction reporting among healthcare workers in a tertiary Centre in Northern Nigeria. Trop J Pharm Res. 2011;10(3):235–42.
55. Ferber R. Research by convenience: The University of Chicago Press; 1977.
56. Hashmi FK, Hassali MA, Khalid A, Saleem F, Aljadhey H, Bashaar M. A qualitative study exploring perceptions and attitudes of community pharmacists about extended pharmacy services in Lahore, Pakistan. BMC Health Serv Res. 2017;17(1):500.
57. Nishtar. S. Health and the 18th Amendment- Retaining national functions in devolution.
58. Prochaska JO, Velicer WF. The transtheoretical model of health behavior change. Am J Health Promot. 1997;12(1):38–48.
59. DAWN. One pharmacist needed for 50 hospital beds: expert. 2016. https://www.dawn.com/news/1289197.
60. Nation T. Govt urged to fill 6,000 vacancies of pharmacist. 2017. https://nation.com.pk/14-Mar-2017/govt-urged-to-fill-6-000-vacancies-of-pharmacists.
61. GOP. SO (ND) 10–6/2007. In: Department H, editor. Punjab: Government of Punjab; 2010.
62. UMC. Communication in pharmacovigilance. Uppsala Monitoring Centre. 2018. https://www.who-umc.org/global-pharmacovigilance/communication-in-pharmacovigilance/patient-centered-communications/. Accessed April 15 2018.
63. Banerjee AK, Ingate S. Web-based patient-reported outcomes in drug safety and risk management. Drug Saf. 2012;35(6):437–46.
64. WHO. The Role of the Pharmacist in the Health Care System. 2017. http://apps.who.int/medicinedocs/en/d/Jh2995e/1.3.html. Accessed April 20 2018.
65. Herdeiro MT, Figueiras A, Polónia J, Gestal-Otero J. Influence of pharmacists' attitudes on adverse drug reaction reporting. Drug Saf. 2006;29(4):331–40.
66. Sharrad AK. Pharmacists'knowledge, attitude and practice about adverse drug reaction in Basra/Iraq. Int J Pharm Sci Res. 2017;8(5):2309.
67. Vallano A, Cereza G, Pedròs C, Agustí A, Danés I, Aguilera C, et al. Obstacles and solutions for spontaneous reporting of adverse drug reactions in the hospital. Br J Clin Pharmacol. 2005;60(6):653–8.
68. Hazell L, Shakir SA. Under-reporting of adverse drug reactions. Drug Saf. 2006;29(5):385–96.
69. Organization WH. Pharmacovigilance: ensuring the safe use of medicines. 2004.

22

Investigation of prescribing behavior at outpatient settings of governmental hospitals in eastern Ethiopia: an overall evaluation beyond World Health Organization core prescribing indicators

Tigist Gashaw[1], Mekonnen Sisay[1*], Getnet Mengistu[2] and Firehiwot Amare[3]

Abstract

Background: Rational prescribing remains an important component of rational drug use. The World Health Organization (WHO) standardized and validated core prescribing indicators for evaluating prescribing pattern of drugs. The prescribing practice has been shown to deviate from national and WHO guidelines in Ethiopia. The aim of this study was; therefore, to investigate the overall prescribing behavior of four governmental hospitals: Hiwot Fana Specialized University Hospital (HFSUH), Federal Harar Police Hospital (FHPH), Jugel Hospital (JH) and Southeast Command III Hospital (SECIIIH), Harar, eastern Ethiopia.

Methods: Hospital based retrospective cross-sectional study was employed to evaluate outpatient prescriptions dispensed from January 1 – December 31, 2016. A total of 2400 prescriptions (600 from each hospital) were assessed. A combination of prescription completeness and prescribing indicator forms were used to collect the data.

Result: From a total of 2400 prescriptions reviewed, only HFSUH and FHPH were using standard prescription at prevalence of 92.5 and 99.8%, respectively. Name and weight of the patient were the most and the least commonly recorded information, respectively. A total of 5217 drugs were prescribed with an average number of drugs per encounter to be 2.17 (±0.39) and the highest value (2.60) was observed at FHPH. The frequency of administration was the most commonly written component (85.0%) with an average of 1.85 per prescription. Among all prescriptions analyzed, the percentage of encounters with antimicrobials and injectables prescribed were 66.9 and 26.5%, respectively. The prevalence of drugs prescribed with generic name and from essential drug list were 4644 (89.01%) and 4613 (88.42%), respectively. Among health professional related information, dispenser name was the least documented in all hospitals with the prevalence being 3.9%.

Conclusion: JH and SECIIIH were not using standard prescriptions at all during the review period. Besides, some important components of the prescription such as age, sex and diagnosis were not properly recorded or missed at all in the selected hospitals. The tendency of prescribing drugs with dose and dosage form was very poor. Overall, none of the core prescribing indicators was in line with the WHO standards. These and other related problems should be investigated in-depth to find out the underlying problems for which interventional strategies can be designed to reverse this worrying practice.

Keywords: Prescribing behavior, WHO, Prescribing indicators, Eastern Ethiopia

* Correspondence: mekonnensisay27@yahoo.com
[1]Department of Pharmacology and Toxicology, School of Pharmacy, College of Health and Medical Sciences, Haramaya University, P.O. Box 235, Harar, Ethiopia
Full list of author information is available at the end of the article

Background

Medicines play a crucial role in the delivery of healthcare service across the globe. Nevertheless, not only is the availability of medicines important, but also rational prescribing remains an important component of treating patients as this may be a reflection of the quality of care delivered to them and the community at large [1, 2]. Appropriate use of medicines plays a pivotal role in reducing global morbidity and mortality. However, the World Health Organization (WHO) has reported that around 50% of all medicines are prescribed, dispensed or sold inappropriately and more than half of all patients fail to take their medicines as prescribed or dispensed. Such inappropriate use is wasteful of resources and causes patient harm in terms of lack of satisfactory outcome, serious adverse events and increased antimicrobial resistance (AMR) [2, 3]. To minimize these problems, WHO developed and validated core drug use indicators for prescribing, patient care and facility specific studies. The prescribing indicators measure the performance of prescribers in five key areas (average number of drugs per prescription, percentage of drugs prescribed by generic name, percentage of prescriptions containing antibiotics, percentage of prescriptions containing injectable drugs, and percentage of drugs prescribed from the latest edition of national Essential Drug Lists (EDL) or formulary) [4]. Even if several studies have been conducted on the area of prescribing practice with the aid of such five core prescribing indicators in various parts of Ethiopia [5–10], none of these findings holistically addressed the overall features of prescription beyond assessing prescribing practice with the usual indicator studies. This study attempted to combine the prescription features and completeness with WHO prescribing indicator forms to generate a cumulative body of evidence for decision making. Prescribing indicators are useful for investigating major problem areas of prescribing practice in quantitative basis. These core indicators, however, failed to address the nature of the prescription, its standards, and presence of essential components (patient, drug and health professional related details), among others [4]. Moreover, a study of prescribing behavior is an important tool to determine rational drug therapy and maximize utilization of resources [9]. Drug utilization reports that assess drug consumption and prescribing patterns should be done on regular basis for monitoring and evaluation of drug use and national drug policy at large [11]. So, this study aimed to investigate the prescribing behavior in outpatient settings of four government hospitals of Harar town, Eastern Ethiopia.

Methods

Study area, design and period

Harar is located 526 km away from the capital of Ethiopia, Addis Ababa to the East. Harari region is one of the nine national regional states of Ethiopia, with the town of Harar as its capital. Harar is one of the most popular historical towns in the eastern part of Ethiopia. The town has a projected total population of 203,438 with male to female ratio of 1.01:1 in 2010. Harar town is divided in to 19 kebeles. In the town, there are four governmental hospitals, two private hospitals, and eight health centers [12]. The study was conducted in four governmental hospitals: Hiwot Fana Specialized University Hospital (HFSUH), Jugel Hospital (JH), Federal Harar Police Hospital (FHPH) and South-East command III Hospital (SECIIIH). HFSUH is a tertiary care teaching hospital of Haramaya university and hosts majority of patient attendees per day from the Harar town and nearby areas. JH is a regional hospital of Harari regional state. Whereas, FHPH and SECIIIH are special government hospitals in which the service is primarily delivered to police and military clients and their relatives. Hospital based retrospective cross-sectional study was employed to investigate the overall prescribing behavior of the year 2016 in the above-mentioned hospitals from July 1 to September 30, 2017.

Population and inclusion/exclusion criteria

All out-patient prescriptions dispensed from January 1 to December 31, 2016 from each hospital were taken as study populations. However, prescriptions that contained only medical supplies like glove, and syringe; those prescriptions contained drug which were found illegible and prescriptions which were brought from outside of the selected hospitals were excluded from the study.

Sample size determination and sampling technique

Based on the current WHO criteria [4], 600 prescriptions were taken from each hospital (a total of 2400 prescriptions) to assess completeness of the prescription and prescribing pattern in the hospitals. A systematic random sampling technique was employed to collect 600 eligible prescriptions from each hospital once the annual prescriptions had been arranged in the chronological order. The sampling interval was 150, 119, 28 and 43 for HFSUH, JH, FHPH and SECIIIH, respectively.

Data collection tools and methods

Data were collected by using data collection tool (observational checklist) containing two components: 1) prescription completeness assessment form customized from manuals developed and validated by Food, Medicine and Healthcare Administration and Control Authority (FMHACA) of Ethiopia and WHO [13, 14]. The manuals emphasized that prescriptions should be standardized (the paper should have the name of the local health facility, contact details and serial numbers (if any) as well as all essential components of the prescription in preprinted form). In addition, the prescription should be considered complete if it contains patient, drug and prescriber and dispenser related directions prepared in preprinted form and with sufficient space for hand filling. 2) prescribing indicator form developed and validated by WHO for assessing prescribing practice at outpatient settings of health facilities [4]. The prescribing indicators include average number of drugs per prescription, percentage of drugs prescribed by generic name, percentage of prescribing encounters containing antibiotics, percentage of prescribing encounters containing injectable drugs, and percentage of drugs prescribed from the latest edition of national EDL or formulary. Data were collected retrospectively from individual prescription and filled in structured observational check list accordingly.

Data quality control

To ensure the data quality, data collectors (pharmacy technicians) and supervisors (pharmacists) were trained by the principal investigators for 3 days. The data collection tool was pretested at HFSUH (data not included in the actual study and solely used for amendment) and necessary modifications were undertaken in the tool. The principal investigators and supervisors underwent frequent checks on the data collection process to ensure the completeness and consistency of the collected data. Data were cleaned to remove inconsistencies and missing values on daily basis.

Data analysis and presentation

Data were entered to EPI-Data Version 3.1 and exported to and analyzed with Statistical Package for Social Sciences version 20.0 (IBM statistics, Armonk, NY, United States). Univariate analysis was employed to summarize the findings. Prescribing indicators were computed using the formula adopted by the WHO for prescribing indicators assessment [4, 15]. Finally, the data were evaluated against WHO standards and presented in tabular way.

Result

Patient related information on a prescription

A total of 2400 prescriptions (600 from each hospital) were analyzed in the study. The analysis showed that standard prescriptions were used in HFSUH and FHPH at a prevalence of 555 (92.5%) and 599 (99.8%), respectively. Almost all prescriptions had a medical registration number in HFSUH ($n = 598$, 99.7%) and FHPH ($n = 599$, 99.8%) whereas lowest recording practice was observed in JH ($n = 332$, 55.3%). The overall prevalence of registration number in prescription was found to be 2082(86.8%). Moreover, the examination of patient related information on the prescription revealed that name of the patient was the most commonly recorded information ($n = 2254$, 93.9%) while weight and address of the patient were the least commonly recorded components obtained from 0.9 and 1.1% prescriptions, respectively (Table 1).

Number of drugs and drug related information on prescriptions

As shown in Table 2, a total of 5217 drugs were prescribed from 2400 prescriptions giving an average value of 2.17 (±0.39) drugs per prescription. The highest and the lowest number of drugs per encounter were observed at FHPH and HFSUH, respectively. Generally, large proportion of the prescriptions contained two drugs ($n = 874$, 36.4%) followed by a single drug ($n =$ 733, 30.5%). Moreover, analysis of drug-regimen information indicated that the route and frequency of administration were the most commonly recorded components with a frequency of 4435 (85.0%) and 4270 (81.8%), respectively. In contrary, drugs prescribed with dose and dosage forms were found to be 1429 (27.4%) and 1708 (32.7%), respectively (Table 2). The mean value of components of drug regimen per encounter showed that the frequency of drug administration had the highest value (mean = 1.85) whereas the dose of the drug had a value of 0.59 (Table 3).

Distribution of antimicrobials and antibacterial agents per encounter

Among the 2400 prescriptions reviewed, the magnitude of antimicrobial (s) and antibacterial (s) containing prescriptions were 1605(66.9%) and 1473(61.4%), respectively. Almost half of the prescriptions contained a single antimicrobial and/or antibacterial agent. From the 5217 drugs prescribed, 2082 (39.9%) were antimicrobial agents from which 1671 (80.25%) were antibacterial agents and the average values per encounter were found to be 1.29(±0.03) and 1.13(±0.08) for antimicrobial and antibacterial agents, respectively (Table 4).

WHO core drug use indicators

The evaluation of prescribing practice using WHO core prescribing indicators revealed that the percentage of encounters with injection (s) and antimicrobial (s) prescribed were 636 (26.5%) and 1605 (66.9), respectively. The percentage of drugs prescribed with generic name and EDL of Ethiopia were 4644(89.01%) and 4613 (88.42%), respectively (Table 5).

Health professional related information

From all prescriptions included in the study, 2133 (88.9%) prescriptions contained the signature of the prescriber and 1083(45.1%) contained the prescriber name. Dispenser related information was found very low with the

Table 1 Patient related information in prescriptions dispensed from Jan - Dec 2016 at four governmental hospitals of Harar town (n = 2400)

Patient related information	HFSUH (n = 600)	FHPH (n = 600)	JH (n = 600)	SECIIIH (n = 600)	Total (2400)
Use of standard prescription	555 (92.5)	599 (99.8)	0(0)	0(0)	1154(48.1)
Medical registration number	598 (99.7)	599 (99.8)	332(55.3)	553(92.2)	2082(86.8)
Date of prescription	367 (61.2)	497(82.8)	497(82.8)	590(98.3)	1951(81.3)
Name of patient	599 (99.8)	600 (100.0)	577(96.2)	478(79.7)	2254(93.9)
Age	527 (87.8)	117 (19.5)	343(57.2)	58(9.7)	1045(43.5)
Weight	18 (3.0)	3 (0.5)	2(0.3)	0(0)	23(0.9)
Sex	522 (87.0)	206 (34.4)	357(59.5)	32(5.3)	1117(46.5)
Patient Address	18 (3.0)	7 (1.2)	2(0.3)	0(0)	27(1.1)
Diagnosis	236 (39.3)	20 (3.3)	26(4.3)	0(0)	282(11.8)

*Abbreviations***:** *HFSUH* Hiwot Fana Specialized University Hospital, *FHPH* Federal Harar Police Hospital, *JH* Jugel Hospital, *SECIIIH* Southeast command III Hospital

prevalence being 94 (3.9%) and 152 (6.3%) prescriptions for dispensers' name and signature, respectively (Table 6).

Frequently prescribed drugs

From all drugs (n = 5217) prescribed, the most commonly prescribed classes of drugs were antimicrobial agents (n = 2036, 39.2%) followed by analgesics and anti-inflammatory agents (n = 1548, 29.67%) and gastrointestinal agents (n = 555, 10.64%). Looking at the individual drugs, amoxicillin (n = 497, 24.41%), diclofenac (n = 594, 38.37) and omeprazole (n = 206, 37.11%) were the top prescribed drugs under antimicrobials, analgesics and anti-inflammatory drugs and gastrointestinal agents, respectively (Table 7).

Discussion

In this study, a total of 2400 prescribing encounters were reviewed from four government hospitals (600 prescriptions for each hospital). Compared to previous studies, this study tried to holistically address the prescribing behavior with better sample size and annual coverage of prescriptions in the four government hospitals of Harar town. In the review process, the general feature of prescriptions and its completeness was assessed. The prescribing practice was evaluated against the WHO

Table 2 Drug related information on prescriptions dispensed from Jan 1 - Dec 31, 2016 at four governmental hospitals of Harar town

Drug related information	Frequency (%)				
	HFSUH	FHPH	JH	SECIIIH	Overall
Drugs per prescription (n = prescription in each hospital)	(n = 600)	(n = 600)	(n = 600)	(n = 600)	(n = 2400)
One	309 (51.5)	129 (21.5)	139 (23.2)	156 (26.0)	733 (30.5)
Two	201 (33.5)	169 (28.2)	209 (34.8)	295 (49.2)	874 (36.4)
Three	64 (10.7)	177 (29.5)	170 (28.3)	129 (21.5)	540 (22.5)
Four	15 (2.5)	76 (12.7)	61 (10.2)	19 (3.2)	171 (7.1)
Five	9 (1.5)	39 (6.5)	17 (2.8)	1 (0.2)	66 (2.7)
Six and above	2 (0.4)	10 (1.7)	4 (0.7)	0 (0)	16 (0.6)
Average number of drugs per encounter	1.70	2.60	2.37	2.02	2.17 (± 0.39)
Drug regimen related information (n = drugs per hospital)	(n = 1021)	(n = 1560)	(n = 1422)	(n = 1214)	(n = 5217)
Dose	317 (31.04)	502 (32.18)	234 (16.5)	376 (30.9)	1429 (27.4)
Strength	661 (64.74)	1039 (66.60)	1161 (81.6)	1036 (85.3)	3897 (74.7)
Dosage Form	153 (14.99)	302 (19.36)	169 (11.9)	1084 (89.3)	1708 (32.7)
Route	816 (79.92)	1098 (70.38)	1208 (84.9)	1148 (94.6)	4270 (81.8)
Frequency	716 (70.13)	1414 (90.64)	1171 (82.3)	1134 (93.4)	4435 (85.0)
Duration	478 (46.82)	409 (26.21)	981 (68.9)	868 (71.5)	2736 (52.4)
Quantity	474 (46.43)	1087 (69.68)	515 (36.3)	1130 (93.1)	3206 (61.5)

Abbreviations HFSUH Hiwot Fana Specialized University Hospital, *FHPH* Federal Harar Police Hospital, *JH* Jugel Hospital, *SECIIIH* Southeast command III Hospital

Table 3 Mean-value of components of drug regimen per prescribing encounter dispensed from Jan 1-Dec 31, 2016

Components	Mean value				
	HFSUH ($n = 600$)	FHPH ($n = 600$)	JH ($n = 600$)	SECIIIH ($n = 600$)	Overall ($n = 2400$)
Dose	0.53	0.84	0.39	0.63	0.59
Strength	1.10	1.73	1.91	1.73	1.62
Dosage Form	0.26	0.50	0.28	1.81	0.71
Route	1.36	1.84	2.01	1.75	1.78
Frequency	1.19	2.36	1.95	1.89	1.85
Duration	0.80	0.84	1.64	1.45	1.14
Quantity	0.79	1.81	0.86	1.88	1.34

Abbreviations: HFSUH Hiwot Fana Specialized University Hospital, *FHPH* Federal Harar Police Hospital, *JH* Jugel Hospital, *SECIIIH* Southeast command III Hospital

standard [4]. Rational prescribing can have significant impact on the drug utilization process. Prescribers have become using substandard prescription papers and have also been practicing the standard format in the wrong way. Missing the drug regimens including the dosage, and duration of therapy might have contributed for emergence of drug resistance, toxicological issues, and poor treatment outcomes, among others [16]. Such baseline survey can be taken as a good input for designing and implementation of interventional studies. Most interventions undertaken to combat inappropriate use of medicines have been educational in nature, have had a relatively small impact and have not taken into account the determinants of behavior. A combination of interventions, involving managerial as well as educational components, appears to be more effective than a single intervention [3].

Regarding the general feature of prescription and its completeness, only HFSUH and FHPH were using standard prescriptions with nearly 100% practice observed in FHPH. However, JH and SECIIIH didn't use standard prescriptions at all. Instead, they were using a piece of paper printed somewhere else and without containing essential components in the preprinted form. Such act of negligence observed throughout the review period is a good indication of how much irrational prescribing has becoming a huge concern. Almost all prescriptions had a medical registration number in HFSUH and FHPH whereas lowest recording practice was observed in JH. It is imperative that all prescription papers, irrespective of its content and form, would have contained the name of a patient to whom the drug was prescribed. Oddly enough, patient name was recorded in 79.7% prescription indicating the absence of this essential component in one out of five prescriptions in SECIIIH. Missing the name of the patient might create a room for the dispensers to issue the drug (s) without adequate counseling and even to the wrong patient. Even if the importance is not that much profound, the overall recording practice of the weight of patients was less than 1%. Considering drug therapy in pediatric patients, age and weight are among the essential components for ease of calculating dosage and correcting regimen errors [17, 18]. Nearly one-tenth of prescriptions contained diagnosis with the lowest (zero) value observed in SECIIIH. Recording diagnosis not only shows the transparency and confidence of the prescriber but also guides the dispenser and the patients about the disease condition being

Table 4 Distribution of antimicrobials and antibacterial agents per encounter in prescriptions dispensed from Jan 1 - Dec 31 2016 at four governmental hospitals of Harar town

No. per encounter	HFSUH ($n = 600$)		FHPH ($n = 600$)		JH ($n = 600$)		SECIIIH ($n = 600$)		Overall ($n = 2400$)	
	AMA	ABA	AMA	ABA	AMA	ABA	AMA	ABA	AMA	ABA
One	267 (44.5)	292 (43.5)	300 (50.0)	319 (53.2)	274 (35.7)	303 (50.5)	390 (65.0)	374 (62.3)	1231 (51.29)	1288 (53.67)
Two	85 (14.2)	46 (7.7)	96 (16.0)	61 (10.2)	97 (16.2)	50 (8.3)	55 (9.2)	17 (2.8)	333 (13.87)	174 (7.25)
Three	10 (1.7)	1 (0.2)	11 (1.8)	3 (0.5)	13 (2.2)	6 (1)	1 (0.2)	0 (0.0)	35 (1.45)	10 (0.41)
Four	1 (0.2)	0 (0.0)	2 (0.3)	0 (0.0)	2 (0.3)	0 (0.0)	0 (0.0)	0 (0.0)	5	0
Five	0 (0.0)	0 (0.0)	1 (0.2)	1 (0.2)	0(0.0)	0 (0.0)	0 (0.0)	0 (0.0)	1	1
Total Rx[a]	363	339	410	384	386	359	446	391	1605 (66.9%)	1473 (61.4%)
Total drugs	471	387	538	455	515	421	558	408	2082	1671
Average drug per encounter	1.30	1.14	1.31	1.18	1.33	1.17	1.25	1.04	1.29 (±0.03)	1.13 (±0.08)

Abbreviations AMA antimicrobial agent, *ABA* antibacterial agent, *HFSUH* Hiwot Fana Specialized University Hospital, *FHPH* Federal Harar Police Hospital, *JH* Jugel Hospital, *SECIIIH* Southeast command III Hospital

[a]Prescriptions containing antimicrobial and/or antibacterial

Table 5 WHO core prescribing indicators in four governmental hospitals of Harar town from Jan 1 – Dec 31, 2016

WHO core prescribing indicators	HFSUH	FHPH	JH	SECIIIH	Total	WHO standard
Encounters with injection(s) prescribed ($n = 600$)	262 (43.67)	123 (20.5)	219 (36.5)	32 (5.3)	636 (26.5)	< 25% (13.4–24.1%)
Encounters with antimicrobial (s) prescribed ($n = 600$)	363 (60.5)	410 (68.33)	386 (64.33)	446 (74.3)	1605 (66.9).	< 30% [a](20.0–26.8%)
Encounters with antibacterial (s) prescribed ($n = 600$)	339 (56.5)	384 (64.0)	359 (59.8)	391 (65.2)	1473 (61.4)	–
Percentage of drugs with generic name (n = total drugs per hospital)	960 (94.02)	1350 (86.53)	1260 (88.60)	1074(88.46)	4644 (89.01)	100%
Percentage of drugs from EDL (n = total drugs per hospital)	960 (94.02)	1352 (86.67)	1103 (77.57)	1198 (98.68)	4613 (88.42)	100%

Abbreviations: *HFSUH* Hiwot Fana Specialized University Hospital, *FHPH* Federal Harar Police Hospital, *JH* Jugel Hospital, *SECIIIH* Southeast command III Hospital
[a]indicates the maximum acceptable value in tropical countries where infectious diseases are highly prevailing

treated. Moreover, such poor recording practice might open a way for extravagant and overprescribing without justifiable reason [13, 14]. This and related gaps might create loss of trust and confidence among healthcare providers and patients in the healthcare system at large.

In contrary to our findings, Alkot et al. reported better results indicating the presence of name and age of the patients in all prescriptions and omission of diagnosis in only 1.56% of prescriptions [18]. In concordant with our findings, Admassie et al. indicated that the address of the patient and diagnosis were omitted in 97.29 and 99.99% prescriptions, respectively. Besides, patients' age, sex and card number were only written in 86.64, 67.93 and 73.54% prescriptions, respectively [10].

Coming to drug related information, 5217 drugs were prescribed from all prescribing encounters reviewed. The average number of drugs per encounter was found to be 2.17(±0.39). Generally, larger proportion of prescription contained two drugs. Looking at the components of drug regimen, the most and least commonly recorded components were frequency and dose, respectively. Similarly, the mean value of frequency and dose per prescribing encounter were found to be 1.85 and 0.59, respectively. Almost similar behavior was observed across hospitals in recording the dose of medications. Even if dose should have been written in simple terms such as one tablet, two capsules, two teaspoons and the like, we had observed a significant mix up of strengths and doses and/or omitting or replacing doses with the strength of drugs. This might be partly ascribed to act of negligence or else lack of trainings on good prescribing practice. Overall, route of administration was the second most commonly recorded component of drug regimen. Nearly half of the drugs were prescribed without specified duration with poorest practice seen in FHPH. However, this hospital compensated such gap by having better record of total quantity of drugs for ease dispensing and inspection. In contrary to our finding, Alkot et al. reported that the dose and duration of therapy were missed only in 1.01 and 14.9% prescriptions, respectively [18]. Missing the duration of therapy might have resulted profound health realted problems including AMR, treatment failure and toxicological issues [4, 15, 19, 20]. The average number of drugs per encounter falls outside of the upper boundary of WHO standard which mandates the average value to be less than or equal to two (ideally, 1.6–1.8) in outpatient settings [4, 21].The average value was obtained low in HFSUH as it is a tertiary care teaching hospital of Haramaya University and hence limited number of drugs might be expected per prescription. The overall practice was not actually far from the WHO cut-off point and may be appreciated considering the context of developing countries like Ethiopia where healthcare delivery has become often erratic and empirical. The finding is also better than previous studies conducted in different settings within

Table 6 Healthcare professional's information in prescriptions dispensed from Jan 1 - Dec 31 2016 at four governmental hospitals of Harar town

Health professional related information	HFSUH ($n = 600$)	FHPH ($n = 600$)	JH ($n = 600$)	SECIIIH ($n = 600$)	Total ($n = 2400$)
Prescriber name	360 (60.0)	327 (54.5)	171(28.5)	225(37.5)	1083(45.1)
Prescriber signature	582 (97.0)	586 (97.7)	396(66.0)	569(94.8)	2133(88.9)
Dispenser name	86 (14.3)	0 (0.0)	1(0.2)	7(1.2)	94(3.9)
Dispensers signature	146 (24.3)	1 (0.2)	1(0.2)	4(0.7)	152(6.3)

Abbreviations: HFSUH Hiwot Fana Specialized University Hospital, *FHPH* Federal Harar Police Hospital, *JH* Jugel Hospital, *SECIIIH* Southeast command III Hospital

Table 7 Common pharmacological classes of drugs prescribed and top three individual drugs per class in prescriptions dispensed from Jan 1-Dec 31, 2016

Top drug classes	N (%)	Top three drugs per class	N (%)
Antimicrobial agents	2036 (39.02)	Amoxicillin	497 (24.41)
		Ciprofloxacin	276 (13.56)
		Metronidazole	202 (9.92)
Analgesics	1548 (29.67)	Diclofenac	594 (38.37)
		Paracetamol	388 (25.06)
		Tramadol	239 (15.44)
Gastrointestinal drugs	555 (10.64)	Omeprazole	206 (37.11)
		Cimetidine	115 (20.72)
		Plasil	104 (18.74)
Cardiovascular drugs	260 (4.98)	Furosemide	62 (23.85)
		Nifedipine	56 (21.54)
		Spironolactone	26 (10.0)
Vitamins & Minerals	253 (4.85)	Multivitamin	84 (33.20)
		Pyridoxine	28 (11.06)
		Vitamin B complex	21 (8.30)
Antihistamines	200 (3.83)	Chlorpheniramine	104 (52.0)
		Almetamin	52 (26.0)
		Diphenhydramine	10 (5.0)
Respiratory drugs	122 (2.33)	Salbutamol	58 (47.54)
		Cough syrup	49 (40.16)
		Theophydrine	9 (7.38)
Antidiabetic agents	119 (2.28)	Glibenclamide	45 (37.82)
		Metformin	40 (33.61)
		Insulin	25 (21.0)
Central nervous system drugs	86 (1.65)	Amitriptyline	33 (38.37)
		Fluoxetine	17 (19.77)
		Chlorpromazine	14 (16.28)
Others	38 (0.73)		
Total drugs	5217 (100)		

Ethiopia and abroad [18, 22–31]. However, lower average numbers of drugs per encounter (1.8, 1.9, 2.1, 1.9, 1.76 and 1.84) was reported from different settings [5, 6, 8, 10, 32, 33]. Two decades review report of 104 countries (in all WHO regions) indicated that average number of drugs prescribed per patient increased from 2.1 to 2.8 from 1900 to 2009 [34]. High average value can be associated with adverse consequences including drug-drug interactions, adverse drug reactions, and wastage of resources for the patient and healthcare system. Evidence based- and/or definitive therapy is mandatory to reduce the burden of drugs prescribed for the patient at a time [2].

Among the core prescribing indicators, WHO gives special emphasis for antimicrobials and injection prescribing practice as they have been mostly utilized but commonly misused class of drugs [4, 21]. In this study, the percentage of encounters with antimicrobial (s) and antibacterial (s) prescribed were found to be 66.9% (60.5% in HFSUH to 74.3% in SECIIIH) and 61.4% (56.5% in HFSUH to 65.2% in SECIIIH), respectively. This study revealed that the prevalence of antimicrobial containing prescription was more in police and military hospitals than the public hospitals (JH and HFSUH) had. These special government hospitals might have empirically prescribed antimicrobials without sufficient clinical evidence or the competency and experience of the prescribers might have also contributed for such difference. Apart from this, what makes all hospital in common is that there is no both culture and antimicrobial susceptibility (antibiogram) testing. Antimicrobial prescribing is solely based on clinical not microbiological evidence. Moreover, the highest number of antibacterial agents (per prescription) was observed in FHPH (1.18). For countries like Ethiopia where the infectious diseases are considered highly prevalent, prescribing antibiotics has become a prevailing practice. WHO set a maximum cut-off point on percent encounter of antibiotics in the outpatient settings of such countries (30%; ideal range, 20–26.8%) [4]. Our finding is more than twice the upper limit of WHO standard. Values that are lower than the present finding were reported from various healthcare settings including 30.3 and 24.27% in Indian tertiary-care hospitals [23, 31], 52.8% in Dessie referral hospital [5], 28.1% in Nigerian army hospital [35], 52.% in Bahawal Victoria hospital, Pakistan [26], and 29.14% in Gondar University referral hospital [10]. In contrary, even more deviation were presented from several studies such as 70.6% in Bule Hora hospital, southern Ethiopia, [22] and 78% in tertiary-care hospital of Bangladesh [25]. Summoro et al. also reported that the percent encounters with antibiotics ranged from 46.7 to 85% in four hospitals of southern Ethiopia [9]. In broader sense, Holloway et al. reported the pecenatge of patients receiving antibiotics had increased from 45 to 54% in drug utilization review of 104 countries included from all WHO regions [34]. Empirical use of antimicrobial agents has come with emergence of AMR in several healthcare settings [4, 15]. If the current practice continues without any intervention, we are running to a post-antibiotic era where all the current antimicrobial agents will become historical. WHO (2014) report on global surveillance of AMR indicated that AMR is no longer a prediction for the future; it is an event happening right now, across the world, and is putting at risk the ability to treat common infections. Legitimate and responsible use of antimicrobials is, therefore, necessary to prevent selection of AMR and to minimize unnecessary wastage of scarce resource in developing countries [15, 19, 20, 36, 37]. It is imperative that antimicrobial stewardship programs should be established to preserve the existing antimicrobials and to contain AMR.

Concerning the injection practice, nearly one-fourth (26.5%) of prescribing encounters had at least one injectable with the highest (43.67%) and lowest (5.3%) values recorded in HFSUH and SECIIIH, respectively. In outpatient settings, WHO limits the prevalence of prescribing encounters with injectables to be less than 25% (ideal range, 13.4–24.1%) [4]. Injection prescribing practices of HFSUH (43.67%) and JH (36.5%) were too far from the upper limit of WHO standard. This might be related to the public nature of these hospitals (patients irrespective of their socio-demographic status could come to these settings unlike police and military hospitals) and the hence the injection demand was found higher. In addition, patient attendees who visited these hospitals might come with severe illness and/or complications to which injections were a primary choice. The overall injection practice is higher than previous studies conducted in Ethiopian healthcare settings and abroad [18, 22, 23, 27, 30, 31]. Comparable injection practices were also reported in different settings as 31% in Dilchora Referral Hospital (DRH) [5], 28.3% in selected hospitals of west Ethiopia [6], 38.1% in Hawassa university teaching and referral hospital [8], and 28.5% in Gondar university teaching and referral hospital [10]. In developing countries, up to 56% of primary care patients received injections. From this, over 90% injections deemed medically unnecessary. Globally, 15 billion injections were given to patients, but half of these injections were not sterilized, which might result in the transmission of potentially infectious diseases. Potential infections attributable to unsafe injection are hepatitis B (33%), hepatitis C (42%), and HIV (2%) [38, 39]. Frequent and impropriate use of injections might be attributable to psychological dependence of both patients and healthcare professionals. Despite the presence of safer, cheaper and more convenient oral alternatives, patients may preferably seek injections for treating their healthcare conditions assuming that injections are more effective than any other agents. Indeed, injections are important formulations in certain clinical conditions including emergency situations, and when other alternatives are not feasible. However, they are not without potential limitations. Frequent use of injections can result in physiological and psychological pain during injection; risk of transmission of potentially infectious biohazards and wastage of resources, among others [4].

In this study, the prevalence of drugs prescribed with generic name and from EDL of Ethiopia were 89.02% (86.53–94.02%) and 88.42% (77.56–94.02%), respectively. In this regard, the ideal WHO standard to which healthcare setting should achieve is 100% [4]. Even if the overall prescribing practice seems appreciable, there is a need to invest more efforts to meet the ideal targets of WHO. Being a tertiary care teaching hospital, HFSUH had a higher generic prescribing practice than the rest hospitals. In contrary to our findings, Prakash et al. reported that the percentage of drugs prescribed by generic name and from EDL were 0.5 and 53%, respectively [23]. There was also 0.0% generic prescribing practice as reported from tertiary hospital of Bangladesh [25]. This gap might be, in part, related to variation in the healthcare system, knowledge and experience of prescribers, healthcare policies and regulations (e.g. generic substitutions) and the sociodemographic indices of the countries. In concordant with the present finding, comparable generic prescribing practices were reported from different directions as 89.88% in tertiary hospital of rural India [31], 93.9% in

DRH [5], and 90.61% in eastern Ethiopia [27]. Better than the present practice were also reported from previous findings [7, 8, 28, 40]. Being generic version is one of the criteria of essential drugs selection. In low-income countries like Ethiopia where resources are often scarce, prescribing with generic name has a multitude of advantages: generic drugs are relatively affordable, accessible, and recallable compared to brand counterparts [4]. It also reduces the likelihood of perverse financial incentives among healthcare workers of private and public healthcare settings.

Regarding the percentage of drugs prescribed from EDL, the overall finding did not meet the ideal target set by WHO (100%) [4]. Closely related findings were reported in previous studies [7, 8, 26, 28]. Prescribing from the EDL has several advantages. Essential drugs are the one that are selected by criteria including generic version, consideration of drugs of choice for the prevailing disease condition in the catchment area or country, cost-effectiveness ratio, quality, safety, risk-benefit aspect, and other pharmacokinetic considerations. Therefore, prescribing from EDL maximizes affordability and availability of drugs, reduces the possibility of drug interactions and adverse drug reactions and ultimately promotes patient therapeutic outcome [4, 38, 39]. To this end, WHO essential medicines policies are associated with improved quality use of medicines, particularly in low income countries. Low income countries reporting implementation of such policies have showed much better medicine use [41].

Concerning the healthcare professional's information, the prevalence of dispenser name or signature was found less than 10%. This practice can vividly show the act of negligence and avoidance of accountability for drug related problems. This poor recording practice might be attributable to high patient load per dispenser and lack of strict rules and regulations governing the prescribing practice.

Looking at the distribution of drug classes and individual agents, antimicrobial drugs were the most frequently prescribed classes of drugs followed by analgesics and gastrointestinal agents. This result is in line with the high prevalence of antimicrobial containing prescriptions in the indicator study. Besides, amoxicillin and ciprofloxacin were the top two drugs prescribed under antimicrobials. In concordant with the present findings, the most common categories of drugs, reported by Pathak et al., were antibiotics (24.64%) followed by anti-diabetic drugs (12.38%), analgesics (12.23%), and cardiovascular agents (11.82%) [31]. Besides, the most commonly prescribed forms of antibiotics were amoxicillin (16.4%), ampicillin (15%), gentamicin (14.9%) and chloramphenicol (11 .6%) [8]. Sisay et al also reported that the most common antibiotic prescribed was amoxicillin followed by ciprofloxacin [27].

Strength and limitation

This study tried to address several aspects of prescription beyond the usual indicator studies. A data abstraction format included general features of prescription and its completeness form as well as WHO prescribing indicator form to generate sufficient data. However, this study was not without potential limitations. It is a retrospective cross-sectional study, and hence some degree of documentation gap might be expected. This is also a quantitative descriptive study which could not answer the underlying causes why this problem exists. It simply highlighted the major problem areas for further action.

Conclusion

Generally, JH and SECIIIH were not using standard prescriptions and the overall prevalence of standard prescriptions was less than 50%. Nearly one in ten prescription papers had a written clinical condition (diagnosis) with nil recording practice in SECIIIH. The tendency of prescribing drugs with dose and dosage form was very poor. Overall, none of the core prescribing indicators was in line with the WHO standard. These and other related problems should be investigated in-depth to find out the underlying problems. As drug use is highly vexed, a multitude of strategies (educational, economic, managerial and regulatory) should be designed to reverse the existing trends of drug use pattern (prescribing pattern in particular) in low and middle-income countries like Ethiopia. Evidence-based and/or definitive therapy reduces the burden of antimicrobial drugs prescription thereby contains the emergence and spread of AMR; limits adverse drug reactions, and contraindications, and possibly avoids unnecessary direct and indirect healthcare costs.

Abbreviations

AMR: Antimicrobial Resistance; DRH: Dilchora Referral Hospital; EDL: Essential Drug List; FHPH: Federal Harar Police Hospital; FMHACA: Food Medicine and Healthcare Administration and Control Authority; HFSUH: Hiwot Fana Specialized University Hospital; JH: Jugel Hospital; SECIIIH: Southeast Command III Hospital; WHO: World Health Organization

Acknowledgments

Authors thank data collectors and staffs of all hospitals, without them this research would not be realized.

Funding

Authors disclosed reception of financial support from Haramaya University for conducting this research work.

Authors' contribution

MS, TG, GM and FA conceived the study and drafted the proposal. All authors had substantial contribution in the study design and development of data collection checklist. All authors were also involved in data acquisition, analysis, interpretation and write up. MS drafted the manuscript, critically revised it and prepared the final version for publication. All authors read and approved the final version of the manuscript.

Competing interest

The authors have declared that there is no competing interest.

Author details

[1]Department of Pharmacology and Toxicology, School of Pharmacy, College of Health and Medical Sciences, Haramaya University, P.O. Box 235, Harar, Ethiopia. [2]Department of Pharmacy, College of Medicine and Health Sciences, Wollo University, Dessie, Ethiopia. [3]Department of Pharmacy Practice, School of Pharmacy, College of Health and Medical Sciences, Haramaya University, P.O. Box 235, Harar, Ethiopia.

References

1. Ofori-Asenso R. A closer look at the World Health Organization's prescribing indicators. J Pharmacol Pharmacother. 2016;7(1):51.
2. Lu Y, Hernandez P, Abegunde D, Edejer T. The world medicines situation 2011. Geneva: Medicine expenditures World Health Organization; 2011.
3. Holloway KA. Combating inappropriate use of medicines. Expert Rev Clin Pharmacol. 2011;4(3):335–48.
4. WHO. How to investigate drug use in health facilities: selected drug use indicators. 1993. Available at: http://apps.who.int/medicinedocs/en/d/Js2289e/. Accessed on 25 May 2018
5. Assen A, Abrha S. Assessment of drug prescribing pattern in Dessie referral hospital, Dessie. Int J Pharm Sci Res. 2014;5(11):777–81.
6. Lenjisa J, Fereja T. A retrospective analysis of prescribing practice based on WHO prescribing indicators at four selected hospitals of West Ethiopia: policy implication. East Central Afri J Pharm Sci. 2013;16(3):69–74.
7. Bilal AI, Osman ED, Mulugeta A. Assessment of medicines use pattern using World Health Organization's prescribing, patient care and health facility indicators in selected health facilities in eastern Ethiopia. BMC Health Serv Res. 2016;16(1):144.
8. Desalegn AA. Assessment of drug use pattern using WHO prescribing indicators at Hawassa University teaching and referral hospital, South Ethiopia: a cross-sectional study. BMC Health Serv Res. 2013;13(1):170.
9. Summoro TS, Gidebo KD, Kanche ZZ, Woticha EW. Evaluation of trends of drug-prescribing patterns based on WHO prescribing indicators at outpatient departments of four hospitals in southern Ethiopia. Drug Des Dev Ther. 2015;9:4551.
10. Admassie E, Begashaw B, Hailu W. Assessment of drug use practices and completeness of prescriptions in Gondar University teaching referral hospital. Int J Pharm Sci Res. 2013;4(1):265.
11. Roughead EE, Lhazeen K, Socialine E, Bahri S, Park BJ, Holloway K. Monitoring medicines use to support national medicines policy development and implementation in the Asia Pacific region. WHO South East Asia J Public Health. 2013;2(2):113.
12. HRHB. Harari region health bureau. Harari reginal state. In: Annnual bulletin; 2014.
13. FMHACA. Manual for Medicines Good Prescribing Practice. Food, Medicine and Healthcare Administration and Control Authority of Ethiopia, Addis Ababa. 2012. Available at: http://apps.who.int/medicinedocs/documents/s22353en/s22353en.pdf. Accessed 15 May 2018.
14. WHO. Guide to good prescribing - a practical manual:World Health Organization action Programme on essential drugs. In: WHO/DAP/94.11 Geneva; 1994.
15. WHO. Antimicrobial resistance: global report on surveillance, Geneva: World Health Organization; 2014. Available at: http://www.who.int/drugresistance/documents/surveillancereport/en/. Accessed 25 May 2018.
16. West SL, Strom BL, Freundlich B, Normand E, Koch G, Savitz DA. Completeness of prescription recording in outpatient medical records from a health maintenance organization. J Clin Epidemiol. 1994;47(2):165–71.
17. Kumari R, Idris M, Bhushan V, Khanna A, Agrawal M, Singh SK. Assessment of prescription pattern at the public health facilities of Lucknow district. Indian J Pharmacol. 2008;40(6):243.
18. Alkot M, Shaheen H, Hathout H. Prescribing patterns and errors in family practice; a retrospective study of prescribing records. J Amer Sci. 2011;7(11):186–90.
19. Roca I, Akova M, Baquero F, Carlet J, Cavaleri M, Coenen S, Cohen J, Findlay D, Gyssens I, Heure O. The global threat of antimicrobial resistance: science for intervention. New Microbes New Infect. 2015;6:22–9.
20. Harbarth S, Samore MH. Antimicrobial resistance determinants and future control. Emerg Infect Dis. 2005;11(6):794.
21. Ghei P. How to investigate drug use in health facilities. Selected drug use indicators: WHO Publications, Geneva; 1993. p. 87. Health Policy 1995, 34(1):73
22. Mariam AH, Raghavendra Y, Bobasa EM. Evaluating rational drug use with the help of World Health Organization's core indicators in Bule Hora hospital, Southern Ethiopia. Encounters. 2015;7(8):11.
23. Prakash P, Rao VU, Kokiwar PR, Sowmya S, Vishweshwaran G. A study to evaluate rationality behind prescription patterns using world health organization prescribing indicators. Indo Am J Pharmaceut Res. 2016;6.
24. Bachewar NR, Choudhari SR, Dudhgaonkar S. Assessment of prescription pattern using WHO drug prescribing indicators in medicine wards of a tertiary care teaching hospital: a retrospective observational study. Int J Basic Clin Pharmacol. 2018;6(8):2070–7.
25. Sultana F, Rahman A, Paul TR, Sarwar MS, Islam MAU, Rashid M. Prescribing pattern and prescription errors: a study at a tertiary care hospital of Bangladesh. Bangladesh Pharm J. 2015;18(1):20–4.
26. Atif M, Azeem M, Sarwar MR, Shahid S, Javaid S, Ikram H, Baig U, Scahill S. WHO/INRUD prescribing indicators and prescribing trends of antibiotics in the accident and emergency Department of Bahawal Victoria Hospital, Pakistan. SpringerPlus. 2016;5(1):1928.
27. Sisay M, Mengistu G, Molla B, Amare F, Gabriel T. Evaluation of rational drug use based on World Health Organization core drug use indicators in selected public hospitals of eastern Ethiopia: a cross sectional study. BMC Health Serv Res. 2017;17(1):161.
28. Mezgebe HB, Tadesse B, Legesse B. Antibiotics prescribing pattern in pediatric unit of Ayder referral hospital, Tigray region, Northern Ethiopia. JSIR. 2015;4(2):57–60.
29. Charles NM: Patterns of prescribing practices in Makueni County referral hospital, Kenya. Unpublished, University of Narobi 2014.
30. Prasad PS, Rudra JT, Vasanthi P, Sushitha U, Sadiq MJ, Narayana G. Assessment of drug use pattern using World Health Organization core drug use indicators at secondary care referral Hospital of South India. CHRISMED J Health Res. 2015;2(3):223.
31. Pathak A, Gupta VK, Maurya A, Kumar A, Singh A. Assessment of drug prescribing pattern using who indicators in hospitalized patients at a tertiary care teaching hospital in rural area of India. Int J Basic Clin Pharmacol. 2016;5(3):651–5.
32. Lenjisa JL, Fereja TH. A retrospective analysis of prescribing practices through WHO prescribing indicators at four selected hospitals of West Ethiopia. J Bioanalysis Biomed. 2014;6(2):29.
33. Chandelkar UK, Rataboli PV. A study of drug prescribing pattern using WHO prescribing indicators in the state of Goa, India. Int J Basic Clin Pharmacol. 2017;3(6):1057–61.
34. Holloway KA, Ivanovska V, Wagner A, Vialle-Valentin C, Ross-Degnan D. Have we improved use of medicines in developing and transitional countries and do we know how to? Two decades of evidence. Tropical Med Int Health. 2013;18(6):656–64.
35. Adebayo E, Hussain N. Pattern of prescription drug use in Nigerian army hospitals. Ann Afr Med. 2010;9(3).
36. Ndihokubwayo JB, Yahaya AA, Dester A, Ki-Zerbo G, Asamoah-Odei E, Keita B. Antimicrobial resistance in the African region: issues, challenges and actions proposed. Afr Health Mon. 2013;16:27–30.
37. Prestinaci F, Pezzotti P, Pantosti A. Antimicrobial resistance: a global multifaceted phenomenon. Pathogens and Global Health. 2015;109(7):309–18.

38. MSH. Management sciences for health (MSH) (1997) managing drug supply. 2nd ed. USA: Kumarian Press; 1997.
39. Jonathan. Essential drugs and medicines policy. Geneva. Switzerland: World Health Organization International Pediatrics Association; 2001.
40. Srikanth BA. A prospective study on evaluation of use of drugs at prescriber, dispenser and patients level based on "who" core drug use indicators in ethiopia. Editorial Board. 2013;6(1):21–32.
41. Holloway KA, Henry D. WHO essential medicines policies and use in developing and transitional countries: an analysis of reported policy implementation and medicines use surveys. PLoS Med. 2014;11(9):e1001724.

Access to innovative cancer medicines in a middle-income country

Daniela Moye-Holz[1*], Rene Soria Saucedo[2], Jitse P van Dijk[1], Sijmen A Reijneveld[1] and Hans V Hogerzeil[1]

Abstract

Background: Cancer has become the third cause of death in Mexico. Treatment for cancer is often complex and lengthy. New and better medicines enter the market at high prices, which may limit access. Like most Latin American countries, Mexico has an essential cancer medicines list that includes innovative medicines. Their accessibility and use in the public sector remains unknown. Therefore, we describe the use, as a proxy of access, of innovative and essential cancer medicines in the public sector in Mexico, by insurance institution, and by five regions between 2010 to 2016.

Methods: We used drug utilization research methods to assess the use of eight patented cancer medicines. Through the national transparency platform, we obtained data on the quantities of these medicines used in all public health facilities and social health insurance institutions and recalculated those figures into defined daily dose (DDD) per 1000 population per year.

Results: Overall, the use of all medicines increased over the years, especially for trastuzumab, rituximab and imatinib. The use of innovative medicines was higher per population covered in social health insurance institutions than in governmental facilities. Throughout the study period, the Central region (including Mexico City) has used more medicines per population than the other regions.

Conclusions: The use and access of some essential innovative cancer medicines has increased over the years, but remains unequal across insurance schemes and regions. Particularly, the Ministry of Health Insurance scheme and Northern and Western regions in the country would benefit from additional efforts to increase access to essential cancer medicines.

Keywords: Access, Drug utilization, Essential cancer medicines, Mexico, Insurance schemes access, Regional access

Background

Cancer has become a leading cause of disability and mortality in the world, particularly in low and middle-income countries (LMIC) [1–3]. Such health care systems are not yet prepared to handle this burden [4]. In 2013, 12.8% of all deaths in Mexico were due to cancer [5]. Although Mexico has introduced specific health policies to tackle non-communicable diseases, like tobacco control, obesity control, and breast cancer screening, cancer remains the third leading cause of death in the country [5]. Like other Latin American (LATAM) countries, Mexico has invested significant resources to enhance preventive efforts - as many cancer cases are diagnosed at advanced stages - which typically have poor prognosis and high mortality [5]. Yet, factors such as lack of awareness on the importance of screening, poor distribution of screening programs, delays in pathology assessment and referrals, poverty, geographic barriers, lack of access to healthcare systems, financial barriers and stigma related to cancer have negatively impacted the improvement of cancer treatments and its outcomes [1, 4–7]. In addition, cancer cases diagnosed at later stages of the disease consume more resources, as treatments tend to be more complex [1, 5, 8].

In Mexico, the public sector provides most of the cancer care including cancer medicines [9]. This sector consists of five different social health insurance (SHI) institutions, each with their independent facilities and managerial styles, responsible for providing health coverage and care

* Correspondence: danymoyeholz@gmail.com
[1]Department of Community and Occupational Medicine, University Medical Center Groningen, University of Groningen, Hanzeplein 1, 9713 GZ Groningen, The Netherlands
Full list of author information is available at the end of the article

to the formal sector (employees and their families). The Mexican Social Security Institute (IMSS) is the main SHI institution, providing coverage to employees of private companies, approximately 46% of the population. The Institute for Social Security and Services for State Workers (ISSSTE) provides coverage to state employees, approximately 10% of the population. The National Defense Ministry (SEDENA), the Navy Ministry (SEMAR) and the National Oil Company (PEMEX) provide coverage to their employees, approximately 2% of the population [10]. These institutions cover cancer treatment according to their own guidelines, policies and medicine formularies. The population without SHI (roughly 42%) can receive healthcare at the Ministry of Health (MoH) facilities; each facility has its own policies and managerial style. Most of this population is affiliated to the People's Health Insurance (Seguro Popular de Salud, SPS), which is a governmental insurance that reimburses health institutions according to a catalogue of interventions [11]. SPS covers all child cancer types and some of the most prevalent adult types, following its own guidelines and protocols. The MoH facilities have a list of selected medicines based on the national formulary and/or according to the list of medicines covered by SPS as described in its catalogue of interventions, which is also based on the national formulary [11–13].

The innovation field for cancer medicines is growing [14, 15]. New and better medicines are coming into the market, forcing constant updates of treatment protocols and formularies. Yet, most of the time, the high prices tagged to these innovations keep newer treatments unaffordable for individual patients [4] and burdensome for health systems, thus limiting patient's access to new cancer medicines [16, 17]. As a result, prices rather than efficacy become a decisive factor for inclusion of these medicines in national or institutional formularies and ultimately, for reimbursement [1, 18].

Access to new cancer medicines is a challenge in all LMIC [19]. Most LATAM countries – including Mexico – utilize essential medicines lists for procurement purposes [1], which should guarantee proper access in health centers [20]. However, differences in access to these medicines across insurance schemes and country regions is not well known [21]. For example, some European countries and Australia have performed drug utilization studies to describe the availability and utilization of these medicines across regions and countries. These methodologies can inform about the distribution and the uptake of resources (e.g. cancer medicines); but these methodologies have rarely been used in middle-income countries (MIC), including Mexico [19, 22–24]. Therefore, this study describes the use of patented cancer medicines in the Mexican public sector, comparing five SHI schemes and the MoH in five geographic regions, and changes between 2010 and 2016.

Methods

Cancer medicines studied

We selected medicines based on the following criteria: inclusion in the national formulary, coverage by the SHI institutional lists, coverage by SPS, inclusion in the national clinical guidelines and SPS treatment guidelines (protocols), patent protection in Mexico until after 2017. We narrowed our selection of medicines based on the criterion that medicines should have gone through price negotiations every year from 2010 to 2016 by the Mexican Coordinating Commission for Negotiation of Prices of Medicines (CCNPMIS) [25]). The CCNPMIS is a commission that negotiates directly with pharmaceutical companies the public procurement prices applicable for the public sector only. The CCNPMIS determines which medicines will be considered for negotiations taking into consideration their relevance, estimated demand and procurement volume [25, 26]. The latter characteristics indicate that these medicines are considered both innovative and essential in Mexico, and that they could have been procured in the public sector during that period of time. Following these criteria, we selected the following medicines: bevacizumab, dasatinib, imatinib, nilotinib, rituximab, sorafenib, sunitinib, and trastuzumab. Some of these medicines (nilotinib and sorafenib) are not covered by SPS; furthermore, some of these are covered by SPS only for children or could be covered in case of disease progression (bevacizumab, dasatinib, sunitinib). We decided to include them because they had been negotiated by the CCNPMIS and included in the national clinical guidelines.

This range of medicines reflects some of the main cancers prevalent in Mexico. Imatinib, dasatinib and nilotinib are indicated for leukemia [27], the most prevalent cancer in children in Mexico [28]. Rituximab is indicated for non-Hodgkin lymphoma (NHL) treatment in addition to leukemia. Trastuzumab is indicated for breast cancer, one of the most common causes of dead among women in Mexico [29]. Bevacizumab, one of the most frequently used anti-cancer medicines worldwide, is indicated as a first line treatment for advanced colorectal cancer [30, 31], which has an increasing incidence in Mexico [32]. Sorafenib and sunitinib are both indicated for renal cancer; sunitinib is covered by SPS only for children.

Measures and procedure

Procurement data (volume and value) from the public sector were retrieved through the National Transparency Platform (PNT) [33]. Procurement data from all possible public health institutions providing cancer care in the country were obtained from the various institutions that provide this type of care (see Table 1).

We used the defined daily dose (DDD) as the unit of measurement of use, in order to standardize and add the

Table 1 Public Health Institutions and Social Health Insurance Institutions providing cancer care in Mexico

Ministry of Health (MoH)
Each states' Ministry of health and/or state health services (SESA)
Mexican Social Security Institute (IMSS)
Institute for Social Security and Services for State Workers (ISSSTE)
National Defense Ministry (SEDENA)
Navy Ministry (SEMAR)
National Oil Company (PEMEX)
National Institute of Cancerology (INCAN)
National Nutrition Institute (INNSZ)
National Institute of Pediatrics (INP)
Federal Hospitals
Regional high specialty hospitals (HRAE)

quantities procured and allow for proper comparisons. Because the WHO has not yet defined DDDs for most cancer medicines we used DDD values as reported by the German national Anatomic-Therapeutic-Chemical classification [34].

To measure the use or utilization rates of these medicines among the five SHI institutions and the MoH, population numbers affiliated to each type of health provider were used, as reported by the National Institute of Statistics and Geography (INEGI) [10]. To measure access among geographic regions, state population affiliated to SPS data were used, as reported by the SPS [35].

Data analysis

Standard drug utilization research methods were used [36]. First, we analyzed the data on the eight medicines from 2010 to 2016 separately, in order to assess their individual use rates in DDDs/1000 inhabitants. Secondly, we expressed differences in access according to health insurance schemes as DDDs/1000 persons covered. We also compared access between the regions for MoH channels only, regrouping 32 states into five regions [37] (Fig. 1) and expressing overall access to all products together as total DDDs/1000 inhabitants per region. We regrouped the country into 5 geographical regions following our own discretion into northern, center, western, eastern and southern regions, derived from the Ministry of Education's classification [38].

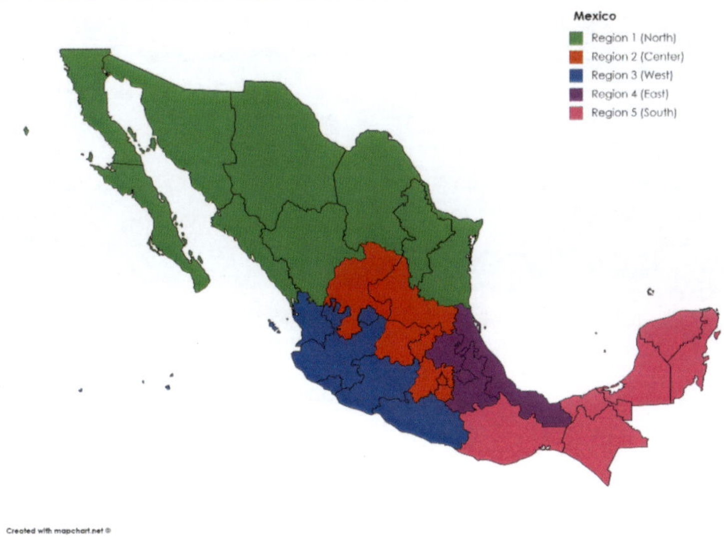

Region 1 (North): Baja California, Baja California Sur, Chihuahua, Coahuila, Durango, Nuevo León, Sinaloa, Sonora, Tamaulipas

Region 2 (Center): Guanajuato, Mexico City, Mexico State, Morelos, Queretaro, San Luis Potosi, Zacatecas

Region 3 (West): Aguascalientes, Colima, Guerrero, Jalisco, Michoacan, Nayarit

Region 4 (East): Hidalgo, Puebla, Tlaxcala, Veracruz

Region 5 (South): Campeche, Chiapas, Oaxaca, Quintana Roo, Tabasco, Yucatan

Fig. 1 Mexico – the five regions of study. Region 1 (North): Baja California, Baja California Sur, Chihuahua, Coahuila, Durango, Nuevo León, Sinaloa, Sonora, Tamaulipas. Region 2 (Center): Mexico City, Mexico State, Guanajuato, Morelos, Querétaro, San Luis Potosí, Zacatecas. Region 3 (West): Aguascalientes, Colima, Guerrero, Jalisco, Michoacan, Nayarit. Region 4 (East): Hidalgo, Puebla, Tlaxcala, Veracruz. Region 5 (South): Campeche, Chiapas, Oaxaca, Quintana Roo, Tabasco, Yucatan.

Results

Differences in access to innovative cancer medicines in Mexico

Figure 2 shows quantities procured of the eight selected cancer medicines from 2010 to 2016 in public facilities in Mexico. Overall, the annual quantities procured have increased for all medicines under study. The most commonly used medicines were imatinib, rituximab and trastuzumab. The quantities of rituximab and imatinib have remained high throughout the years, while trastuzumab shows a considerable increase since 2012 and a decrease between 2015 and 2016. The quantities of bevacizumab, dasatinib, nilotinib, sorafenib and sunitinib have remained steadily increasing, but in much lower quantities.

Access to innovative cancer medicines in the public sector

Figure 3 shows that quantities of innovative cancer medicines procured by different SHI institutions and the MoH have increased over the years (especially since 2013). The quantities of medicines procured by IMSS and the MoH have remained lower than by other SHI institutions in the period of study. Among SHI institutions, ISSSTE has procured larger quantities than all other institutions. IMSS procured the largest volume of medicines, but when adjusted to quantities procured per population covered (approximately 50%), it has the lowest rates among the five SHI institutions. The SHI for the oil company (PEMEX), the army (SEDENA), and the navy (SEMAR) have increased their use the most since 2011, and have had constantly higher quantities per population covered than IMSS and MoH.

Regional quantities of innovative cancer medicines

Figure 4 shows that quantities of innovative cancer medicines procured by the MoH remained lower in the northern, western, eastern and southern regions than in the central region (including Mexico City). In all regions, quantities have remained largely the same from 2010 to 2013. From 2013 to 2015, most regions experienced an increase, particularly the central region. However, the western and the southern region experienced a decrease in the quantities of medicines procured since 2014 and 2015 respectively.

Discussion

To our knowledge, this is the first study to describe the use of cancer medicines across the Mexican public sector. Reporting use of medicines provides a proxy measure of access to medicines and allows for comparisons between different settings (e.g. insurance schemes, geographical regions). First, the amount of DDDs of rituximab, imatinib and trastuzumab account for more than 70% of the total of DDDs of all procured medicines under study. Second, SHI institutions provide larger quantities per insured population than the MoH. Third, the central region (including Mexico city) reports, on average, a constantly higher use of cancer medicines than the other regions, which continued to have a low level of use.

Access barriers to individual medicines

All medicines under study showed an increase in quantities procured throughout 2010–2016. For most of them, this increase was slow and only for some medicines, in particular imatinib, rituximab and trastuzumab, the increase was larger. These three medicines were

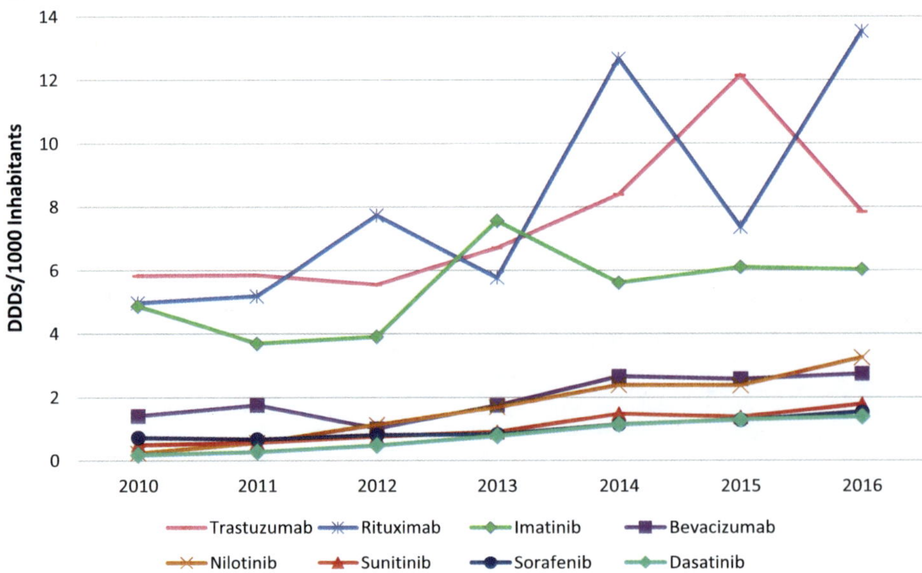

Fig. 2 Annual quantities of eight essential cancer medicines procured in the public sector (SHI institutions and MoH) in Mexico (2010–2016)

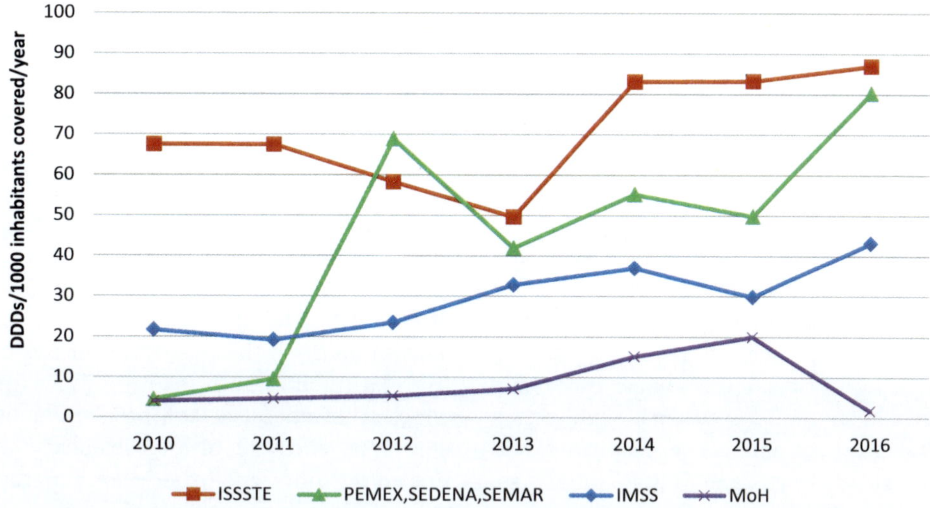

Fig. 3 Total annual quantities of eight essential cancer medicines, procured in the Mexican public sector (SHI institutions and MoH) per insurance scheme (2010–2016). *1000 inhabitants covered per SHI institution and by the MoH/SPS; for abbreviations see Table 1

covered by all SHI institutions and by the SPS. These medicines have demonstrated improved health outcomes [21], which has been recognized by the WHO and justifies their inclusion in the WHO-EML since 2015 [21]. However, only SPS does not fully cover dasatinib, nilotinib, bevacizumab, sunitinib and sorafenib [27]. Low accessibility of effective innovative medicines could limit adequate cancer care [16], particularly for the most vulnerable populations with colorectal and renal cancer.

Use and access to new cancer medicines is low in Mexico, with levels similar to those reported from other developing regions such as, for example, Africa, South-East Asia and Latin America [39, 40]. Studies performed on the use of some innovative medicines in the USA, Russia, Turkey, Brazil and Mexico [41, 42], have reported that barriers to access and use of innovative cancer medicines link to limited coverage by public insurance schemes, inclusion in the EML, availability of the medicine at the facilities, and updated clinical guidelines. The lack of availability in the public sector has pushed patients in Mexico, Russia and Brazil to get these medicines in the private sector and pay out of pocket [41, 42].

Access barriers by health coverage

We found large differences in use linked to the type of health coverage. For example, all eight medicines studied were covered by all SHI institutions (IMSS, ISSSTE, PEMEX, SEDENA, SEMAR) but only three were covered by the governmental SPS for children and adults (imatinib, rituximab, trastuzumab), and another two

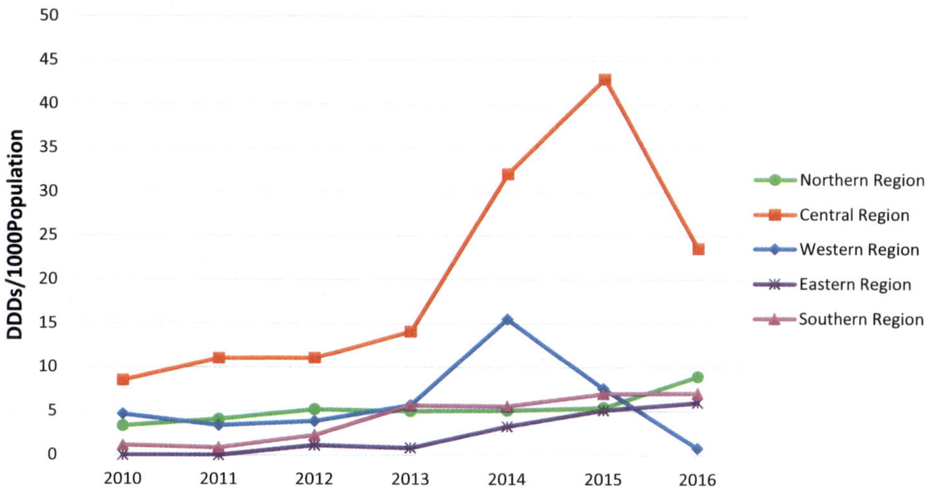

Fig. 4 Total annual quantities of eight essential cancer medicines, purchased in MoH facilities, per region (2010–2016). *1000 inhabitants covered by SPS per region

medicines where covered by SPS only for children (dasatinib and sunitinib), therefore limiting use of the other medicines in the MoH facilities [27]. Other studies have consistently reported higher availability and accessibility rates for essential medicines at the IMSS than other institutions in the public sector [43–47]. Previous research reported that MoH and IMSS are the largest providers of cancer care in the country [9]; despite this, access to the medicines of study at these two institutions [32] remained lower than at the other SHI institutions when expressed as quantities used per population insured. High prices of medicines, financial barriers, budget constraints, and the lack of prioritization of cancer care could explain the differences among institutions, highlighting the inequalities in access to innovative medicines and health care [16, 32]. This is worrisome as it could indicate that over 80% of the population experiences barriers to innovative medicines that could provide them with better outcomes of their treatment against cancer.

Access barriers by geographic location

We found regional variations in the use of the studied medicines, in line with previous findings from other countries [24, 31, 48–50]. These variations could be due to differences in the burden of disease, budget and resource allocation, purchasing power, differences in capacity within the health care system and disease priorities [16, 36, 51]. Like other LATAM countries, Mexico concentrates resources and health care in big cities (e.g. Mexico City, Monterrey and Guadalajara in the central, northern and western region respectively). Such a policy generates an "overwhelming influx of patients" [1, 52], which may have led to the relatively large increase in provision in recent years. Based on the number of hospital discharges, these three regions report high proportions of cancer patients attended by the MoH [9, 53]. Yet, use is far greater in the central region than in all other regions. In addition, distance to health facilities and traveling costs prevent patients from seeking health care and getting treatment [32, 54–56]. Thus, decentralization of health care is needed to bring treatment closer to patients, and improve access and health outcomes in regions currently lagging behind.

We also found a decrease in the quantities of medicines procured at MoH facilities in 2016, particularly in the central and western regions, largely explained by decreased quantities of trastuzumab. Trastuzumab had experienced constant increases in use particularly from 2012 to 2015 and had a sudden drop in 2016 (Fig. 2). This finding is unexpected, since Mexico has invested efforts in the control of breast cancer [29, 57]. The reasons for this decrease and the possible barriers that MoH facilities face when procuring trastuzumab need to be further explored.

Research in the US, Australia, China, Canada and Sweden suggest that geographic variations in access to innovative medicines [23, 24, 31, 48–50] could be explained by differences in coverage, insurance guidelines and management of the disease, professional disagreement and prescription preferences, budget issues and local policies. Heterogeneity in the burden of disease can also influence allocation of resources to a specific type of medicines [16, 23]. In the case of China, regional differences were also attributable differences in access to health care [48].

Strengths and limitations

The strength of this study lies in the collection of data from all public health institutions in the whole country, which allowed for a comprehensive overview on procurement and use of the selected medicines and for presenting differences between geographic regions and insurances schemes. Potential limitations include that we were unable to retrieve data from some states (e.g. Michoacan) while some other states provided incomplete data (e.g. Nayarit, Quintana Roo, Nuevo Leon, Guerrero), particularly before 2014. Our regional results (particularly northern, western and southern regions) may therefore underestimate the real quantities. Another limitation is that we did not take into account any regional variations in cancer burden, which could affect the quantities of medicines needed. Furthermore, this study focused on a selected number of innovative cancer medicines and does not account for a whole treatment scheme and does not differentiate use according to burden of each disease. Further research should focus on complete treatment schemes and weigh the use of these medicines against the burden of diseases (e.g. using mortality, incidence and/or morbidity data).

Implications

At the organizational level, use of medicines through IMSS and the MoH was lower than through other SHI institutions. Since IMSS and the MoH together cover most of the population, a more detailed analysis is needed to identify the barriers preventing adequate use and access to cancer essential medicines. Differences between regions continue to reflect a concentration of resources in the center of the country and limited infrastructure to manage specialized health care needs in the rest of the regions.

Previous research on access to innovative cancer medicines in LMIC has focused on whether these are included in national EMLs [20, 58]. Further research should now focus on use and actual access to comprehensive treatment schemes of the most prevalent types of cancer [20], in order to inform stakeholders and policy makers on the current situation and identify potential barriers to be addressed. Public health institutions and the government need to reflect on how resources can be allocated more equally and efficiently to ensure universal access to the most cost-effective level of care. Improving access and use of innovative treatments of which the effectiveness, safety and cost-effectiveness have been established, will provide better quality of cancer care, better health outcomes and fewer deaths due to cancer [49, 51]. The government should monitor the needs for these medicines along with their actual use and access to guarantee the best level of care. Efforts on improving access to cancer medicines need to go along with better access to screening, prevention and other types of treatment.

Conclusions

Over the last 6 years, the use of eight innovative essential cancer medicines has increased in Mexico, particularly of imatinib, rituximab and trastuzumab. The use of five other essential cancer medicines has remained low due to insufficient insurance coverage. Regional differences in the use of innovative cancer medicines highlight inequalities in access to cancer care. Providing access to essential innovative cancer medicines remains a challenge in Mexico. Further decentralization of cancer care is warranted to improve equitable access and use of effective and affordable cancer treatments.

Abbreviations

CCNPMIS: Coordinating Commission for Negotiation of Prices of Medicines; CONAPO: Population National Council; DDD: Defined daily dose; EML: Essential Medicines List; HRAE: Regional high specialty hospitals; IMSS: Mexican Social Security Institute (Insituto Mexicano del Seguro Social); INCAN: National Institute of Cancerology; INEGI: National Institute of Statistics and Geography; INNSZ: National Nutrition Institute; INP: National Institute of Pediatrics; ISSSTE: Institute for Social Security and Services for State Workers (Instituto de Seguridad y Servicios Sociales de los Trabajadores del Estado); LATAM: Latin America; LMIC: Low- and Middle-Income countries; MIC: Middle Income Countries; MoH: Ministry of Health; NHL: Non-Hodgkin Lymphoma; PEMEX: National Oil Company (Petróleos Mexicanos); PNT: National Transparency Platform; SEDENA: National Defense Ministry (Secretaría de la Defensa Nacional); SEMAR: Navy Ministry (Secretaría de la Marina); SESA: State health services; SPS: People's Health Insurance (Seguro Popular de Salud); WHO: World Health Organization

Acknowledgements

This work was supported by CONACYT (National Council of Science and Technology Mexico) (DMH scholarship 217161).

Authors' contributions

DMH carried out the planning of the study, the data collection, data analysis and discussion and interpretation of the results. She carried out the writing of the manuscript. RSS contributed to the planning of the study, carried out revisions of the data analysis, revisions and editing of the manuscript. JPvD carried out revisions and editing of the manuscript. SAR carried out revisions and editing of the manuscript. HVH contributed to the planning of the study, carried out revisions and editing of the manuscript. All authors read and approved the final manuscript.

Authors' information

DMH is a PhD candidate at the Global Health Research Unit of the University Medical Center Groningen. This research article is part of the PhD research project that focuses on access to innovative essential medicines in Mexico. HVH is professor at the Global Health Research Unit of the University Medical Center Groningen. HVH was director of the Essential Medicines Department at the WHO, is a Co-Chair of the Lancet Commission on Essential Medicines Policies, and is part of the supervisory board of the Access to Medicines Foundation. JPvD is an associate professor at Public Health Research group at the University Medical Center Groningen and scientific director of the Graduate School 'Kosice Institute for Society and Health' (KISH), Safarik University in Kosice, Slovak Republic. SAR is professor of Community and Occupational Medicine and Head of the department of Health Sciences and Head of the Public Health Research program at the University Medical Center Groningen. RSS is a research associate at the Department of Health Policy and Health Services Research at the Boston University.

Competing interests

The authors declare that they have no competing interests.

Author details

[1]Department of Community and Occupational Medicine, University Medical Center Groningen, University of Groningen, Hanzeplein 1, 9713 GZ Groningen, The Netherlands. [2]Boston University School of Public Health, Boston, USA.

References

1. Goss PE, Lee BL, Badovinac-Crnjevic T, Strasser-Weippl K, Chavarri-Guerra Y, St Louis J, et al. Planning cancer control in Latin America and the Caribbean. Lancet Oncol. 2013;14(5):391–436.
2. Knaul FM, Frenk J, Shulman L, for the Global Task Force on Expanded Access to Cancer Care and Control in Developing Countries.: Closing the Cancer Divide: A Blueprint to Expand Access in Low and Middle Income Countries. 2011.
3. Cancer. Fact Sheet. http://www.who.int/mediacentre/factsheets/fs297/en/. Accessed 6 July 2017.
4. Farmer P, Frenk J, Knaul FM, Shulman LN, Alleyne G, Armstrong L, et al. Expansion of cancer care and control in countries of low and middle income: a call to action. Lancet. 2010;376(9747):1186–93.
5. Reynoso-Noveron N, Meneses-Garcia A, Erazo-Valle A, Escudero-de Los Rios P, Kuri-Morales PA, Mohar-Betancourt A. Challenges in the development and implementation of the National Comprehensive Cancer Control Program in Mexico. Salud Publica Mex. 2016;58(2):325–33.
6. Sharma K, Costas A, Shulman LN, Meara JG. A systematic review of barriers to breast cancer care in developing countries resulting in delayed patient presentation. J Oncol. 2012;2012:121873.
7. Olver I. Cancer control-A global perspective. Eur J Cancer Care (Engl). 2017; 26:1. https://doi.org/10.1111/ecc.12654.
8. Gomez-Dantes H, Lamadrid-Figueroa H, Cahuana-Hurtado L, Silverman-Retana O, Montero P, Gonzalez-Robledo MC, et al. The burden of cancer in Mexico, 1990-2013. Salud Publica Mex. 2016;58(2):118–31.
9. Hernandez-Avila JE, Palacio-Mejia LS, Gonzalez-Gonzalez L, Morales-Carmona E, Espin-Arellano LI, Fernandez-Nino JA, et al. Utilization of hospital services for cancer care in Mexico. Salud Publica Mex. 2016;58(2):142–52.
10. Derechohabiencia y uso de servicios de salud. Población protegida por los servicios de salud, 2000 a 2014. http://www3.inegi.org.mx/sistemas/sisept/default.aspx?t=msoc01&s=est&c=22594. Accessed 10 July 2017.
11. Gómez Dantés O, Sesma S, Becerril VM, Knaul FM, Arreola H, Frenk J. Sistema de Salud de México [the health system in Mexico]. Salud Publica Mex. 2011;53(supplement 2):s220–32.
12. OECD: Reviews of health care systems: Mexico 2016. 2016.

13. Servan-Mori E, Montanez-Hernandez J, Avila-Burgos L, Wirtz VJ, Heredia-Pi I. Access to medicines by Seguro popular beneficiaries: pending tasks towards universal health coverage. PLoS One. 2015;10(9).
14. Lewis LD. Cancer pharmacotherapy: 21st century 'magic bullets' and changing paradigms. Br J Clin Pharmacol. 2006;62(1):1–4.
15. Buckland D. New drug treatments for cancer: what the future holds. Prescriber. 2016;27(1):17–21.
16. Kos M, Obradovic M, Mrhar A. Accessibility to targeted oncology drugs in Slovenia and selected European countries. Eur J Cancer. 2008;44(3):408–18.
17. Meropol NJ, Schulman KA. Cost of cancer care: issues and implications. J Clin Oncol. 2007;25(2):180–6.
18. Shulman LN, Wagner CM, Barr R, Lopes G, Longo G, Robertson J, Forte G, Torode J, Magrini N. Proposing essential medicines to treat Cancer: methodologies, processes, and outcomes. J Clin Oncol. 2016;34(1):69–75.
19. Wilking N, Jönsson B. A pan-European comparison regarding patient access to cancer drugs. Sweden: Karolinska Institutet; 2005.
20. Bazargani YT, de Boer A, Schellens JH, Leufkens HG, Mantel-Teeuwisse AK. Selection of oncology medicines in low- and middle-income countries. Ann Oncol. 2014;25(1):270–6.
21. Robertson J, Barr R, Shulman LN, Forte GB, Magrini N. Essential medicines for cancer: WHO recommendations and national priorities. Bull World Health Organ. 2016;94(10):735–42.
22. Wilson A, Cohen J. Patient access to new cancer drugs in the United States and Australia. Value Health. 2011;14(6):944–52.
23. Vitry AI, Thai LP, Lu CY. Time and geographical variations in utilization of endocrine therapy for breast cancer in Australia. Intern Med J. 2011;41(2):162–6.
24. Wilking U, Jonsson B, Wilking N, Bergh J. Trastuzumab use in breast cancer patients in the six health care regions in Sweden. Acta Oncol. 2010;49(6):844–50.
25. Gomez-Dantes O, Ortiz M, Terrazas P, Reich MR, Wirtz VJ. A new entity for the negotiation of public procurement prices for patented medicines in Mexico. Bull World Health Organ. 2012;90(10):788–92.
26. Bañuelos F: Mexico's Coordinating Commission for Negotiating the Price of Medicines and other Health Inputs. 2016. https://publications.iadb.org/handle/11319/7987. Accessed 10 Oct 2017.
27. Secretaría de Salud: LINEAMIENTOS para la adquisición de medicamentos asociados al Catálogo Universal de Servicios de Salud y al Fondo de Protección contra Gastos Catastróficos, por las entidades federativas con recursos transferidos por concepto de cuota social y de la aportación solidaria federal del Sistema de Protección Social en Salud. Mexico: Diario Oficial de la Federación; 2016.
28. Perez-Cuevas R, Doubova SV, Zapata-Tarres M, Flores-Hernandez S, Frazier L, Rodriguez-Galindo C, et al. Scaling up cancer care for children without medical insurance in developing countries: the case of Mexico. Pediatr Blood Cancer. 2013;60(2):196–203.
29. Chavarri-Guerra Y, Villarreal-Garza C, Liedke PE, Knaul F, Mohar A, Finkelstein DM, Goss PE. Breast cancer in Mexico: a growing challenge to health and the health system. Lancet Oncol. 2012;13(8):e335–43.
30. Wilking N, Jönsson B. Market uptake of new oncology drugs. Ann Oncol. 2007;18(Supplement 3):iii31–48.
31. Fu AZ, Tsai H, Marshall JL, Freedman AN, Potosky AL. Utilization of bevacizumab in US elderly patients with colorectal cancer receiving chemotherapy. J Oncol Pharm Pract. 2014;20(5):332–40.
32. Verastegui E, Mohar A. Colorectal cancer in Mexico: should a middle income country invest in screening or in treatment? Eur J Health Econ. 2010; 10(Suppl 1):S107–14.
33. Sistema Nacional de Transparencia: Plataforma Nacional de Transparencia. https://www.plataformadetransparencia.org.mx/web/guest/inicio. Accessed 26 Nov 2016.
34. Wissenschaftliches Insitut der AOK, Deutschen Institut für Medizinsche Dokumentation und Information: Anatomisch-therapeutisch-chemische Klassifikation mit Tagesdosen. 2017.
35. Seguro Popular: Beneficiarios de Protección Social en Salud de Seguro Popular. https://datos.gob.mx/busca/dataset/beneficiarios-de-proteccion-social-en-salud-de-seguro-popular. Accessed 17 July 2018.
36. Elseviers M. Drug utilization research: methods and applications. Chichester: Wiley; 2016.
37. Jönsson B, Wilking N. New cancer drugs in Sweden: assessment, implementation and access. J Cancer Policy. 2014;2(2):45–62.
38. CONEVYT: Regiones de México [Regions of Mexico]. https://www.conevyt.org.mx/colaboracion/colabora/objetivos/libros_pdf/sso1_u3lecc2.pdf. Accessed 29 Jan 2017.
39. Alwan AD, Maclean D, Mandil A; World Health Organization. Noncommunicable Diseases and Mental Health Cluster: Assessment of national capacity for noncommunicable disease prevention and control: the report of a global survey. Geneva: World Health Organization; 2001.
40. Lopes Gde L, Jr, de Souza JA, Barrios C. Access to cancer medications in low- and middle-income countries. Nat Rev Clin Oncol. 2013;10(6):314–22.
41. Lammers P, Criscitiello C, Curigliano G, Jacobs I. Barriers to the use of Trastuzumab for HER2+ breast Cabcer and the potential impact of Biosimilars: a physician survey in the United States and emerging markets. Pharmaceuticals. 2014;7:943–53.
42. Baer Ii WH, Maini A, Jacobs I. Barriers to the access and use of rituximab in patients with non-Hodgkin's lymphoma and chronic lymphocytic leukemia: a physician survey. Pharmaceuticals. 2014;7(5):530–44.
43. Wirtz V, Serván Mori E, Dreser A, Heredia-Pi I, Avila Burgos L. Surtimiento y gasto en el acceso a medicamentos en instituciones pública: asignaturas pendientes [Supply and spending on access to medicines in public institutions: pending issues]. ENSANUT. 2012;4.
44. Sesma-Vázquez S, Gomez-Dantes O, Castro-Tinoco M, Wirtz VJ. Abasto, surtimiento y gasto de bolsillo en medicamentos en hospitales públicos de México en 2009 [supply prescription filling and out-of-pocket expenditures on medicines in public hospitals in Mexico in 2009]. Salud Publica Mex. 2011;53:470–9.
45. Garrido-Latorre F, Gomez-Dantes O, Hernandez-Llamas H, Garrido-Latorre F. Surtimiento de recetas a los afiliados al Seguro popular de Salud de México [dispensing prescriptions to persons affiliated with the Seguro popular de Salud de México]. Salud Publica Mex. 2008;50:429–36.
46. Barraza Llórens M, Guajardo Barrón V: Descripción del Sector Farmacéutico en México, 2012. 2013.
47. Gutierrez JP, Rivera-Dommarco J, Shamah-Levy T, Villalpando-Hernández S, Franco A, Cuevas-Nasu L, et al.: *Encuesta Nacional de Salud y Nutrición 2012. Resultados Nacionales:* 2nd ed. Cuernavaca: Instituto Nacional de Salud Pública; 2013.
48. Yu-Wen H, Mei-Bian Z, Xiang X, Xiao-Hua X, Quan Z, Le J. Socioeconomic inequality in the use of rituximab therapy among non-Hodgkin lymphoma patients in Chinese public hospitals. Asia Pac J Public Health. 2014;26(2):203–14.
49. Wahlster P, Scahill S, Lu CY, Babar Z. Barriers to access and use of high cost medicines: a review. Health Policy and Technology. 2015;4(3):191–214.
50. Menon D, Stafinski T, Stuart G. Access to drugs for cancer: does where you live matter? Can J Public Health. 2005;96(6):454–8.
51. Torres Vigil I, Aday LA, De Lima L, Cleeland CS. What predicts the quality of advanced cancer care in Latin America? A look at five countries: Argentina, Brazil, Cuba, Mexico, and Peru. J Pain Symptom Manag. 2007;34(3):315–27.
52. Curado MP, Pontes T, Guerra-Yi ME, de Camargo Cancela M. Leukemia mortality trends among children, adolescent, and your adults in Latin America. Rev Panam Salud Publica. 2011;29(2):96–102.
53. Bases de Datos sobre Egresos Hospitalarios. http://www.dgis.salud.gob.mx/contenidos/basesdedatos/std_egresoshospitalarios.html. Accessed 19 July 2017.
54. Dorantes-Acosta E, Zapata-Tarres M, Miranda-Lora AL, Reyes-López A, Muñoz Hernández O, Cortés-Gallo G, Garduño Espinosa J. Apoyo de organizaciones no gubernamentales a pacientes pediátricos con leucemia linfoblástica aguda afiliados al Seguro popular en México [support from nongovernmental organizations to pediatric patients with acute lymphoblastic leukemia affiliated with the Seguro popular insurance program in Mexico]. Bol Med Hosp Infant Mex. 2012;69(3):212–7.
55. Knaul FM, Gonzalez-Pier E, Gomez-Dantes O, Garcia-Junco D, Arreola-Ornelas H, Barraza-Llorens M, Sandoval R, et al. The quest for universal health coverage: achieving social protection for all in Mexico. Salud Publica Mex. 2013;55(2):207–35.
56. Gonzalez-Block MA. What is purchased, how and from whom by Seguro popular in Mexico? Experience with strategic purchasing at national level and in a pioneer institution. Salud Publica Mex. 2017;59(1):59–67.
57. Nigenda G, Gonzalez-Robledo MC, Gonzalez-Robledo LM, Bejarano-Arias RM. Breast cancer policy in Latin America: account of achievements and challenges in five countries. Glob Health. 2016;12(1):39 -016-0177-5.
58. Barr R, Robertson J. Access to cytotoxic medicines by children with Cancer: a focus on low and middle income countries. Pediatr Blood Cancer. 2016; 63(2):287–91.

Permissions

All chapters in this book were first published in JPPP, by BioMed Central; hereby published with permission under the Creative Commons Attribution License or equivalent. Every chapter published in this book has been scrutinized by our experts. Their significance has been extensively debated. The topics covered herein carry significant findings which will fuel the growth of the discipline. They may even be implemented as practical applications or may be referred to as a beginning point for another development.

The contributors of this book come from diverse backgrounds, making this book a truly international effort. This book will bring forth new frontiers with its revolutionizing research information and detailed analysis of the nascent developments around the world.

We would like to thank all the contributing authors for lending their expertise to make the book truly unique. They have played a crucial role in the development of this book. Without their invaluable contributions this book wouldn't have been possible. They have made vital efforts to compile up to date information on the varied aspects of this subject to make this book a valuable addition to the collection of many professionals and students.

This book was conceptualized with the vision of imparting up-to-date information and advanced data in this field. To ensure the same, a matchless editorial board was set up. Every individual on the board went through rigorous rounds of assessment to prove their worth. After which they invested a large part of their time researching and compiling the most relevant data for our readers.

The editorial board has been involved in producing this book since its inception. They have spent rigorous hours researching and exploring the diverse topics which have resulted in the successful publishing of this book. They have passed on their knowledge of decades through this book. To expedite this challenging task, the publisher supported the team at every step. A small team of assistant editors was also appointed to further simplify the editing procedure and attain best results for the readers.

Apart from the editorial board, the designing team has also invested a significant amount of their time in understanding the subject and creating the most relevant covers. They scrutinized every image to scout for the most suitable representation of the subject and create an appropriate cover for the book.

The publishing team has been an ardent support to the editorial, designing and production team. Their endless efforts to recruit the best for this project, has resulted in the accomplishment of this book. They are a veteran in the field of academics and their pool of knowledge is as vast as their experience in printing. Their expertise and guidance has proved useful at every step. Their uncompromising quality standards have made this book an exceptional effort. Their encouragement from time to time has been an inspiration for everyone.

The publisher and the editorial board hope that this book will prove to be a valuable piece of knowledge for researchers, students, practitioners and scholars across the globe.

List of Contributors

Jaden Brandt
College of Pharmacy, Rady Faculty of Health Sciences, University of Manitoba, Winnipeg, MB, Canada

Brenna Shearer
College of Pharmacy, Rady Faculty of Health Sciences, University of Manitoba, Winnipeg, MB, Canada
Pharmacists Manitoba, Winnipeg, MB, Canada

Steven G. Morgan
School of Population and Public Health, Faculty of Medicine, University of British Columbia, Vancouver, BC, Canada

Xavier Nsabagasani and Herbert Muyinda
Child Health and Development Center, College of Health Sciences, Makerere University, Kampala, Uganda

Japer Ogwal-Okeng
Department of Pharmacology and Therapeutics, Gulu University, Gulu, Uganda

Ebba Holme Hansen
Section for Social and Clinical Pharmacy, Department of Pharmacy, Faculty of Health and Medical Sciences, University of Copenhagen, Copenhagen, Denmark

Anthony Mbonye
Department of Community Health, Ministry of Health Uganda, Kampala, Uganda
Department of Health, Uganda Christian University, Mukono, Uganda

Freddie Ssengooba
School of Public Health, College of Health Sciences, Makerere University, Kampala, Uganda

Kebede Beyene, Trudi Aspden and Janie Sheridan
The School of Pharmacy, Faculty of Medical and Health Sciences, the University of Auckland, Private Bag 92019, Auckland 1142, New Zealand

Muhammad Atif, Muhammad Rehan Sarwar, Muhammad Azeem, Danial Umer, Abdul Rauf, Arslan Rasool and Muhammad Ahsan
Department of Pharmacy, The Islamia University of Bahawalpur, Bahawalpur, Pakistan

Shane Scahill
School of Management, Massey University, Auckland, New Zealand

Jessica L. Killen
College of Pharmacy, Dalhousie University, 5968 College Street, Halifax, Nova Scotia B3H 4R2, Canada

Jennifer E. Isenor
College of Pharmacy, Dalhousie University, 5968 College Street, Halifax, Nova Scotia B3H 4R2, Canada
Canadian Center for Vaccinology, IWK Health Centre and Nova Scotia Health Authority, Dalhousie University, 5850/5980 University Ave, Halifax, Nova Scotia B3K 6R8, Canada
Faculty of Medicine, Dalhousie University, 1459 Oxford St, Halifax, Nova Scotia B3H 4R2, Canada

Susan K. Bowles
College of Pharmacy, Dalhousie University, 5968 College Street, Halifax, Nova Scotia B3H 4R2, Canada
Canadian Center for Vaccinology, IWK Health Centre and Nova Scotia Health Authority, Dalhousie University, 5850/5980 University Ave, Halifax, Nova Scotia B3K 6R8, Canada
Faculty of Medicine, Dalhousie University, 1459 Oxford St, Halifax, Nova Scotia B3H 4R2, Canada
Department of Pharmacy, 1796 Summer St, Nova Scotia Health Authority- Central Zone, Halifax, Nova Scotia B3H 3A6, Canada

Shelly A. McNeil
Canadian Center for Vaccinology, IWK Health Centre and Nova Scotia Health Authority, Dalhousie University, 5850/5980 University Ave, Halifax, Nova Scotia B3K 6R8, Canada
Faculty of Medicine, Dalhousie University, 1459 Oxford St, Halifax, Nova Scotia B3H 4R2, Canada

Donna MacDougall
Canadian Center for Vaccinology, IWK Health Centre and Nova Scotia Health Authority, Dalhousie University, 5850/5980 University Ave, Halifax, Nova Scotia B3K 6R8, Canada
School of Nursing, St.Francis Xavier University, Antigonish, Nova Scotia B2G 2W5, Canada

Beth A. Halperin
Canadian Center for Vaccinology, IWK Health Centre and Nova Scotia Health Authority, Dalhousie University, 5850/5980 University Ave, Halifax, Nova Scotia B3K 6R8, Canada
School of Nursing, Dalhousie University, 5869 University Avenue, Halifax, Nova Scotia B3H 4R2, Canada

Kathryn L. Slayter
Canadian Center for Vaccinology, IWK Health Centre and Nova Scotia Health Authority, Dalhousie University, 5850/5980 University Ave, Halifax, Nova Scotia B3K 6R8, Canada
IWK Health Centre, 5850/5980 University Avenue, Halifax, Nova Scotia B3K 6R8, Canada

Beverly A. Billard
Nova Scotia Department of Health and Wellness, Halifax, Nova Scotia B3J 2R8, Canada

Shahrzad Salmasi
Collaboration for Outcomes Research and Evaluation (CORE), Faculty of Pharmaceutical Sciences, The University of British Columbia, Vancouver, British Columbia, Canada

Long Chiau Ming
Unit for Medication Outcomes Research and Education (UMORE), Pharmacy, School of Medicine, University of Tasmania, Hobart, Tasmania, Australia

Tahir Mehmood Khan
School of Pharmacy, Monash University, Sunway City, Selangor, Malaysia
Department of Pharmacy, Abasyn University, Peshawar, Pakistan

N. Athuraliya
Department of Medicine, The Maitland Hospital Clinical School, 550-560 High Street, Maitland 2320, NSW, Australia

E. J. Walkom and J. Robertson
Department of Clinical Pharmacology, School of Medicine and Public Health, The University of Newcastle, Newcastle, Australia

S. Dharmaratne
Medical Education Unit, Faculty of Medicine, University of Peradeniya, Peradeniya, Sri Lanka

Philip O. Anum
National Drug Information Centre, Ministry of Health, Accra, Ghana

Berko P. Anto
Department of Clinical and Social Pharmacy, Kwame Nkrumah University of Science and Technology, Accra, Ghana

Audrey G. Forson
Department of Medicine, School of Medicine and Dentistry, University of Ghana, Accra, Ghana

Tsitsi G. Monera-Penduka and Charles C. Maponga
Drug and Toxicology Information Services (DaTIS), School of Pharmacy, University of Zimbabwe College of Health Sciences, Harare, Zimbabwe

Gene D. Morse
Center for Integrated Global Biomedical Sciences, University at Buffalo, Buffalo, New York, USA

Charles F. B. Nhachi
Department of Clinical Pharmacology, University of Zimbabwe College of Health Sciences, Harare, Zimbabwe'

Niranjan Konduri, Shiou-Chu Judy Wang and Tanya Malpica-Llanos
Systems for Improved Access to Pharmaceuticals and Services (SIAPS) Program, Management Sciences for Health, Arlington, VA, USA

Megan Rauscher
Pharmaceuticals and Health Technologies Group, Management Sciences for Health, Arlington, VA, USA

Muhammad Rehan Sarwar, Muhammad Atif, Anum Saqib and Muhammad Qamar-uz-Zaman
Department of Pharmacy, The Islamia University of Bahawalpur, Bahawalpur, Pakistan

Shane Scahill
School of Management, Massey University, Auckland, New Zealand

Zaheer Babar
Department of Pharmacy, University of Huddersfield, Huddersfield, UK

Syed Masud Ahmed, Nahitun Naher and Tarek Hossain
Centre of Excellence for Universal Health Coverage, James P Grant School of Public Health, BRAC University, 5th Floor, (Level-6), icddr, b Building, 68 Shahid Tajuddin Ahmed Sharani, Mohakhali, Dhaka -1212, Bangladesh

Lal Bahadur Rawal
Health Systems and Population Studies Division, icddr, b, Dhaka 1212, Bangladesh

Amie Bain and Lois Nettleship
School of Applied Sciences, University of Huddersfield, Queensgate, Huddersfield HD1 3DH, United Kingdom

Zaheer-Ud-Din Babar
School of Applied Sciences, University of Huddersfield, Queensgate, Huddersfield HD1 3DH, United Kingdom
School of Pharmacy, Faculty of Medical and Health Sciences, University of Auckland, Private Mail Bag, Auckland 92019, New Zealand

Sallianne Kavanagh
Pharmacy Department, Sheffield Teaching Hospital NHS Foundation Trust, Herries Road, Sheffield S5 7AU, United Kingdom

Ingvild Holdø
Norwegian Centre of Addiction Research (SERAF), University of Oslo, Oslo, Norway

Svetlana Skurtveit
Norwegian Centre of Addiction Research (SERAF), University of Oslo, Oslo, Norway
Domain of Mental and Physical health, Norwegian Institute of Public Health, Oslo, Norway

Jørgen G. Bramness
Norwegian National Advisory Unit on Concurrent Substance Abuse and Mental Health Disorders, Ottestad, Norway

Marte Handal and Leila Torgersen
Domain of Mental and Physical health, Norwegian Institute of Public Health, Oslo, Norway

Ted Reichborn-Kjennerud
Domain of Mental and Physical health, Norwegian Institute of Public Health, Oslo, Norway
Institute of Clinical Medicine, University of Oslo, Oslo, Norway

Hedvig Nordeng
Domain of Mental and Physical health, Norwegian Institute of Public Health, Oslo, Norway
PharmacoEpidemiology and Drug Safety Research Group, School of Pharmacy, University of Oslo, Oslo, Norway

Eivind Ystrøm
Domain of Mental and Physical health, Norwegian Institute of Public Health, Oslo, Norway
PharmacoEpidemiology and Drug Safety Research Group, School of Pharmacy, University of Oslo, Oslo, Norway
Section of Health, Developmental and Personality Psychology, Department of Psychology, University of Oslo, Oslo, Norway

Amer Hayat Khan and Syed Azhar Syed Sulaiman
School of Pharmaceutical Sciences, Universiti Sains Malaysia, Penang, Malaysia

Ammar Ali Saleh Jaber
School of Pharmaceutical Sciences, Universiti Sains Malaysia, Penang, Malaysia
School of Pharmacy, Lebanese International University, Taiz, Yemen

Afia Frimpomaa Asare Marfo and Frances Thelma Owusu-Daaku
Faculty of Pharmacy and Pharmaceutical Sciences, Kumasi, Ghana

Akram Hernández-Vásquez
Universidad Privada del Norte, Lima, Peru

Christoper A. Alarcon-Ruiz
Facultad de Medicina, Universidad Ricardo Palma, Lima, Peru

Guido Bendezu-Quispe
Universidad Peruana Cayetano Heredia, Lima, Peru

Daniel Comandé
Institute for Clinical Effectiveness and Health Policy (IECS), Buenos Aires, Argentina

Diego Rosselli
Departamento de Epidemiología Clínicay Bioestadística, Facultad de Medicina, Pontificia Universidad Javeriana, Bogotá, Colombia

Belinda Blick, Stella Nakabugo and Birna Trap
Management Sciences for Health, Plot 15, Princess Anne Drive, Bugolobi, Kampala, Uganda

Laura F. Garabedian
Harvard Pilgrim Health Care Institute, 401 Park Drive Suite 401, Boston, MA 02215, USA

Morries Seru
Ministry of Health, Pharmacy, Division, Lourdel Road, Wandegeya, Kampala, Uganda

Ramesh Sharma Poudel
Hospital Pharmacy, Chitwan Medical College Teaching Hospital, Bharatpur, Chitwan, Nepal

Shakti Shrestha
Department of Pharmacy, Shree Medical and Technical College, Bharatpur, Chitwan, Nepal

Santosh Thapa
Hospital Pharmacy, Ashwins Medical College and Hospitals Pvt. Ltd, Lalitpur, Nepal

Bhupendra Kumar Poudel
Department of Drug Administration, Ministry of Health, Kathmandu, Nepal

Muniraj Chhetri
School of Public Health, Chitwan Medical College Teaching Hospital, Bharatpur, Chitwan, Nepal

D. Thambavita, P. Galappatthy and R. L. Jayakody
Department of Pharmacology and Pharmacy, Faculty of Medicine, University of Colombo, Kynsey Road, Colombo 08, Sri Lanka

Rabia Hussain and Mohamed Azmi Hassali
School of Pharmaceutical Sciences, Universiti Sains Malaysia, Penang, Malaysia

Furqan Hashmi
University College of Pharmacy, University of the Punjab, Lahore, Pakistan

Maryam Farooqui
Unaizah College of Pharmacy, Qassim University, Buraydah, Saudi Arabia

Tigist Gashaw and Mekonnen Sisay
Department of Pharmacology and Toxicology, School of Pharmacy, College of Health and Medical Sciences, Haramaya University, Harar, Ethiopia

Getnet Mengistu
Department of Pharmacy, College of Medicine and Health Sciences, Wollo University, Dessie, Ethiopia

Firehiwot Amare
Department of Pharmacy Practice, School of Pharmacy, College of Health and Medical Sciences, Haramaya University, Harar, Ethiopia

Daniela Moye-Holz, Jitse P van Dijk, Sijmen A Reijneveld and Hans V Hogerzeil
Department of Community and Occupational Medicine, University Medical Center Groningen, University of Groningen, Hanzeplein 1, 9713 GZ Groningen, The Netherlands

Rene Soria Saucedo
Boston University School of Public Health, Boston, USA

Index